To my parents, whom I will always be indebted to.

To my wife, who gave me unlimited support in all aspects of my life and kept me focused in my career.

To my children, who got used to see me carrying my small laptop and writing the book every time we went out together for the last 5 years.

Preface

During my professional orthopedic career, I had to pass many orthopedic exams: the orthopedic master degree, the orthopedic doctorate degree, the SICOT diploma and finally the American Board of Orthopedic Surgeons exam. During my residency and fellowship training, I had studied from the many text books (Rockwood adult and pediatric fractures, McRae Orthopedics, Campbell orthopedics, Miller Review of orthopedics; to list few). Reading these text books is necessary to build the knowledge needed by every orthopedic surgeon to understand the fundamental of orthopedics; however, due to time restrain and current exams structure, detailed text books may not be the best choice for orthopedic final exam review.

This review book was designed to help the orthopedic surgeons preparing for their final multiple questions orthopedic surgery exam to review the knowledge that they have been acquiring from their previous readings, lectures, and conferences. The bullets format that was used for this book will help the reader better follow the important facts in each topic. Avoiding paragraphs in this book will facilitate reviewing the information included in shorter amount of time compared to other text books with regular book format.

There had been many details in each topic that were intentionally not included in the book as the primary intention of this book is to be a concise a quick review for the final orthopedic multiple choices questions. Despite that these details which were not included may rarely become a target for questions, including every single fact in each topic will not be compatible with main purpose of this book (which is helping busy orthopedic surgeons and trainees to review the most important facts that are frequently tests in the final orthopedic exams). Also, some of the basic information in orthopedics and trauma were not included in this book with the assumption that the orthopedic surgeon who is reviewing his/her final orthopedic exam would be oriented with these facts.

All efforts were done to ensure that information in the book is uptodate and that pertinent knowledge needed to answer most questions is included in the book. This is a "moving target" that will require frequent editions.

I wish you great success in your exam and your professional life.

Amr Abdelgawad, MD, MBA

Contents

Chapter 1:   Basic Sciences

Bone Histology/ Formation:

- Bone structure can be: trabecular or woven (disorganized bone).
  - **Two types of trabecular bone:**
    - Cortical bone (lamellar) and cancellous bone.
    - Cortical bone is denser (less porous), stiffer and stronger than cancellous bone.
    - Cortical bone has less surface area, a slower metabolic rate, and remodels slower than cancellous bone.
- **Bone structure chemistry:**
  - **Extra cellular matrix:**
    - 60-70% mineral component, 25-30% organic component, water 5-8%.
  - Bone is a composite of both inorganic and organic materials.
  - The inorganic component (Calcium and phosphate) of bone comprises 60% to 70% of the tissue (responsible for the hardness of bone),
    - Calcium hydroxyapatite structure: $Ca_{10}(PO4)_6(OH)_2$
  - Water accounts for 5% to 8%.
  - The organic matrix is about 30%.
    - Collagen type I accounts for 90% of the organic component and thus 20% to 25% of bone weight.
- **Bone cells:**
  - Osteoclast, osteoblast, osteocyte.
  - **Osteoclast:**
    - They are multinucleated giant cells with ruffled border on the cell periphery.
    - Their function is to resorb bone.
    - Originates from hematopoietic cells from a monocyte/macrophage lineage (not mesenchymal stem cells).
    - The osteoclasts have two prominent findings — a **ruffled border and a sealing (clear) zone (See Fig 1)**.
      - In the sealing zone, the osteoclast seals off the area of bone to be resorbed by attaching to the bone surface with the assistance of proteins called integrins (through Vitronectin receptor)
      - The ruffled border is an area found in the infoldings of the cell membrane. At the area of the ruffled border, the osteoclasts lower the pH with hydrogen ions through the carbonic anhydrase system. This lowered pH increases the solubility of the apatite crystals so that the mineral can be removed from the matrix. The organic components of the bone are then

hydrolyzed through activity of the enzymes **cathepsin K**, matrix metalloproteinase, and carbonic anhydrase.

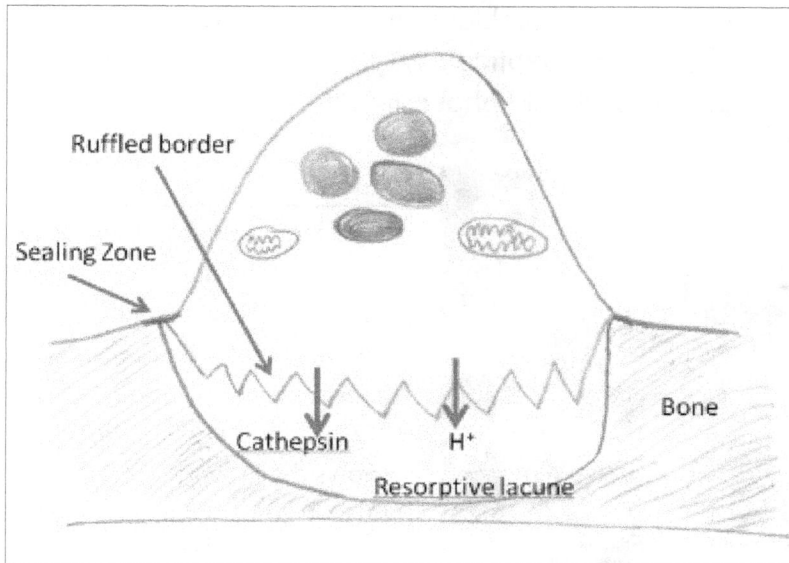

Fig 1: showing osteoclast cell attached to the bone with sealing zone and ruffled border. The resorption lacuna has low pH to absorb the apatite crystals.

- They can be found in small depressions on the bone's surface, called Howship's lacunae.
- It is the final pathway for all causes of bone resorption (eg normal bone turnover, remodeling, polyethylene-related osteolysis, metastasis, seconday hyperparathyroidism, etc). *(Question: What is final pathway for wear osteolysis? for metastasis bone destruction? for multiple myeloma?)*
- Stimulated by **RANK-L** (receptor activator of nuclear factor Kappa β ligand) and **IL-1,** tumor necrosis factor (TNF)-related activation induced cytokine.
- Inhibited by Osteoprotegerin (OPG) (see below), calcitonin.
  - Factors that increase RANKL expression will increase osteoclast activity (see below) (see osteoporosis in systemic conditions chapter).
- Receptors on the osteoclast include tartrate-resistant acid phosphatase (**TRAP**), and calcitonin receptor. Other factors (including PTH, RANK-L) work through the relation between osteoblast and osteoclast.
- **Osteopetrosis:**
  - An enzymatic mutation leading to abnormal carbonic anhydrase function in osteoclasts leading to loss of the ruffled border.
  - Two types: Infantile form (autosomal recessive) severe; adult form (tarda) (autosomal dominant), less severe.

- XR: femur will appear as: "Erlenmeyer flask"; lateral spine: "rugger jersey spine" (See Fig 2).
- The markers of osteoclastic activity are:
  - Serum and urine C-terminal telopeptide of type I collagen
  - Urine cross-linked N-telopeptides of type I collagen
  - Serum tartrate resistant acid phosphatase

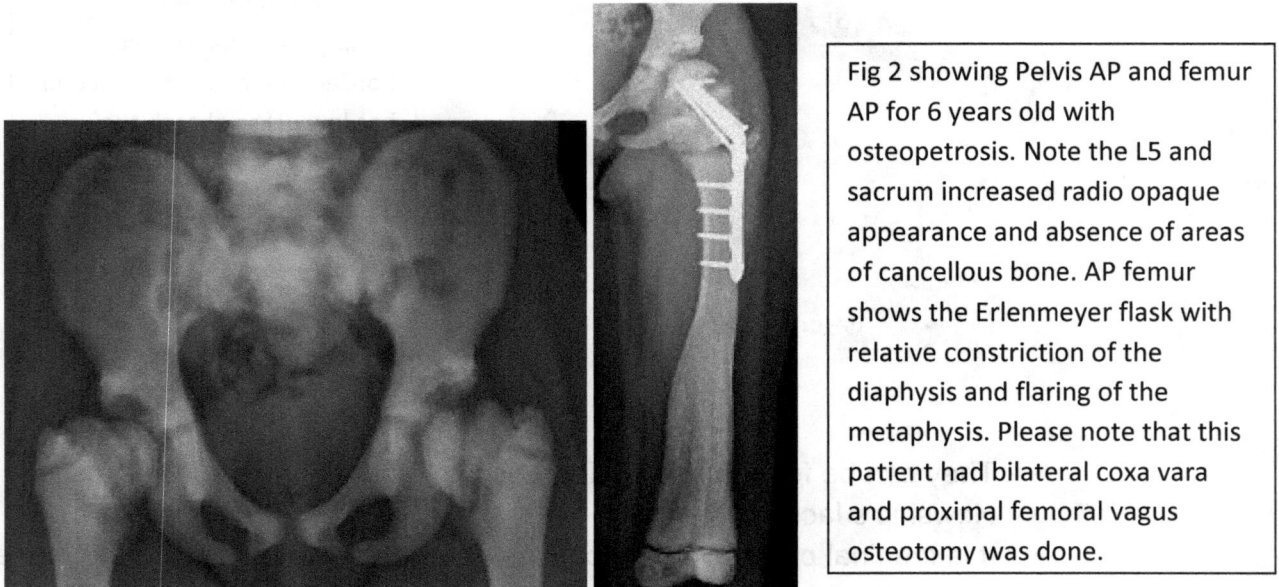

Fig 2 showing Pelvis AP and femur AP for 6 years old with osteopetrosis. Note the L5 and sacrum increased radio opaque appearance and absence of areas of cancellous bone. AP femur shows the Erlenmeyer flask with relative constriction of the diaphysis and flaring of the metaphysis. Please note that this patient had bilateral coxa vara and proximal femoral vagus osteotomy was done.

- **Osteoblast:**
  - They line the bone surface and rim immature bone. They produce the bone matrix.
  - Originates from mesenchymal stem cell.
  - Produce RANKL.
  - Release **Osteocalcin** (bone Gla protein) by mature osteoblast:
    - Gamma-carboxyglutamic acid-containing protein.
    - Marker for differentiation of osteoblast (produced by mature osteoblast and not immature osteoblast)
    - Because it has Gla domains, its synthesis is vitamin K dependent.
    - Most prevalent non-collagenous protein in mature bone.
    - Increased in serum level with increase of bone mineral density.
    - It has a role in bone mineralization (mineral proliferation and maturation) and calcium homeostasis.
  - Osteoblasts have receptors for parathyroid hormone, prostaglandins, 1,25 dihydroxyvitamin D3, glucocorticoids, and estrogen and

androgens. *(Question: intermittent PTH does its effect through receptor on which cell?)*

- Tumors and Inflammatory stimuli can stimulate osteoblasts to express RANKL, which is a key molecule in the proliferation of osteoclasts. *(Question: mechanism by which a metastatic tumor cause osteolysis?).*
- The markers of osteoblastic activity are:
  - Serum bone specific alkaline phosphatase.
  - Serum osteocalcin.
  - Serum type I procollagen C-propeptide.
- Core binding factor alpha 1 (Cbfa1 or RUNX2) is a transcription factor that induces genes involved in differentiation **mesenchymal stem cells** into osteoblasts and chondrocyte during enchondral bone formation (see genetics section).

o **Osteocytes:**

- Osteocyte are osteoblast that becomes impeded in the bone matrix.
- They become less metabolically active than osteoblast (not producing the same amount of protein, and have less organelle), so they have higher nucleus to cytoplasm ratio.
- Osteocytes are connected to each other by cell processes in the bone canaliculai and sends signals to other cells in response to mechanical stimuli to increase bone remodeling in areas of maximum mechanical stress.

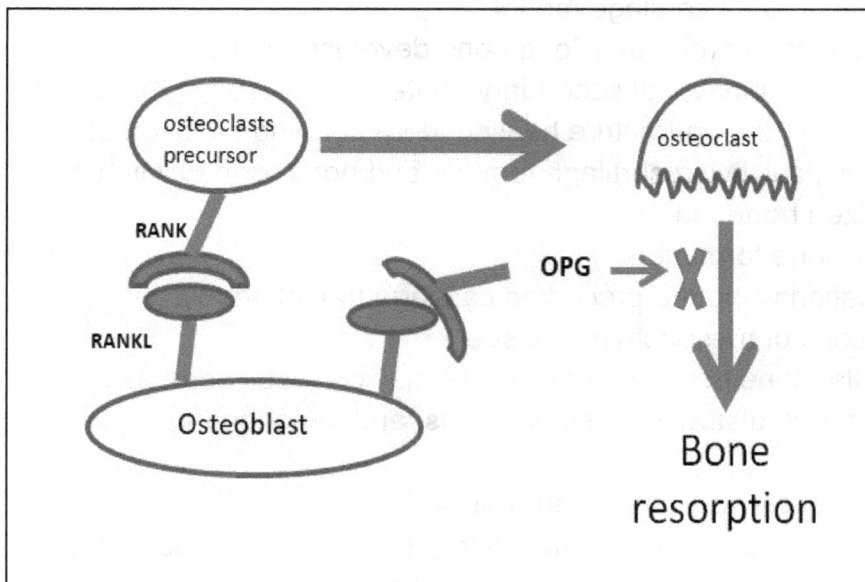

Fig 3: Interaction between RANKL and RANK will stimulate differentiation of osteoclast precursor to osteoclast. OPG can inhibit this process

- **RANK and RANKL:**
  o RANKL exists on the osteoblasts and RANK exists on osteoclasts precursor.

- o Osteoblast has RANKL on the surface. This can interact with RANK on osteoclast precursor to stimulate its differentiation to osteoclast (see Fig 3).
- o Up regulation of RANKL by osteoblast will cause increase in osteoclast differential and hence activity. This is the mechanism of increase osteolysis-related different conditions (e.g. tumors, hyperparthyoidism, etc) *(Scenario: elderly patient with history of cancer presenting with osteolytic lesion, what is the responsible mediator?) (Question: multiple myeloma bone resorption is mediated by?) (Scenario: patient with multiple myeloma, osteolysis is mediated by what type of cell?) (Scenario: Breast cancer metastasis secreting PTHrP causes osteolysis by which mechanism? (increase RANKL expression by osteoblast)).*
- o Osteoprotegerin (OPG) (similar structure to RANK) can block the RANKL and prevent the activation of osteoclast:
    - This will lead to decrease osteoclast activity, protect against bone resorption.
    - Denosumab is human monoclonal antibody that performs the same function as OPG. It can be used for treatment of osteoporosis and other osteolytic conditions (see osteoporosis in systemic conditions chapter).
- o Substances increasing RANKL expression: IL-1, IL-6, PTH (continuous expression), PGE2, Vit D, Glucocorticoids, TNF.
- **Bone formation**
    - o Enchondral ossification
        - Bone formation on a cartilage model.
        - Occurs in cases of embryonic long bone development (primary center of ossification), epiphyseal secondary center of ossification formation, callus formation during fracture healing, degenerating cartilage of osteoarthritis, calcifying cartilage tumors, and bone formed with use of demineralized bone matrix
    - o Intramembranous bone formation
        - Bone formation without a preceding cartilage model, from condensations of mesenchymal tissue.
        - Occurs in flat bone development (pelvis, clavicle, skull bones), bone formation during distraction osteogenesis, and perichondrial bone formation
    - o First bone to ossify is clavicle (intra membranous)
    - o Primary center of ossification: osteoblast changes the cartilaginous diaphysis to calcified bone.
        - Occurs in the embryo. First primary center to appear is the humerus shaft.

- o Wnt molecule binds to lipoprotein receptor-related protein 5/6 (LRP5/6) which results in stimulation of osteoblast differentiation (by increase in the unphosphorylated β-catenin):
    - Dkk-1 and sclerostin inhibit the binding of the Wnt molecule to receptors LRP5/6 (resulting in inhibition of bone formation).
    - Inhibiting or blocking sclerostin or Dkk-1 will result in increased bone formation by increasing osteoblast differentiation.
- **Blood supply to the bone:**
    - o There are three mechanism of blood supply for the bone:
        - Nutrient vessel passing through the diaphysis supplying the inner two thirds of the cortex (enodsteal system) (can be injured during nailing) (inside-out) (high pressure system).
        - Periosteal vessels supply the outer 20% to 30% of the cortex (can be injured by stripping the periosteum during ORIF) (low pressure system).
        - Metaphyseal vessels from the peri-articular vessels.
- **Bone mineralization:**
    - o Mineralization starts at the site of hole zones between the collagen fibrils.
    - o Enzymes within the extracellular matrix vesicles degrade inhibitors such as adenosine triphosphate, pyrophosphate, and proteoglycans found in the surrounding extracellular matrix.
    - o Macromolecules facilitate formation of the critical nucleus and increasing local concentrations of necessary ions.
        - Once the crystals are formed and proliferating, macromolecules bind to the surface and block the growth of the crystal, regulating size, shape, and number of crystals.
    - o Bone sialoprotein: initiation of mineralization of collagen, while osteocalcin: proliferation and maturation of mineralization.

Fracture healing:

- Fracture Healing:
    - o Stages: hematoma formation, inflammation, hypertrophic cartilage formation, new bone formation, and remodeling to mature bone.
    - o Healing occurs by a combination of enchondral and intramembranous bone formation.
        - Motion at the fracture site will stimulate healing by endochondral ossification, while increased stability at the fracture site will result in more direct intramembranous ossification.

- - Callus formation (sign of micro motion) is a form of enchondral ossification.
- The most important factor in determining fracture healing in adults is the blood supply.
  - The vascular response and the blood flow rate to the fracture area reaches maximum around 2 weeks after the fracture.
- Peripheral callus forms around the shaft during healing. This increased diameter of the callus area (compared to the rest of the shaft) will help to increase resistance to bending by the forth power (minimizing the stress on fracture healing).
- Concurrent head injury results in an increased osteogenic response during healing.
- Following a fracture, local release of PGs occurs early as a result of the acute aseptic inflammatory response. COX-2 plays a critical role in this phase and its induction in osteoblasts is essential for bone healing.
  - Nonsteroidal anti-inflammatory (both non selective and selective COX-2): will delay or inhibit fracture healing.
- Factors that inhibit healing:
  - NSAIDs, **smoking**, bisphophsonate (inhibit osteoclasts thus decrease remodeling), Vit D deficiency, alcohol.
- The predominant cell type found in fracture callus just prior to calcification of the chondroid callus is hypertrophic chondrocytes (not proliferative).
  - Collage type X is expressed by hypertrophic chondrocytes as the extracellular matrix which undergoes calcification (see collagen types).
  - If hypertrophic nonunion develop (failure of healing), there will be abundance of type II collage.
  - Collagens type II and X are cartilage specific (see collage section) and would be present in cases of enchondral ossification (not intramembranous ossification)

Coagulation, DVT and Pulmonary Embolism:

- Clotting cascade (See Fig 4):
  - Extrinsic pathway starts with VII, measured by PT. With damage to the blood vessel, VII leaves the circulation and comes into contact with tissue factor (TF) expressed from stromal fibroblasts and leukocytes, forming TF-VIIa. This is quicker than intrinsic pathway.
  - Intrinsic pathway starts with factor XII, measure by PTT. It is activated by by exposed endothelium and collagen. It is slower than extrinsic pathway.
- Risk factor for Venous thromboembolism (VTE):
  - Prior history of VTE, family history of VTE, obesity, smoking, prolonged immobilization, intimal injury, estrogen use, Factor V Leiden, protein C and

protein S deficiency, SLE, type of surgery (total joint arthroplasty are risk), bilateral knee arthroplasty, DM and high blood glucose level, myocardial infarction, congestive heart failure and hormonal replacement therapy.
- Hypercholesterolemia is not a risk factor for VTE.
- Factor V Leiden: mutation of factor V which will make it less susceptible for degradation by protein C.
  o Virchow's triad: Endothelial injury, stasis, and hypercoagulability.

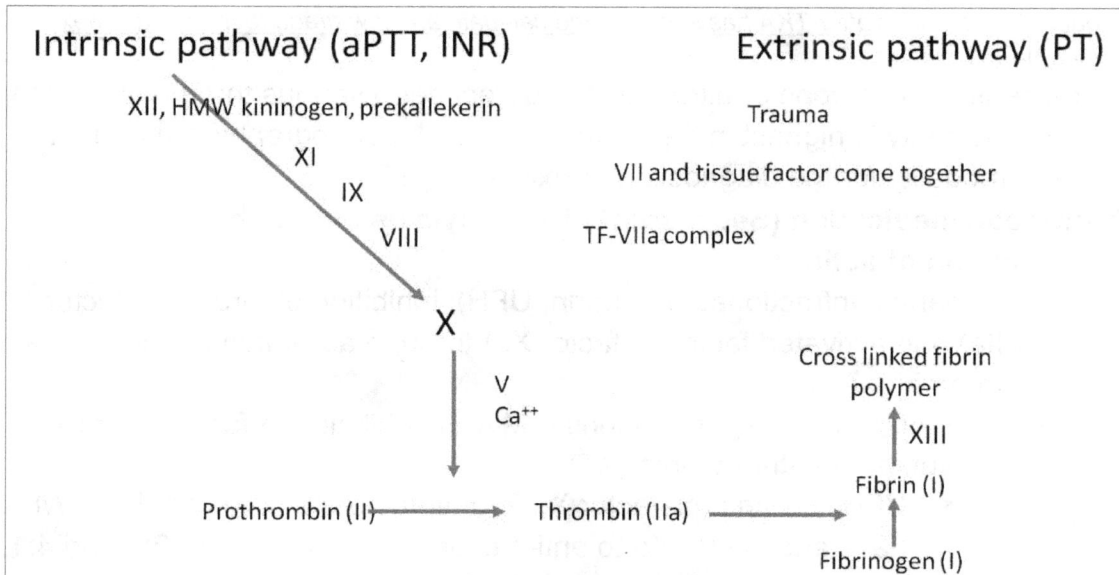

Intrinsic pathway (aPTT, INR)

XII, HMW kininogen, prekallekerin

XI

IX

VIII

X

V
Ca⁺⁺

Prothrombin (II) ⟶ Thrombin (IIa)

Extrinsic pathway (PT)

Trauma

VII and tissue factor come together

TF-VIIa complex

Cross linked fibrin polymer

XIII

Fibrin (I)

Fibrinogen (I)

Fig 4: Clotting cascade. Both intrinsic and extrinsic pathways will end in the "common" pathway. Formation of the fibrin clot is the end product of the clotting cascade

- Pulmonary embolism:
  o Clinical presentation: tachypnea and tachycardia
  o Lab results in cases of PE:
    - Arterial blood gas (not very specific): hypoxemia (decrease PaO_2), hypocapnia (decreased $PaCO_2$), and respiratory alkalosis.
    - Pulse oximetry is not an adequate alternative to arterial blood gas measurements on room air because patient hyperventilation can maintain adequate oxygenation in the pulse oximetry.
    - Increased alveolar-arterial (A-a gradient) gradient.
    - Massive PE can have hypercapnia and combined respiratory and metabolic acidosis.
    - EKG: New onset right bundle branch block
    - Elevated D-dimer levels and brain natriuretic peptide (BNP).
  o Imaging study:

- Computed tomography angiography (CTA) is the initial imaging modality of choice for stable patients with suspected PE.
- Ventilation perfusion scan: V/Q mismatch.
  - Initial evaluation of the patient suspected of PE includes:
    - Arterial blood gas on room air, a chest radiograph, and EKG to rule out alternative diagnoses.
- DVT:
  - If suspecting mid-calf DVT, venous ultrasound should be obtained. _(Scenario: patient seven days after TKA has swelling and calf pain and low grade fever, what is next step?)_
  - The sensitivity of Doppler ultrasound to detect deep venous thrombosis in the lower extremity is highest in the thigh. Venous ultrasonography is the most useful modality for the diagnosis of proximal thigh DVT.
- **Antithrombotic medication (See also: DVT prophylaxis in hip chapter):**
  - **Mechanism of action:**
    - Heparin (Unfractionated heparin, UFH): inhibition of thrombin (factor IIa) and activated factor X (factor Xa) through activation of anti-thrombin (AT).
    - Low molecular weight heparins (LMWH): inhibition of factor Xa through activation of anti-thrombin (AT).
      - UFH has an anti–factor Xa to anti–factor IIa ratio of 1:1. LMWHs have anti–factor Xa to anti–factor IIa ratios between 2:1 and 4:1, depending on their molecular size distribution.
    - Warfarin (Coumadin): inhibiting vitamin K 2, 3-epoxide reductase, leading to decrease carboxylation of factors II, VII, IX, X (vitamin K dependent factors) (Warfarin replaces normal clotting factors with decarboxylated factors).
    - Aspirin is a cyclooxygenase inhibitor (for details: see pharmacology section later)
    - Selective Xa inhibitor (will end with the Xa-ban): Rivaroxaban and Apixaban.
    - Argatroban (IV agent) and Dabigatran (oral agent): a direct thrombin inhibitor (factor IIa).
    - LMWH, fondaparinux, apixaban and rivaroxaban: inhibit factor Xa activity (LMWH and fondaparinux through antithrombin stimulation; Apixaban and rivaroxaban by direct inhibition).
  - Rivaroxaban, and Apixaban:
    - Oral medication, selective direct factor Xa inhibitor.
    - No anti-dote available.
  - Fondaparinux:

- Similar structure and mechanism of action to LMWH.
- Advantage of fondaparinux over LMWH: lower risk for heparin-induced thrombocytopenia (HIT)
- Disadvantage: cannot be used in patients with renal dysfunction.
  - o Dabigatran:
    - Oral agent, reversible (antidote is idarucizumab).
    - Does not require monitor (in contrast to warfarin).
    - Decrease the dose in renal dysfunction.
  - o Warfarin (Coumadin):
    - The plasma half-life in about 40 hours.
    - Metabolized in the liver, Phenobarbital may antagonize the anticoagulation effect of warfarin (by increasing the degradation of the medication in the liver through enzyme induction)
  - o Heparin and LMWH overdose is reversed by Protamine.
  - o Both LMWH and fondaparinux are metabolized in the kidney.
  - o Warfarin, argatroban and rivaroxaban are metabolized primarily in the liver.
  - o If a patient is diagnosed with DVT or PE:
    - LMWH is used until the INR is between 2 and 3 then use oral medication (e.g warfarin or dabigatran) for 3-6 months.
- **Bleeding:**
  - o Tranexamic acid (medication to help decrease bleeding) acts as a competitive inhibitor of plasminogen and interferes with fibrinolysis.

Growth Plate (Physis) (See Fig 5)
- Characters:
  - o Proliferative zone has highest rate of extracellular matrix synthesis.
  - o Reserve zone has the lowest oxygen concentration.
- Perichondrial artery is main blood supply to the growth plate.
- Mechanical support of the growth plate is by the perichondrial ring of La Croix.
- Appositional growth of the growth plate (growth by addition at the periphery) is performed by the groove of Ranvier.
- Pathology affecting certain growth plate layer:
  - o Reserve zone: Gaucher's and diastrophic dysplasia.
  - o Proliferative zone of growth plate
    - Both Gigantism and Achnodroplais affect the proliferative zone of growth plate (overgrowth and undergrowth).
- Appositional growth of the growth plate (growth by addition at the periphery) is performed by the groove of Ranvier.
- Pathology affecting certain growth plate layer:

- o Reserve zone: Gaucher's and diastrophic dysplasia.
- o Proliferative zone of growth plate
  - ▪ Both Gigantism and Achnodroplais affect the proliferative zone of growth plate (overgrowth and undergrowth).

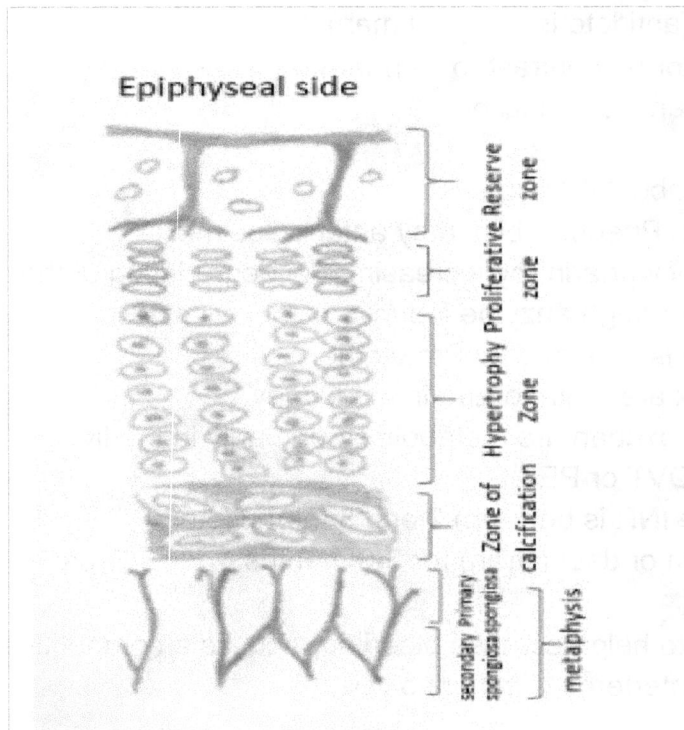

Epiphyseal side

Fig 5: The composition of growth plate.

- • Pathology affecting certain growth plate layer:
  - o Reserve zone: Gaucher's and diastrophic dysplasia.
  - o Proliferative zone of growth plate
    - ▪ Both Gigantism and Achnodroplais affect the proliferative zone of growth plate (overgrowth and undergrowth).
  - o Provisional calcification (part of the hypertrophic zone):
    - ▪ SCFE and Salter Harris Type I and II fractures occur through the zone of provisional calcification (part of hypertrophic zone). The reserve and proliferative zone remain intact and growth can proceed normal after healing of the fracture (distal femur physeal fractures occur through multiple layer making it more prone to growth disturbance, see pediatric fracture chapter).
    - ▪ Scurvy affects the zone of provisional calcification. It is caused by a vitamin C deficiency with a resultant decrease in chondroitin sulfate and collagen synthesis.

- o Metaphysis: Bacterial hematogenous osteomyelitis.
- The mechanism of premature closure of the physis after trauma is invasion of the physis by blood vessels connecting between the metaphysis and epiphysis. This will provide an access for osteoblasts to form a bony bar that prevents further longitudinal growth.
- The Heuter-Volkmann principle:
  - o The rate of epiphyseal growth is affected by pressures applied to its axes:
    - Longitudinal tension will stimulate longitudinal growth of growth plate, and compressive forces inhibit longitudinal growth of growth plate *(question: what is the principle of using staples or growth modulation plate for treatment of Blount's. disease?)*
- Wolff's law:
  - o Bone will adapt to the applied loads (remodels in response to mechanical stress).
    - If loading on a particular part of the bone increases, the bone will remodel itself over time to so that part becomes stronger to resist the loading and if the loading on a bone decreases, the bone will become less dense and weaker (increased stresses cause increased bone gain, and decreased stresses lead to bone loss).
- Effects of various hormones on the physis:
  - o IGF-1 (somatomedin-C) induce proliferation without maturation of the growth plate and thus induce linear skeletal growth.
  - o Growth hormone effect on the physis is by stimulation of production of IGF-1.
  - o Thyroid hormone and steroids stimulate both proliferation and maturation of the growth plate.

Radiation Exposure:

- Less radiation exposure with:
  - o Imaging smaller body part, position the body part further away from the source of radiation (closer to the intensifier).
  - o Using mini C arm (compared to standard fluoroscopy). *(Question: How to decrease the radiation exposure? (Imaging the thumb (rather than hand or forearm) positioned against the image intensifier (rather than source of XR) with the mini C-arm (rather than regular C arm)))*
  - o Exposure to radiation decreases as an inverse square of the distance from the source. If you double distance from the beam of irradiation, your exposure is going to be lowered by about 4 times.
  - o Distance at which no significant radiation exposure is expected is 6 feet from the beam (0.025%).
  - o Pedicle screw insertion has the highest exposure to radiation.

- o Orienting the source of irradiation (cathode ray tube) beneath the patient and placing the image intensifier as close as clinically possible to the patient will minimize the scatter radiation exposure to the personnel.

irradiated part	average dose of irradiation (mrem)
XR Pelvis	70
XR Lumbar spine AP/LAT	70/30
XR Chest	10-20
XR Hand/Foot	0.5
CT Chest	700

- Amounts of radiation received from a chest radiograph is about 10-20 mrem (less than 1/3 from the radiation for spine XR).
- CT delivers the highest radiation dosage of all imaging modalities.
- Irradiation from mini C arm is about 120 mrem/min, regular C arm 1200 mrem/min.
- IM nailing (tibia and femur) average per case is 100 mrem
  - o Surgeon can safely perform up 400 cases/year, limited by exposure to the hands.
- The principle of "as low as reasonably achievable" (ALARA) dosing is recommended for children and pregnant women.
- Radiation accidents:
  - o Low energy injuries (0.5-10 Gy) transient erythema, pruritis, and hair loss.
  - o Moderate energy injuries (10-20 Gy) desquamation, swelling.
  - o High energy wounds (>20Gy): Extensive scarring and ulceration over a period of weeks to months

Pharmacology:
- Botulinum A injections reduce spasticity by **irreversible** blocking of presynaptic acetylcholine release (despite being irreversible inhibition, it works only for 6 months, due to regeneration of new pre synapses).
- Ginkgo and ginseng (two common supplements for possible benefits related to memory, mental performance, and brain function) can inhibit platelet function resulting in bleeding during surgery.
- Intra-articular steroid injection that is accidentally injected extra-articular can lead to fat atrophy, local flare in surrounding tissues and skin pigmentation.

- Iontophoresis is a physical therapy modality to deliver a medication (e.g. steroid) through the skin with electrical current
- Inflammatory pathway (see Fig. 6):

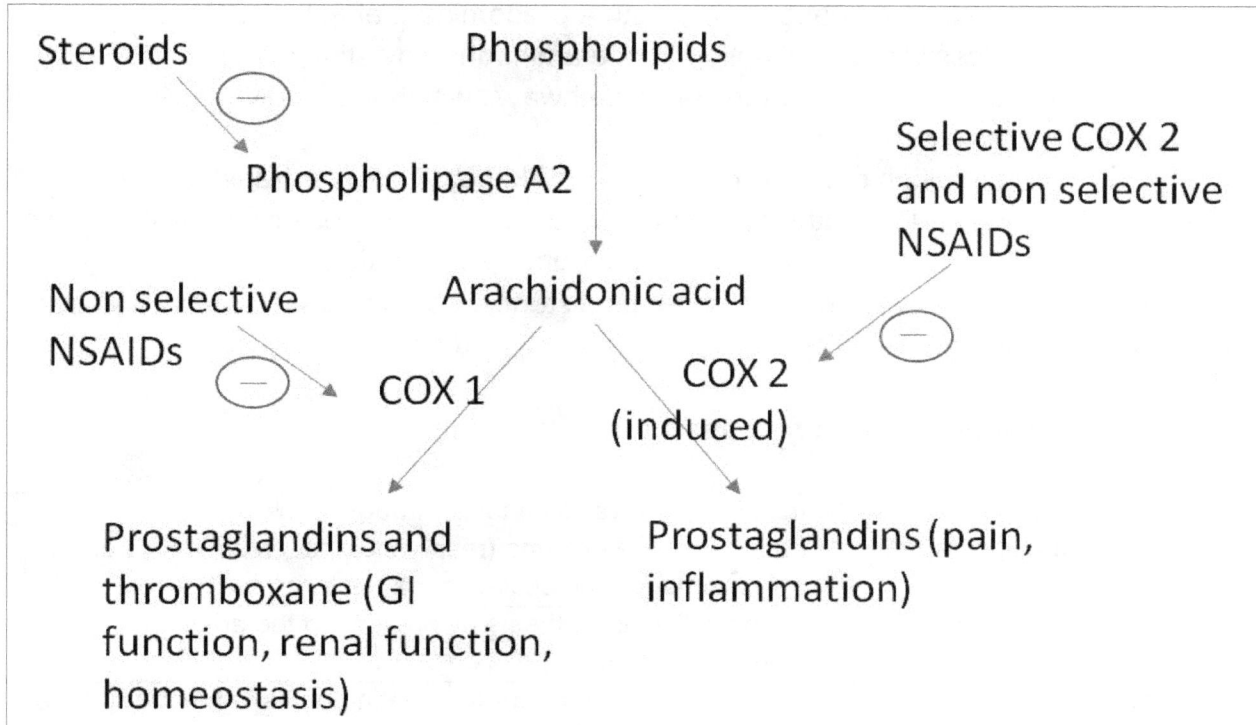

Fig 6: Mechanism of action of Steroid, COX-2 selective and non-selective NSAIDs

- o Phosophlipids are converted to Arachidonic acid by phospholipase A2 enzyme. Corticosteroids inhibit this step.
- o Arachidonic acid is converted to Prostaglandins (PG) by cyclooxygenage (COX) enzyme. NSAID inhibits this step. There are two types of COX. COX-2 is the one which is induced by inflammation. COX-1 is the one responsible for protection of the stomach and platelet function.
- o COX-2 is necessary for fracture healing (inflammation is part of fracture healing process), inhibiting COX-2 will result in inhibition or delay of fracture healing (see fracture healing section).
- o For patients above 65 years old, NSAIDs are better prescribed with proton pump inhibitors to protect against GI ulcers and bleed.
- o The anti-platelet effect of aspirin is due irreversible inhibition of platelet cyclo-oxygenase 1 (COX-1), which is responsible for the formation of PG (which is then converted to thromboxane (TX) A2 by thromboxane synthetase). This leads to blocking of platelet aggregation.

- Its effect on bleeding lasts for about 7 days (this is half-life of platelets until new ones are formed).
  o Acetaminophen mechanism of action is not well defined:
    - The primary mechanism of action is believed to be inhibition of cyclooxygenase (COX), with a predominant effect on COX-2.
    - Possible central action of acetaminophen by stimulating effect on descending serotoninergic pathways, which are involved in inhibition of pain sensations.
    - Inhibition of IL-1 β-dependent NF-kappa β nuclear translocation (signaling pathways to the pathogenesis of various rheumatic diseases including osteoarthritis and rheumatoid arthritis).
- Nistrous oxide is associated with gaseous distension of the bowel, this may hinder visualization for image guided procedures performed on spine and pelvis
- **Antibiotics:**
  o **Mechanism of action of antibiotics:**

Beta lactam antibiotics (penicillins, cephalosporins)	Inhibit of Cell wall synthesis through blocking the transpeptidase enzyme (responsible for cross-linking of polysaccharide molecules in the bacterial cell wall.)
Glycopeptides (vancomycin)	Inhibit cell-wall synthesis by preventing the addition of new cell-wall subunits.
Daptomycin	Binds to the cell membrane creating holes in the membrane causing rapid depolarization and cell death.
Aminoglycosides (e.g. gentamycin, topramycin)	Bind ribosomal RNA **30S** subunits (causing Inhibition of bacterial protein synthesis (Inhibit translation))
Linezolid (see below)	Binds to a 50S ribosomal subunit (preventing formation of the 70S initiation complex) (causing inhibition of bacterial protein synthesis (Inhibit translation)).
Macrolides (e.g. erythromycin, azithromycin)	Bind the 50S ribosomal subunits RNA (inhibition of protein synthesis).
Clindamycin	Bind the 50S ribosomal subunits RNA (inhibition of protein synthesis).
Quinolones/ Fluoroquinolones	Inhibit DNA gyrase and DNA replication
Rifampin	Inhibit DNA-dependent RNA polymerase
Trimethoprim/sulfamethoxazole (TMP/SMX))	Block folic acid metabolism.
Metronidazole (Flagyl)	Forms oxygen radicals that are toxic to anaerobic organisms
Amphotericin and nystatin	Increase cell membrane permeability by disrupting the functional integrity of the cell membrane.

- o **Linezolid**
  - Member of oxazolidinone group of antibiotics.
  - Used to treat methicillin-resistant staphylococcus aureus (MRSA). It has NO effect against gram negative bacteria
  - Their mechanism of action is inhibition ribosomal activity (prevent formation of the 70S ribosomal translation complex).
  - Linezolid is a reversible nonselective monoamine oxidase inhibitor (MAOI) and can induce serotonin syndrome (headache, diaphoresis, nausea, dilated pupils, tachycardia, hypertension, tremor, and possibly clonus) in combination with other serotonergic medications (e.g. selective serotonin reuptake inhibitor (SSRI), monoamine oxidase inhibitor (MAOI), tricyclic antidepressants (TCAs)). Treatment is to discontinue the medication and administration of benzodiazepines.
- o Bacitracin is poorly absorbed from the intestinal tract; its only use is for topical application. Bacitracin is mainly bactericidal for gram-positive bacteria, including penicillinase-resistant staphylococci.
- o Fluoroquinolones can lead to increased rates of tendinitis and non-traumatic rupture of Achilles tendon.
  - Quinolones-associated tendinosis: stop antibiotic, boot with lift to relax the Achilles tendon
- o Tetracyclin should not be given to children less than 8 years old because it causes teeth discoloration.
- o **MRSA:**
  - Resistance to penicillinase-stable antibiotics through genetic mutation (the mecA gene) encoding for an altered penicillin binding protein (PBP) which has a low affinity for these antibiotics (known as penicillin-binding protein 2a (PBP2a))
- o **D-Test for "inducible" resistance for clindamycin:**
  - Some bacteria strains express a positive susceptibility tests to clindamycin, but in vivo the bacteria will display resistance to the antibiotic.
  - D-test: an agar plate is inoculated with the bacteria with two drug-impregnated disks (one with erythromycin, one with clindamycin) placed near each other. If the area of inhibition around the clindamycin disk is "D" shaped, the test result is positive and clindamycin should not be used due to the possibility of resistant pathogens and therapy failure. If the area of inhibition is round, the antibiotic can be used.
- o **Antibiotic prophylaxis**

- Cefazolin (1st generation) or cefuroxime (2nd generation) within one hour before skin incision. Patients with an allergy should be given vancomycin 10 to 15 mg/kg or clindamycin 600 to 900 mg.
      - Intravenous antibiotic administration within 1 hour of surgical incision is the most effective measure to reduce surgical site infection.
    - Patients with penicillin allergy demonstrate cross-reactivity with cephalosporins in about 10% of cases.
- **Chemotherapeutic agent complications:**
    - Doxorubicin is associated with cardiotoxicity (the most severe side effect).
    - Methotrexate is associated with mucositis and hepatic toxicity.
    - Ifosfamide is associated with cystitis. *(Scenario: 30 years old, history of Ewing 10 years ago, treated with Doxurubicin, now needs TKA, what pre op test to do? (Echocardiography for possible cardiac complication))*
- **Blood transfusion/blood borne carriers:**
    - Hepatitis B virus carries the highest risk of transmission following allogeneic blood transfusion.
    - Routine screening of donated blood includes: Hepatitis B, Hepatitis C, syphilis, HIV-l , HIV-2, and West Nile virus.
    - Risks of blood transfusion:
      - Incorrect blood transfusion (wrong blood unit by mistake) which can cause acute hemolysis (1 in 12,000 to 1 in 50,000 transfusions).
      - Anaphylactic reactions (1 in 150,000 transfusions).
      - Hepatitis B transmission (1 in 205,000 transfusions).
      - HIV transmission (1 in 2,000,000 transfusions)
      - Hepatitis C (1 in 2,000,000 transfusions).

Bone grafting/ Osteobiologics:

- Bone grafts may be osteogenic, osteoinductive, and/or osteoconductive:
    - Osteogenic: capability to provide bone forming cells.
    - Osteoinductive: the ability to stimulate local bone formation (growth-factor-mediated differentiation of MSCs into osteoblasts).
    - Osteoconductive: the ability to permit in-growth of new bone tissue and sprouting of capillaries and perivascular tissue (acting as a scaffold).
      - Cancellous allograft (bone chips) is predominantly osteoconductive.
      - Bone marrow aspirates provide osteogenic mesenchymal precursor cells.
      - BMP 2, 7 (TGF-β superfamily) are osteoinductive factors (they do not have osteoconductive properties) (see below).

- DBMs (demineralized bone matrix) have variable amounts of BMPs (depending on harvesting and preparation).

- **Bone morphogenetic proteins (BMPs):**
  - Part of (transforming growth factor beta) (TGF-beta) superfamily of molecules.
  - Extra-cellular proteins that use transmembrane serine-threonine kinase cell surface receptor to transduce intracellular signal molecules called SMADs.
    - This will lead to of many cellular functions including osteogenesis (differentiation of MSCs into osteoblasts) and cell differentiation.
  - rh MBP-7 is comparable to autogenous bone graft for treatment of tibial nonunions.
  - Adding rhBMP-2 to the treatment of open tibial fracture was found to reduce the need for secondary interventions.

- **Bone graft substitutes:**
  - Calcium sulfate has the fastest rate of resorption among synthetic bone substitutes.
  - Calcium phosphate (NOT tricalcium phosphate) has the strongest compressive strength among synthetic bone substitutes.
    - It is composed calcium and phosphate that hardens in situ and cures by a crystallization. When hardened, has a much higher compressive strength than other forms of bone graft substitutes and 4 to 10 times greater than cancellous bone. *(Question: in depressed tibial plateau fractures, after elevating the depressed fragment, what bone substitute gives the least loss of reduction?)*
  - Both calcium sulfate and calcium phosphate cements resist tension and shear stresses poorly
  - Bone ceramics:
    - Tricalcium phosphate (TCP) and hydroxyapatite (HA) or combination of both.
    - TCP undergoes biologic resorption 10 to 20 times faster than HA. TCP partially convert to hydroxyapatite, thus slowing its resorption rate.
    - TCP more readily remodels because of its larger porosity.
    - TCP is weaker in compression than HA.
    - Both are converted to bone through: vascular in growth (neovascularization), differentiation of osteoprogenitor cells, and graft resorption (foreign body giant cell reaction, not osteoclast) with host bone ingrowth into voids left behind during resorption (appositional new bone growth).

- **Bone healing stimulators**

- o Low-intensity pulsed ultrasound (LIPUS) and Pulsed ElectroMagnetic Field (PEMF).
- o Low-intensity pulsed ultrasound (LIPUS):
  - $30mW/cm^2$ pulsed-waves is the most effective dose for the healing of fractures.
  - It reduces the time to healing for fractures treated non-operatively.
- **Allograft bone**
  - o In allograft, bone cells surface glycoproteins are the primary responsible factor for the antigenicity of the graft.
    - Freezing, freeze-drying, or chemical sterilization and antigen extraction of the bone allograft can all reduce the antigenicity of the graft.
  - o **FDBA (Freezed dried bone allograft):**
    - The impaction of FDBA is harder than that of fresh-frozen bone, so it may be mechanically more efficient than the fresh-frozen bone in surgical conditions.
  - o Osteoarticular allografts:
    - Host chondrocytes are lost during processing. The cartilage architecture is preserved in the first 2 to 3 years after transplantation.
  - o Well-fixed bulk allografts heal with bridging external callus at the host bone junction site.
    - External callus is annealed to the surface of the allograft. There is very little penetration of the allograft (bulk bone allografts do not remodel).
    - About 25% of structural cortical allografts will develop insufficiency fracture.

Collagen

- Structure of collagen:
  - o Triple helical structure (three alpha chains (2 alpha one and one alpha 2) forming fibril)
  - o Covalent cross-links between glysine residues.
  - o Glycine occurs as the third amino acid in the collagen chain.
    - The chain has the structure of glycine-X-Y (where X and Y are frequently proline or hydroxyproline).
- Type I: main collagen in the bone, menisci, and annulus fibrosis.
- Types II, IX, and XI: main cartilage collagens.
  - o Type II: about 90% of the collagen content of the cartilage is type II.
  - o Type XI collagen form thin fibrils that act as nuclei for deposition of type II collagen in articular cartilage.

- Type X: main collagen of hypertrophying chondrocytes and endochondral ossification.
- Bone sialoproteins are important in the initiation of mineralization of collagen.

Cartilage (See Also Osteoarthritis in The Systemic Conditions Chapter):

- Type II collagen is the main of collagen in the cartilage.
- Type II collagen in healthy cartilage is very stable with half-life of about 25 years.
- Glycosaminoglycans:
  - Most of the glycosaminoglycans are in the form of large aggregates called aggrecan (See Fig 7).
    - Aggrecan has a long core protein with multiple keratin sulfate and chondroitin sulfate chains (large aggregating type of proteoglycans).
    - Aggrecan can associate with 50 times its weight in water. The swelling pressure in cartilage is predominantly due to aggrecan.
  - Link protein binds to both the G1 domain of the aggrecan and the hyaluronic chain to form the aggrecan-hyaluronate-link protein complexes, which are called proteoglycan aggregates (extra cellular assembly).
  - Aggrecan is responsible for swelling pressure of the cartilage.

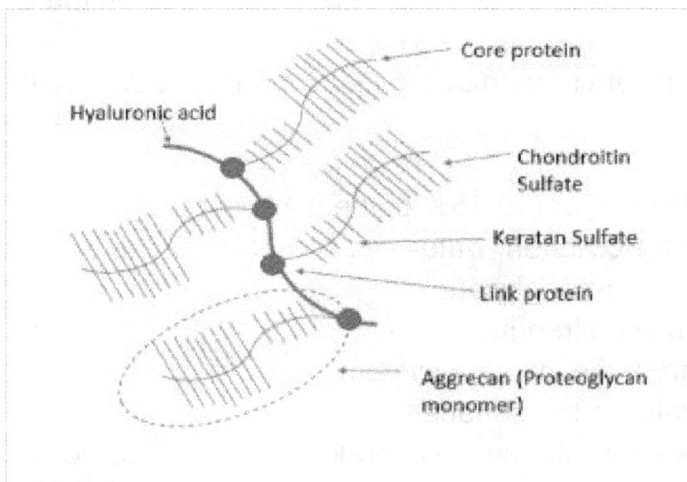

Core protein
Hyaluronic acid
Chondroitin Sulfate
Keratan Sulfate
Link protein
Aggrecan (Proteoglycan monomer)

Fig 7: The structure of proteoglycan aggregates (aggrecan-hyaluronic acid protein complex). Aggrecan is formed of core protein with attached chondroitin sulfate and keratan sulfate. Aggrecan is linked by "link protein" to hyaluronic acid backbone to form the proteoglycan aggregate.

- Chondro-protective agents (anabolic):
  - TGF-β and BMP-2, 7 and their intra cellular signal (SMAD3).
  - Insulin-like growth factor (increase collagen and proteoglycan synthesis).
  - Glucosamine: has anabolic effects on proteoglycan synthesis and prevents IL-1 beta-induced decrease in proteoglycan synthesis (see below).
- Chondro-ablative (catabolic)

- o Interleukin-1:
  - Inhibits proteoglycan synthesis.
  - Stimulates matrix metalloproteinase activity (see below).
  - Stimulates cyclooxygenase 2 (COX-2) and nitric oxide synthetase.
- o Tumor necrosis factor alpha:
  - Inhibits collagen synthesis.
  - Stimulates metalloproteinase activity.
- o COX-2 enzyme.
- o Metalloproteinase (catabolic enzymes that directly degrade cartilage).
- Articular cartilage consists mainly of extra cellular matrix (water, proteoglycans, and collagen) (95-98%) and a small percentage of chondrocytes, which are responsible for the synthesis, maintenance, and homeostasis of cartilage.
  - o Water is the largest constituent, then collagen (type II collagen), then proteoglycan.
  - o In normal adult articular cartilage, only 2% of the total volume is occupied by chondrocytes.
- Cartilage is an avascular structure in adults:
  - o Superficial lacerations that do not cross the tidemark (the region between uncalcified and calcified cartilage) do not heal.
  - o Deeper lacerations may heal with fibrocartilage (type I collagen).
  - o Cartilage lacks undifferentiated cells that can migrate and participate in the repair response.
- Articular cartilage is divided into four layers (superficial, middle, deep, and calcified) (See Fig 8).
  - o The superficial zone
    - Thinnest articular cartilage layer (10-15% of the thickness).
    - Highest concentrations for collagen, water and fibronectin.
    - Lowest concentrations for proteoglycan.
    - Highest tensile stiffness and strength.
    - Seals off the cartilage from the immune system.
    - Collagen fibers are parallel to the surface.
    - Chondrocytes are elongated with the axis parallel to the surface, less cellular than deep layers.
  - o Middle Zone: Transition between superficial and deep layers.
  - o Deep zone
    - Collagen fibers are perpendicular to the articular surface crossing the tide mark.
    - Highest concentration of proteoglycans.
    - Lowest concentration of water.

- Chondrocytes are spherical and arranged in columnar fashion, more cellular than superficial layer.
  - Tide mark.
    - The tidemark in articular cartilage separates between the deep zone and the calcified zone
    - It is seen most prominently in the adult, non-growing joint.
    - Seen only in joint cartilage (not seen in cartilage cap over tumors).
  - Calcified Zone.

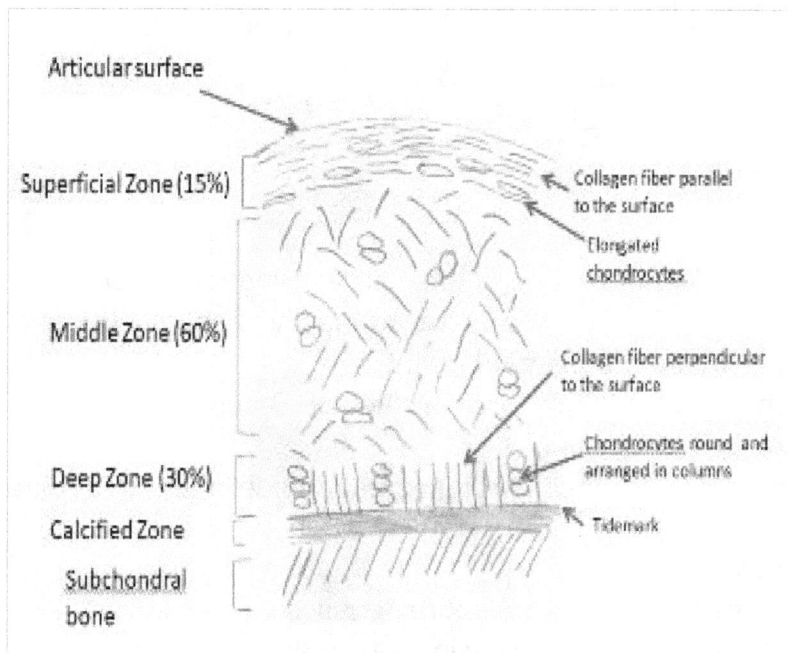

Fig 8: The layers of the articular cartilage. The tidemark separates the deep zone and the calcified zone

- Lubrication co-efficient for normal cartilage is about 0.002 to 0.04.
- Adult articular cartilage has about 5% of the synthesis rate of type II collagen compared to teenagers.
  - In osteoarthrosis, both synthesis and degradation are increased (however, the collagen does not properly incorporate into the matrix)
- **Age changes in cartilage (differs from changes due to OA) (see table below):**
  - Chondroitin 4-sulfate levels progressively decrease.
  - Chondroitin 6-sulfate levels progressively increase.
  - Total chondroitin sulfate level decrease.
  - Keratan sulfate levels progressively increase.
  - Chondrocyte repair response decreases with aging.
- **Comparison** between cartilage changes due to aging and due to OA:

Characteristics	Aging process	Osteoarthritis
Water content	Decreased	Increased
Stiffness	Increased (less soft) (higer modulus of elasticity)	Decrease (softer) (lower modulus of elasticity
Collagen	Unchanged	Decrease in late oa
Proteoglycan content	Deceased	Deceased
Proteoglycan synthesis/degradation	Decreased	Increased
Chondroitin-4-sulfate concentration	Decreased	Increased
Keratin sulfate concentration	Increased	Decreased
Chondrocyte number	Decreased	Increases

Joint:

- Articular joint synovium is composed of two layers: the intimal lining (which contains macrophage-like cells and fibroblast-like cells), and the connective tissue sub-lining.
    - The synovium does not contain a basement membrane.
    - Type A cells are responsible for phagocytosis while type B cells are responsible for synovial fluid production.
- Synovial fluid made of hyaluronic acid, lubricin, proteinases, and collagenases (ultra-filtrate of blood plasma).
    - Secreted from type B cells
    - Synovial fluid exhibits non-Newtonian flow characteristics. The viscosity coefficient is not a constant, and its viscosity increases as the shear rate increases
- **Lubrication:**
    - Elastohydrodynamic lubrication (deformation of articular surfaces occurs and a thin films of joint lubricant separate surfaces) is the **main mode** of dynamic lubrication of articular cartilage.
    - Boundary lubrication:
        - Boundary lubrication occurs with non-deformed surfaces when the fluid film becomes depleted and the bearing surfaces are separated only by a boundary lubricant of molecular thickness; this will prevent excessive bearing friction.
        - Hyaluronic acid diffuses from cartilage with compression and binds to lubricin creating a cross-linked network. (*What protein binds to hyaluronic acid to function as an effective boundary layer?*)
    - Lubricin and superficial zone protein (SZP):

- Share a similar primary structure.
- Both are mainly responsible for boundary lubrication. _(Question: What type of lubrication maintained by lubricin?_

Muscle Tissue (See Also Sports-Basic Science Chapter):
- **Types of muscle fibers:**
  - Type I (Slow twitch):
    - Slow, more vascular (more **red**), uses more aerobic metabolism, more mitochondria and triglycerides.
    - For endurance activity, slow fatigue (fatigue resistant).
    - First to be affected by immobilization.
    - Smaller motor unit (lower strength of contraction).
    - Examples include posture and balance muscles (eg soleus muscle).
  - Type II (Fast twitch):
    - Fast, less vascular (more white), uses more anaerobic metabolism, less triglyceride.
    - Larger motor unit (higher strength of contraction), stronger, for high intensity short duration activities (sprint running), rapid fatigue.
    - Two subtypes (IIA and IIB): IIA has better endurance than type IIB fibers.
- Muscles have 3 layers of connective tissue envelops: epimyseum, perimyseum, endomyeseum.
- Effect of insulin on muscle metabolism:
  - Increased glucose and amino acid entry into the cell, increased glycogen synthesis and protein synthesis.
- Types of contraction:
  - Isometric: muscle length remains constant as tension is generated (muscles not allowed to shorten).
    - For isometric contraction: the force generated varies with starting length (If the length is long, the muscle generates less tension).
  - Isotonic: muscle shortens against a constant load (muscle tension remains constant through the range of motion).
  - Isokinetic: muscle contracts at a constant velocity/speed using submaximal and maximal contraction (muscle tension is generated as the muscle maximally contracts at a constant velocity over a full ROM).
- Types of contraction according to change in length:
  - **Concentric**: muscular contraction results in a decrease in muscle length.

- o **Eccentric**: muscular contraction (activation) with simultaneous increase in muscle length (lengthening of a muscle during active resistance against an opposing force)
  - Eccentric contraction generates the highest tension and greatest risk of musculotendinous injury.
  - Eccentric contraction most efficiently strengthens skeletal muscle

- o **Plyometrics**: eccentric contractions at a rapid rate (muscles exert maximum force in short intervals of time through muscle stretching followed by rapid shortening).
- Maximal force production is proportional to muscle PCSA (physiological cross sectional area).
- Grading of muscle contraction goes from 1-5, with 3/5 strength represents to contract against gravity.
- Physiology of muscle contraction:
  - o Muscles have of two protein filaments: a thick filament composed of the protein myosin and a thin filament composed of the protein actin. Contraction occurs by sliding of myosin over the actin.
  - o Tropomyosin blocks the myosin binding sites on the actin preventing the bonding between myosin and actin.
  - o For sliding to occur, Ca binds to troponin causing tropomyosin to move and the myosin binding sites to be uncovered.
- The sarcomere is organized into bands and lines (see Fig 9).
- The site of action of both depolarizing and nondepolarizing medications is the neuromuscular junction.
- Muscle contusion:
  - o Early mobilization resulted in a progressive increase in myotubule, early nerve regeneration, reduced inflammation, better penetration of regenerative muscle through limited connective tissue scar in line with native surrounding muscle
  - o Prolonged immobilization after muscle contusion will result in increased granulation tissue production (which may lead to myositis ossificans) and decreased tensile strength.
- Complete mid-substance laceration of skeletal muscle in adults will result in dense connective tissue scaring.
- 4 phases of muscle repair after trauma: necrosis, inflammation, repair, and fibrosis.
  - o Fibrosis and scaring after muscle injury are promoted by Transforming growth factor beta 1 (TGF-β1).

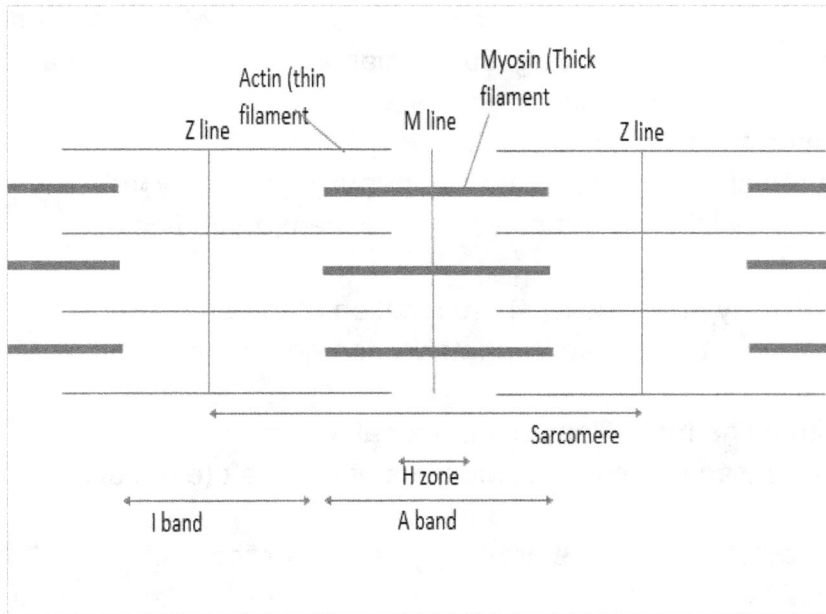

Fig 9: The sarcomere. The sarcomere is the distance between 2 Z lines. H zone has only Myosin, while I band has only Actin. The A band has the Myosin filament (including areas with overlapping actin) . *__With muscle contracture: sarcomere, H zone and I band will all get shorter while the A band will remain the same length.__*

Neurology, EMG and Nerve Conduction Studies:

- The connection tissue surrounding to nerve tissue has 3 layers: endoneurium, perineurium and epineurium.
    - The perineurium is a thin connective-tissue sheath with high tensile strength that surrounds nerve fascicles. It is an extension of the blood-brain barrier of the central nervous system.
- Classification of nerve injury:
    - First-degree (neuropraxia): localized conduction block in a peripheral nerve in which the nerve is intact and full recovery is expected.
    - Second-degree (Axonotmesis) severance of the axon leading to Wallerian degeneration, with continuity of endoneurium sheath.
    - Third-degree: Injury to axons and the endoneurium tube, with perineurium intact.
    - Fourth-degree: Injury to axons, endoneurium and perineurium tube, with intact epineurium. This will lead to neuroma in continuity. Surgical repair of the nerve is necessary (excision and grafting).
    - Fifth-degree (neurotmesis): Loss of nerve trunk continuity (complete cut) (needs surgical repair).
    - In both axonotmesis and neurotmesis, the distal nerve segment will undergo Wallerian degeneration.
- **Neuroma:**
    - Due to previous injury of the nerve leading to "faulty" repair process.

- - Painful neuroma will cause numbness in the distribution of the affected nerve and positive Tinel's sign (e.g. superficial radial nerve neuroma will result in numbness in the first web space.
  - o The pathology is related to ephaptic conduction:
    - Magnification of normal and spontaneous nerve impulses by inducing aberrant nerve impulses within uninvolved adjacent nerve fibers.
- **Nerve repair:**
  - o Nerve repair (neurorrhaphy) involves re-approximation of the ends of a transected nerve, with the fascicles appropriately oriented and under minimal tension.
  - o It should be done with a fine monofilament epineurial suture.
  - o For short gaps (2-3 cm): can use either autologous nerve graft (e.g. sural) or nerve conduit.
  - o For gaps more 3 cm, autologous nerve grafting gives better results.
  - o Good prognostic factors after nerve repair for peripheral nerves: clean wound laceration and early direct repair. Bad prognostic factors: crush injuries, blast injuries, infected wounds and delayed repair.
    - The most important factor in determining recovery after surgical repair of a complete laceration of a nerve is patient's age.
- **Neurotization (nerve transfer):**
  - o Transfer of nerve fascicles to distal part of transected/injured nerve (e.g. low ulnar nerve injury: AIN to the distal ulnar nerve motor fascicles).
  - o An alternative treatment to tendon transfers for irreparable peripheral nerve injury (recently the indications have been expanding with some surgeons using this technique as an alternative to certain nerve repairs).
  - o Can be end-to-end (no potential for recovery of injured nerve) or end-to-side (potential for future recovery of injured nerve).
- The radial, musculocutaneous, and femoral nerves have the best recovery potential followed by median, ulnar, and tibial nerves which have moderate potential. The peroneal nerve has the worst prognosis for motor recovery
- If after nerve repair, the motor recovery is not functional: proceed with tendon transfer. *(Scenario: low median nerve laceration, what surgery can be done few months after repair to enhance function? (opponensplasty using extensor indices as full motor recovery is usually not expected)).*
- Nerve signal transmission:
  - o Myelination accelerates the transmission of action potentials by saltatory conduction occurring at nodes of Ranvier (the impulse transfer from one point to the other).
  - o Temperature, age, demyelination, and loss of axons decrease the rate of impulse transmission through nerves.

- All the peripheral sensory nerves have their cell body in the dorsal root ganglion.
- Neuropathy (e.g. compression neuropathy) causes loss of distal function in the following sequence: motor, proprioception, touch, temperature, pain, and sympathetic activity. Nerve function recovers in the inverse order.
  - Conduction velocity changes seen in peripheral nerve chronic compression syndromes result primarily from Schwann cell affection (cells which are responsible from myelination).
    - Chronic compression syndromes with result in increased both proliferation and apoptosis of Schwann cells.
- Electromyography measures electrical signal activity generated by muscle cells when they are electrically activated. This includes needle insertional activity, resting potential, and muscle activation.
  - Normal muscles exhibit full motor unit recruitment with voluntary contraction, little or no spontaneous activity at rest (absence of sharp waves, and little or no fibrillations).
  - EMG should be done about 6 to 8 weeks following the injury to detect reinnervation
    - Severance of the nerve: positive sharp waves and fibrillation potentials at 2 weeks.
    - Incomplete nerve injury: small amplitude motor unit potentials at 6 to 8 weeks (failure of full motor unit recruitment).
  - Abnormality on EMG in two different muscles supplied by two different peripheral nerves but from the same nerve: indicates radiculopathy as possible pathology (rather than peripheral neuropathy).
- Nerve Conduction velocity (NCV) test:
  - NCV test measures speed at which the nerve impulse travels down the axon of the fastest fibers (which are the large myelinated fibers) (motor and sensory for light touch).
  - Large myelinated fibers are not the first nerve fibers to be affected by compression, so results may not be false negative.
  - Sensory nerve action potentials will be normal in cases of pre-ganglionic injuries (injuries proximal to the dorsal root ganglia).
- Focal nerve compression will lead to focal demyelination and has the following findings in nerve conduction studies:
  - Nerve conduction velocity slowing.
  - Conduction block across the site.
  - Fibrillation potentials.
  - Positive sharp waves.
  - High amplitude-long duration motor unit potentials (chronic denervation).

- Denervation of skeletal muscle due to injury to its nerve supply will show (after about 2-3 weeks):
  - High number of fibrillation potentials (low amplitude short bi- or triphasic deflections), and positive sharp waves (positive deflections followed by a negative wave).
- Myopathy presents as small amplitude-short duration motor unit potentials.
- Fasciculation potentials are spontaneous discharges of the whole motor unit. It occurs in:
  - Anterior motor horn diseases.
  - Cervical myelopathy.
  - Radiculopathy.
  - Demyelinating neuropathy.

Immunology:

- IgG is the most abundant immunoglobulin in adults.
- Antigen presentation by dendritic cells and memory B cells is the most common initial step for a specific immune response mediated by T lymphocytes (cell mediated immunity).

Research:

- Level of evidence:
  - Level I evidence: Well-designed multi-center randomized control studies (and meta-analysis of level one randomized studies).
  - Level II evidence: Randomized control studies with some flaws in the design (e.g. higher percentage of patients dropping form the study) or prospective non-randomized comparative studies.
  - Level III evidence: retrospective, case-control study.
  - Level IV evidence: case series.
  - Level V: expert opinion.
- Bias:
  - Definition: systematic deviation from the true outcome.
  - Randomization, concealment of allocation, and blinding are key methodological principles to limit bias in clinical research.
- Types of studies:
  - Meta-analysis: is a systematic review method to analyze combined results of several independent studies, usually randomized clinical trials (usually using sophisticated statistical methodology).

- Meta-analysis of level one studies has the highest level of clinical evidence.
  - Observational study: studies that assess the prevalence rate, risk factors, prognosis of a condition without intervention by the observer.
  - Experimental: studies that assess intervention by the investigator (always prospective).
  - Case control studies: a study in which the subjects are selected based on whether they have (cases) or do not have (controls) the disease or outcome of interest.
    - Case control studies are **retrospective** as they assess how a certain risk factor may be different between the two groups. _(Scenario: group of patients had bad outcome from procedure are matched to group of patients who had good outcome from the same procedure to identify the risk factors associated with bad outcome, what type of study?)_
  - Cohort studies (prospective) follow a group of individuals over time for studying the incidence, course, and risk factors of a disease.
    - Cohort studies are NOT randomized. It is type of observational study.
  - A randomized clinical trial study design is done to assess if clinical outcome in one treatment group is different from that in another treatment group (comparing two different treatment options, patients will be randomized between these treatment options and reassessed).
    - Parallel design study is one type of randomized clinical studies in which group A receive one certain treatment only and group B receive another treatment with "no crossover" between groups.
- Using Short Form 36 (SF-36) in musculoskeletal conditions:
  - A patient-derived assessment (self-reported and self-administrated). It measures: functional ability, well-being, and overall health.
  - Has potential for "ceiling" and "floor" effects (cannot detect the difference between two good options to detect which is better (ceiling) or two bad options to detect which is worse (floor).
- Evidence-based medicine is the practice of integrating individual clinical expertise with the best available clinical evidence, based on systematic research, for the procedures used in medical practice.

Statistics:
- Confidence interval (CI): the estimated range of values likely to include the unknown population parameter:
  - 95% CI: consists of the range of values that is 95% certain to contain the true value of the variable.
  - If 95% CI for relative risk (RR) cross 1, it means non-significant.

- P value is the probability of type I error (alpha error):
  - Alpha error (type I) is a **false-positive** conclusion by rejecting the null hypothesis when it is actually true.
  - Another definition for alpha error is the finding an effect when, in fact, there is not a one (the observed difference was by a chance on not due to the presence of real difference between the measured parameters) (see the example below).
  - P value is related to significance level.
    - A researcher will often "reject the null hypothesis" when the *p*-value is less than a predetermined significance level, often 0.05 or 0.01 (these values are arbitrary value, chosen by researchers. They do not signify if the observed values are true or false).
    - Example: researcher did a study about difference in weight between males and females in X country, men average was 80Kg, women was 75Kg, P values 0.4; this means that there is 40% chance that there is no actual difference between males and females and that the observer got the difference by chance.
  - P value of less than 0.05 indicates that the result of the study has a high probability (more than 95%) that it is **not** due to chance alone (but p value itself cannot be used to validate the results).
    - The P-value alone, no matter how small, does not establish **clinical** significance or importance.
  - Fragile P value: small size sample will make wide variability in the P value with one change in the data.
    - Minimize fragility by increasing sample size.
- The power of a study:
  - It is the ability to find a difference between various groups when a true difference exists (probability of finding a significant association in a research study when one truly exists).
  - A reasonable probability (typically 80% to 90%) is a minimum sample size (number of patients) required so that if there a statistically significant difference exists between the two populations, there is this probability (80% or 90%) that these sample populations will show the difference at the desired level of statistical significance (usually, but not necessarily, P < 0.05).
  - It is used to estimate the number of subjects needed for this study. *(Question: What type of calculation can assess potential number of sample size for a study to successfully address the effectiveness of an intervention? (power analysis))*
  - A type II (beta) error is the probability of determining that there is no difference in the effects of a treatment or other intervention or variable in a

treatment group and in an untreated control group when there is a difference (false negative results).

- A type II error (Beta error) (false negative), when null hypothesis is false, but erroneously fails to be rejected (failure to reject null hypothesis when it is actually false).
- Power equals 1- probability of beta error (power of 80% means that there is a 20% chance that this sample size can miss a real difference between the two groups).
- Type II errors often occur when the sample size of a treatment group is too small to yield a statistically valid result and leads to a false-negative result.
- To calculate the power of a statistical test, you will need the following parameters: sample size, type I error rate (significance level, P value) and standard deviation (variance) and effect size of the studied variable. *(Question: what affect Power? sample size, variance, p value, effect size).* All these variables are determined by the researcher expect the variance which is calculated from previous similar studies.
- More frequently, you will need to decide on the sample size (and not the power) because you are already determined on your power (e.g. 90%).

	Null hypothesis is true (there is no difference)	Null hypothesis is false (there is difference between the two groups)
Reject null hypothesis	Type I error False positive (researcher found false difference)	Correct outcome (researcher found true difference)
Not rejecting null hypothesis	Correct outcome True negative (researcher found correctly that there is no difference)	Type II error False negative (researcher found there is no difference which is not true)

- **Statistical tests:**
  - Categorical data (eg. gender or the presence/ absence of a parameter) can be compared statistically with a Chi-square test (or Fisher's exact).
  - Both the Student t test and ANOVA are used with parametric variables.
    - Two means (e.g. average weight or average height) are compared with a Student t test.
    - Analysis of variance (ANOVA) is used to compare means of three or more independent groups with continuous variables that are normally distributed (e.g., age, weight, height) (parametric variables).
  - The Mann-Whitney U test used for nonparametric variables (either not normally distributed or variances are not equal among groups).

o Kaplan Meier analysis is used to analyze survivorship of subjects or products in an outcome study.

o Linear regression analysis is used to assess the relationship between a dependent variable and one or more independent variable (by controlling potentially confounding variables). *(Question: what is the test used to assess the relation of patient weight to their ability to weight bear after IM nailing of tibia?)*

o Incidence: number of new cases over a certain period of time (e.g.. year):
  ▪ Measure the risk of developing new cases.
  ▪ Determined by prospective studies.

o Prevalence: number of all cases (old and new) at a one given time.

o Odds ratio and Relative risk:
  ▪ Both measure association between an outcome variable and a predictor variable.
  ▪ The effect of predisposing factor is expressed as relative risk (RR) in prospective cohort study and as odds ratios in a case-control retrospective studies.
  ▪ Odds ratio: the odds that an outcome will occur with a specific exposure compared to the odds of the outcome occurring in the absence of that exposure (comparing two odds) (odds is the probability of an event/ the probability of a non-event).
    • Usually calculated from case control (retrospective).
  ▪ Relative risk: risk in exposed/risk in unexposed (risk is the probability of an event in a the group).
    • Usually calculated from cohort study (prospective).

- **Assessment of a test (See table below):**
  o The sensitivity of a test:
    ▪ The proportion of individuals who have a designated disorder and who are identified by a test as having that disorder (to all diseased individual) (true positive to all disease).
    ▪ Highly sensitive test has low false negative
    ▪ Sensitivity: true positive (A)/ [true positive (A)+ false negative (C)] (small C will lead to high sensitivity).
    ▪ Screening tests should have very high sensitivity.
  o Specificity of a test:
    ▪ The proportion of individuals who are truly free of a designated disorder and who are so identified by a diagnostic test for the disorder (true negative to all non-diseased individual).
    ▪ Highly specific test has low false positive.
    ▪ True negative (D) / [true negative (D)+ false positive (B)] (small B will lead to high specificity).

- Confirmatory test should have very high specificity.
  - Positive predictive value:
    - Proportion of diseased with positive test to all those with positive results.
    - True positive (A) / [True positive (A) + false positive (B)]
  - Negative predictive value:
    - Proportion of individual with a negative test who are free from of the disorder to all negative results.
    - Tr///////u//e negative (D) / [True negative (D) + false negative C)].
    - /Both posit.ive and negative predictive values are affected by the prevalence of the disease in the general population.
  - Accuracy:
    - Overall ability of a test to identify patient with disorder (true positive) and individual free from disorder (true negative) in the study population.
  - Reliability:
    - It is a measure of how reproducible a test is and it is two types:
      - Inter-observer reliability: reliability between different people.
      - Intra-observer reliability: reliability among the same person doing the same outcome measure at different occasions.
  - Validity:
    - The ability of the test to measure what it intends to measure.

	Disease	No disease
Positive test	A (true positive)	B (false positive)
Negative test	C (false negative)	D (true negative)

Microbiology:

- The following organism are grown on specific culture:
  - Kingella Kingae: blood culture.
  - Mycobacterium tuberculosis: Lowenstein Jensen (LJ) medium at a lower temperature 28-32 (stain by Ziehl-Neelsen).
  - Mycobacterium avium: LJ or Middlebrook medium.
  - Neisseria gonorrhea from naturally sterile sources (joint fluid): chocolate agar.
  - Neisseria gonorrhea from naturally contaminated sources (vaginal swap): Thayer-Martin medium.
  - E-coli: Luria Bertani medium.
- Most orthopedic implant-associated bacterial infections are caused by bacteria that had produced and hided in a biofilm:

- o Bacteria proliferating in biofilms are resistant to host defenses and antibiotic therapy.
- o Biofilm formation: 2-stage process.
  - First: **adhesion** of individual bacteria to a substrate.
  - Second: **quorum sensing** (cell-to-cell communication) allows maturation of the biofilm and activation of transcription of genes that activate virulence factors.
- o Infected implants and their adherent biofilms must be removed surgically in order to clear infection.
- Unexplained postoperative leukocytosis, fever, and/or watery **diarrhea** may indicate infection by Clostridium difficile (most patients in the post-operative period will complain of constipation due to narcotics):
  - o Treatment of C. difficile is by oral metronidazole.
- More than half of orthopedic surgical site infections (SSIs) are caused by S aureus.
- *Pseudomonas* infection is responsible for more than 90% of osteomyelitis following nail puncture through tennis shoes (see foot and ankle chapter).
- Mechanisms of Resistance to antibiotic:
  - o Avoidance: e.g. biofilm.
  - o Decreased susceptibility and inactivation (see antibiotic section)
- MRSA:
  - o Panton-Valentine leukocidin (PVL) is a cytotoxin that is usually present CA (community accuired)-MRSA and not in hospital-acquired MRSA. PVL has the ability to lyse white blood cells and cause tissue necrosis, and rapid abscess formation.
    - PVL-positive strains of CA-MRSA are associated with higher incidence of DVT, septic emboli, sepsis, and multisystem organ failure, complex infections, myositis, and chronic osteomyelitis.

Hormones and Calcium (See Systemic Conditions Chapter):
- Mechanism of action of hormones:
  - o **Autocrine** is the process in which cell synthesizes and releases a molecule that influences the same cell leading to changes in the cell.
  - o **Paracrine** is the process in which a cell synthesizes and releases a molecule that binds to a receptor on a nearby cell leading to changes in nearby cells, altering the behavior or differentiation of those cells
  - o **Endocrine** is the process in which a cell synthesizes and releases a molecule that binds to a receptor on a cell located at a distant anatomic site.
- **Vitamin D:**
  - o Liver converts vitamin D3 to 25 hydroxy vitamin D3.

- o Then kidney converts 25 hydroxy vitamin D3 to 1,25 dihydroxy vitamin D3 (the active form).
- o The alpha 1-hydroxylation of vitamin D in the kidney is the rate-limiting step in the formation of the active from of vitamin D3 and is stimulated by parathyroid hormone.
- o The main end organ effect of 1,25 dihydroxy vitamin D is **stimulation of small intestine absorption of calcium and phosphorus**. The indirect effect is promotion of bone mineralization.
- o Increased serum calcium, increased serum phosphate level, and decreased parathyroid hormone will cause 25 OH vitamin D to transform to its inactive from (24,25 dihydroxy vitamin D) instead of the active for 1,25 dihydroxy vitamin D.
- o With aging, requirement of both vitamin D and calcium increase (less vitamin D synthesis skin in response to ultraviolet exposure and decrease conversion of 25 hydroxy vitamin D to 1,25 dihydroxy Vitamin D in the kidney).
- **Calcium:**
  - o Recommended daily intake for elemental calcium:f
    - ▪ 4-8 years old: 750 mg/day.
    - ▪ 9-18 years children: 1200 mg/day.
    - ▪ Pre menopausal female 1200 mg/day.
    - ▪ Post menopausal women: 1500 mg/day.
    - ▪ Pregnancy: 1500mg per day.
    - ▪ Lactating women: 2000 mg/day (highest amount).
    - ▪ Adult male 750-1000.
  - o One glass of milk (8-ounce cup) has about 250-300 mg elemental calcium.
  - o Phosphate administration creates a complex with calcium in the intestine which will decrease calcium absorption.
- **Estrogen** is an important hormone for normal skeletal development and reaching peak bone mass in men and women.
  - o It inhibits osteoclast activity. After menopause (decreased estrogen levels), increased bone resorption occurs leading to increase bone loss and decreased bone mass.
- **Parathyroid hormone (PTH)**
  - o Secreted from the chief cells of the parathyroid gland.
  - o Parathyroid hormone receptor activation primarily stimulates Adenylyl cyclase (intra cellular signal). The hormone utilizes adenylyl cyclase as a mediator for its cellular signaling within osteoclast.
  - o Parathyroid hormone has the following effects:

- Kidney: Stimulates 1,25 dihydroxy vitamin D formation (by stimulation of 1 hydroxylation of 25 hydroxy vitamin D); increases fractional resorption of filtered calcium; increases urinary excretion of phosphorus
        - Bone: Stimulates osteoclast resorption of bone.
        - Net effect of its actions on the kidney and bone is increased serum calcium and decreased serum phosphorus.
    - Teriparatide (see osteoporosis in the systemic conditions chapter):
        - Recombinant N terminal of PTH.
        - In cyclic (intermittent (daily)) application: stimulates bone formation.
- Calcitonin:
    - Inhibits osteoclast resorption of bone (direct signal inhibition).
    - Secreted by the thyroid gland (clear cells).

Ligaments and Tendons:

- Collagen content:
    - The composition of tendons and ligaments is **primarily type I collagen** aligned in the direction of loading.
    - Type III collagen is also present in tendons and ligaments.
    - Fibroblasts detect applied strain to the tendon through deflection of cilia in response to tendon loading.
    - Ligaments have more elastin contents.
- Tendon covering:
    - Paratenon (non sheather): rich capillary supply (e.g. Achilles tendon).
    - Sheathed: the venicula carries blood supply to certain areas and nutrition diffuse from these areas to surrounding parts (e.g. flexor tendons)
- Tendon insertion into the bone: tendon, fibrocartilage, mineralized fibrocartilage (Sharpey's fibers) then bone.
- Ligament insertion into the bone: either indirectly into the periosteum or indirectly (ligament, fibrocartilage, mineralized fibrocartilage, bone).
    - Avulsion of ligaments (common in children) occurs between the unmineralized fibrocartilage and mineralized fibrocartilage.
- Healing ligaments/ tendons:
    - Initially there will be higher portion of type III that will later reach normal concentration at about one year.
    - Increased number of collagen fiber, but with decreased number mature cross link, decrease mass and diameter of collagen fibers.
- Healing tendons:

- o A tendon is thought to be weakest 5 to 10 days after repair (during the inflammatory stage of healing), reach maximum strength around 6 months.
- o Immobilization of tendon decreases its tensile strength, stiffness, and total weight with a decrease in cellularity, overall collagen organization, and collagen fibril diameter.
- Non-sheathed (Paratenon) tendons and extra-articular ligaments have a greater capacity to heal than sheathed tendons and intra-articular ligaments.

Anesthesia, Preoperative Assessment and General Post-Operative Complications:

- Noninvasive cardiac testing is recommended in the presence of the three or more of the following risk factors: history of ischemic heart disease, history of heart failure, history of stroke, and diabetes mellitus or chronic renal disease.
- If there is orthopedic surgery related vascular injury: urgent vascular surgery consultation or interventional radiologist consultation, urgent arteriogram. In certain cases, vascular re-perfusion may be obtained at the time of an arteriogram with the use of a stent. If this fail to re-perfuse the extremity, urgent exploration of the vessel at the level of injury (determined by the arteriogram).
- For regional anesthesia with LMWH:
  - o Puncture at least 10 hours from the dose of last LMWH
  - o Catheter removal at least 10 hours from the dose of last LMWH.

Gait:

- A gait cycle (stride): complete sequence of all the stages of gait of a single limb during walking, from initial contact to initial contact on the same foot.
- The gait cycle is divided into: stance (60%) and swing phases (40%).
- 60% of the gait cycle is spent in stance phase:
  - o The plantar flexors are active in stance (to produce the ankle rockers).
  - o The dorsiflexors muscles are active in swing phase (for foot clearance).
    - The main concentric contraction that occurs during swing phase is that of the anterior tibialis muscle (which dorsiflexes the foot for easier clearance during swing and prepositions the foot for initial contact).
    - During the initial heel contact of the stance phase, the tibialis anterior muscle (dorsiflexor) has the greatest activity to control the rate of ankle plantar flexion.
  - o More muscle activity occurs during stance phase than during swing phase.
    - In swing phase, momentum generated by the gastrocnemius and hip flexors at terminal stance carries the leg forward.

- Knee flexion in early swing and then extension at terminal swing occur passively.
- The Center of Mass (COM) is located anterior to the second sacral vertebra, midway between the hip joints.
- Gait abnormality:
  - Antalgic gait is a nonspecific term that describes any gait abnormality resulting from pain.
  - Weakness of the hip flexors limits limb advancement during swing and results in a shortened step length.
  - A plantar flexion contracture of the ankle results in a knee extension moment (knee extension thrust) at initial contact of the forefoot with the floor (to be able to achieve the heel touching of the floor).
  - With quadriceps weakness, the patient compensates by leaning the trunk forward to keep the COM anterior to the knee joint.
  - Knee extension during gait is mainly achieved by gastrocnemius (planter flexion against the floor causing backward movement of the tibia and knee extension). Ankle plantar flexor weakness causes increased quadriceps activity (to achieve knee extension) which will lead to limiting step length and painful overuse syndromes of the patella and quadriceps.
  - Trendelenburg gait:
    - Due to weakened hip abductors.
    - Patient should hold assistive device on the opposite side of weakness.
    - The affected hip (due to weak abductor) during the stance phase will have increased adduction and the contralateral pelvis will drop on the swing phase of the gait. To decrease the drop of the contra lateral side during gait, the patient will lean his/her torso to the affected side so that the center of gravity comes close to the affected hip decreasing the moment arm of the gravity and the amount of work needed by abductors to balance the patient weight.

Material Characteristics

Load/ Elongation Curve:

- Slope of the curve will represent the **stiffness**
- Stiffness: force /displacement (or load/deformation)

Stress/Strain Curve

- Describe the mechanical property of a particular material.
- Stress = force/area.

- Strain:
    - Deformation of a material by a force acting on the material.
    - Equals change of length/ original length (has no unit).
- The slope of the curve is the **modulus of elasticity.**
    - modulus of elasticity: stress/strain
    - Modulus of elasticity is determined by the slope of the linear portion of the stress-strain curve of a material.
    - Stiffness is directly proportional to modulus of elasticity. *(Question: what is the most important factor affecting stiffness).*
    - The modulus of elasticity measures the ability of a material to maintain its shape under the application of an external load. The higher the modulus of elasticity, the stiffer the material is.
    - The elastic modulus of stainless steel is about double titanium alloy. An advantage of the titanium alloy IM nails is that it will bend more easily, to accommodate the curvature of the femur during insertion.
    - Stainless steel> titanium alloy> cortical bone bone cement;

Biomechanical Definitions (see Fig 10):

- **Stiffness**: the steepness of the slope of the load elongation curve; the steeper the slope the stiffer the material.
- **Yield Point**: the point where the material changes from elastic to plastic deformation.
    - When an implant is loaded below the yield point, it undergoes elastic deformation (the deformation fully recovers when the load is removed).
    - Plastic deformation: change in the length of a material under loading that does not return to the original length after the load is removed. *(Question: a screw is loaded by a machine causing bending, after removing the load, the screw returns to its normal shape. What type of deformation?)*
    - Titanium has more yield strength than stainless steel (higher yield point, see below)
- **Failure Point**: the point at which the material break.

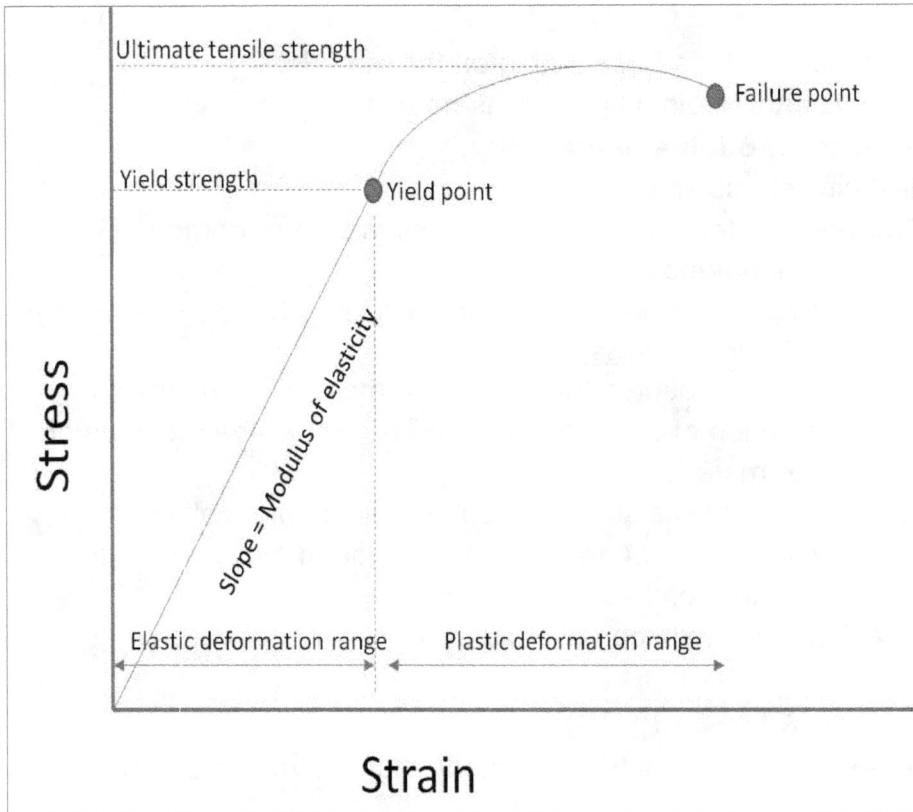

Fig 10: Stress-Strain curve, showing the definitions of Modulus of elasticity, yield point, yield strength, failure point, ultimate tensile strength, elastic and plastic deformation.

- **Strength**:
  - **Yield strength**: magnitude of the load where the material reaches the yield point (point of starting plastic deformation).
  - **Ultimate strength:** magnitude of the load at the point where the material breaks.
  - **Fatigue strength**: magnitude of load need to achieve failure under cyclic loading (see below).
- **Brittle**: material which breaks without significant plastic deformation (narrow range of plastic deformation).
- **Ductile**: material which can have significant plastic deformation before fracture (wide range of plastic deformation).
- **Toughness**:
  - The amount of energy that material can absorb prior to failure.
  - It is represented by the area under the stress strain curve (the larger the area the tougher the material). *(Question: if you want to manufacture a new plate that you want to absorb as much energy before it fails, what material do you chose (the highest toughness))*

- **Fatigue failure**: failure of a material due to repeated cycles of stress (progressive and localized structural damage that occurs when a material is subjected to cyclic loading).
    - The most common cause of mechanical failure of orthopedic materials during clinical use is fatigue failure.
- **Hysteroresis:** when the load and unload stress- strain curves are not identical.
- **A viscoelastic material:**
    - Material which has properties that are rate dependent (time-dependent) for applied forces.
    - Bones, tendons and ligaments are viscoelastic. *(Question: when you test for ligaments, why do you have the control the rate of application of force?)*
    - Creep and stress relaxation are characters of viscoelastic materials:
        - **Creep**: Progressive deformation in response to a constant force applied over an extended period of time.
        - **Stress relaxation:** when deformation is constantly applied to a material, the stress generated in the material will decrease over time
- **An isotropic/ anisotropic material:**
    - Isotropic material: material which has the same mechanical properties in all directions. In general: metals, plastics, and ceramics are isotropic.
    - Anisotropic material has properties that differ depending on the direction of load. Most living tissues (e.g. Bone, muscle, ligament, and tendon) are anisotropic (bone strongest in compression and weakest in torsion). Calcium phosphate cement is also anisotropic (strong in compression and week in shear).

Corrosion:
- Corrosion is the deterioration of a metal because of chemical reactions between it and the surrounding environment. It results in gradual destruction of metal by chemical or electro-chemical reaction with surrounding environment.
- Metals used in orthopedic surgery obtain their corrosion resistance by forming an adherent oxide layer:
    - Titanium alloy form an adherent passive layer of titanium oxide (see later).
    - The addition of chromium to other alloys (stainless steel and cobalt chrome) results in formation of a chromium oxide passive layer that forms on the surface and separates the material from the corrosive body environment.
- **Galvanic corrosion:**
    - Occurs between two different metals in electrical contact (immersed in a conductive medium such as serum or interstitial fluid).

- o Combination of Co-Cr and stainless steel produce the worst galvanic corrosion among the commonly used implants.
- o When using plate- screw- cable construct, they all must be of the same material to avoid corrosion.
- **Crevice corrosion:**
  - o Localized damage on a metal surface at, or immediately adjacent to, the gap or crevice between two joining surfaces.
  - o Stainless steel exhibits the greatest amount of crevice corrosion among commonly used orthopedics materials.

Material in orthopedics:
- **Stainless steel:**
  - o Composition: **Iron, carbon**, molybdenum, chromium, nickel and manganese.
  - o Chrome increases hardness and corrosion resistance (prevent rusting), molybdenum produce fine grain structures with high strength.
- **Cobalt Chrome:**
  - o Composition: cobalt, chromium, nickel and molybdenum.
- **Titanium**
  - o Highly biocompatible.
  - o Has lower modulus of elasticity and higher strength than stainless steel, and is highly resistant to corrosion.
  - o Self-passivation (oxide layer) makes it resistant to surface corrosion.
  - o Commonly used for plates/screws construct and intramedullary nails because of its low modulus of elasticity which can reduce stress shielding.
  - o Can be used for porous-ingrowth coatings. But titanium is not used for cemented hip arthroplasty because it transmits greater stresses to the cement mantel (less stiff than cobalt-chrome and stainless steel).
  - o Cannot be used for femoral head due to its susceptibility to abrasive wear and third-body wear (PMMA fragments, bone chips, metal debris, etc).
- Nickel is present in cobalt-chrome and stainless-steel alloys used in orthopaedic surgery. Adding nickel to metallic alloys adds to strength.
  - o Nickel is not present in titanium alloys or in ceramic components. *(Question: what materials should not be used for nickel-allergic patients?)*
- Chrome helps with corrosion resistance. Not added to titanium alloys as it self-passivate.
- Metal allergy is a type IV (delayed-type) hypersensitivity cell-mediated response.
- **Ceramics:**

- o Ceramics are strong, brittle, and corrosion-resistant materials consisting of elements linked to one another by covalent or ionic bonds, such as alumina (Al_2O_3) and zirconia (ZrO_2),
- o Ceramics are immune to corrosive processes (they are not metals).
- o Ceramics do not undergo fatigue fracture; they fail from a process of slow crack growth.
- o Zirconia has a higher toughness than alumina, making it less susceptible to gross fracture.
- o Zirconia has a metastable phase (tetragonal). High fracture toughness and excellent bending strength.
- o Ceramics have good wettability, allowing lubricating layers between ceramic surfaces to reduce adhesive wear (fretting) of these surfaces.
- **Polymers**
  - o Materials made of atoms of carbon and other elements that are covalently bound to one another to form identical subunits, known as monomers, with the subunits themselves also bound to one another, often in repeating sequences, to form chains or sheets.
  - o **Bioabsorbable polymers:**
    - Polyglycolic acid and Polylactic acid.
    - They have low strength, low elastic modulus and low stiffness.
    - Its main disadvantages is induction of foreign body reactions and joint synovitis.
- **Poly-methyl methacrylate (PMMA) (Bone cement):**
  - o PMMA is an acrylic polymer that is formed by mixing two sterile components: a liquid MMA (methyl methacrylate) monomer (inhibitor) and a powered MMA-styrene co-polymer (initiator).
  - o When the two components are mixed, the liquid monomer polymerizes around the pre-polymerized powder particles to form hardened PMMA.
  - o MMA acts as a space-filler that creates a tight space which holds the implant against the bone and thus acts as a "grout" (not a glue).
  - o Bone cements have no intrinsic adhesive properties, they depend on close mechanical interlock between the irregular bone surface and the prosthesis
  - o Consists of two components: a powder (co-polymer powder,) and a liquid (MMA monomer, stabilizer, inhibitor).
  - o Strong in compression, weak in shear.

Mechanical Principles:

- Torque is associated with the rotational or twisting effect of the applied forces; moment is related to the bending effect.

- **Binding rigidity**
  - o Binding rigidity of cylinder is related to the forth power of the radius.
  - o Binding rigidity of rectangular is related to the third power of the axis of the rectangular along which the bending moment is applied.
  - o **Area** moment of inertia is related to the resistance to bending. **Polar** moment of inertia is related resistance to torsion. **Mass** moment of inertia is related to resistance of rotation.
- When bending load is applied to bone: the maximum stress occurs at the outer (periosteal) surface of bone (the greatest distance from the center of the bone).
  - o The magnitude of the stress is equal to the magnitude of the applied moment multiplied by the distance to the surface (the radius of the bone) divided by the area moment of inertia (resistance to bending).
- Kinematics and Kinetics
  - o Kinematics describes the motion of objects without regard to their mass or how their motion is brought about.
  - o Kinetics involves analysis of the effects of forces and/or moments that are responsible for motion.

Joint Reaction Force:
- Load transferred across the joint.
- Moment: force acting at distance from a point (angular motion)
- For hip joint reaction force is 3-6 times body weight.
  - o To decrease: medialization of the joint, using a cane on the contra-lateral side, decrease the body eight (see hip joint).
- Patella-femoral joint 7-time body weight during running.
- Joint contact pressure/stress: the load transferred across the joint divided by the contact area between the joint surfaces.
  - o Mechanisms that decrease the load across the joint (eg, cane) will decrease the pressure. Mechanisms that increase the contact area will also decrease the stress.

Free-body diagrams
- Show the locations and directions of all forces and moments acting on a body.
- It takes into account the weight and the moment arm (see Fig 11)

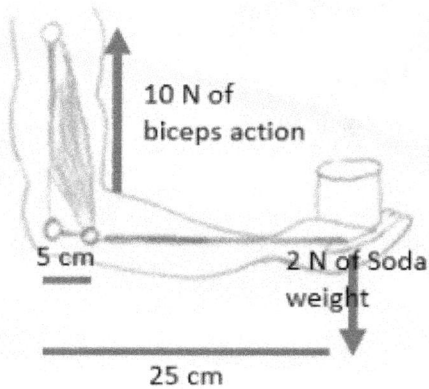

Fig 11: the free body diagram for holding 2 N soda can. The biceps moment arm is 1/5 of the moment arm of soda can to hold it at a transverse level. So, biceps have to do 5 times the weight of Soda

Degree of freedom in movements:

- A body moving in three-dimensional space has six degrees of freedom (three translational and three rotational).
  - Ball-and-socket joint (eg shoulder, hip): rotation in 3 planes.
  - Hinge joint (eg PIP, DIP, elbow) has one rotational plane (about the axis of rotation of the joint).

Chapter 2:   Genetics

Diseases associated with gene mutation

Disease	Gene affected
Osteogenesis imperfecta	COL1A1 (Type I collagen)
Achondroplasia	Fibroblast growth factor (FGF) **receptor** 3
Marfan syndrome	FNB1 (which code for Fibrillin protein).
Diastrophic dysplasia	DTDST (sulfate transporter gene (proteoglycan sulfation).
Pseudoachondroplasia	Cartilage oligomeric matrix protein (COMP)
Multiple Epiphyseal Dysplasia (MED)	COMP (collagen oligomeric matrix protein)
Spondyloepiphyseal dysplasia	Type II collagen
Duchenne muscular dystrophy	Dystrophin
Fibrous dysplasia	Gs alpha (receptor-coupled signaling protein) GNAS1 gene
Osteopetrosis	Carbonic anhydrase type II proton pump (Mutations of CLCN7 and TCIRG 1)
Multiple hereditary exostoses	EXT1, EXT2 genes
Neurofibromatosis type 1	NF1 (neurofibromin) on chromosome 17
Charcot-Marie-Tooth disease	PMP22 (peripheral myelin protein 22) on chromosome 17 (overexpression)
Spinal muscular atrophy	Survival motor neuron protein gene.
Turner's syndrome	Short stature homeobox gene
Vitamin D-dependent rickets Type 1	25(OH) vitamin D hydroxylase gene
Cleidocranial dysplasia	CBFA1/RUNX2
Apert's Syndrome	Fibroblast growth factor receptor (FGFR) 2 gene
X-linked hypophosphatemic rickets	PEX (PHEX) (a cellular endopeptidase)
Friedreich's ataxia	Frataxin gene.
Clubfoot	PITX1-TBX4
Fibular Hemimelia	Sonic hedgehog (SHH) gene

Genes Controlling Bone and Cartilage Development:

- **Runx2** (also called core-binding factor-alpha (CBFA1)) and Osx genes are responsible for bone development and skeletal morphogenesis.
  - o Loss-of-function Mutation in the Cbfa 1 gene causes cleidocranial dysplasia.
- Wnt protein binds and activates the lipoprotein receptor-related protein 5/6 (LRP5/6) during bone development through beta-catenin pathway; this will activate transcription of genes that control osteoblast differentiation (see basic science chapter).
  - o Mutations in the Wnt and Hedgehog (Hh) pathways result in skeletal malformations (as well as osteoarthritis).
- SOX 9: transcription factor which is a major regulator of chondrogenesis. *(Question: what gene control chondrogensis in endochondral ossification?)*.

  - o SOX 9 is a transcription factor associated with chondroblasts differentiation. It is important regulator gene for the differentiation of cells of chondrocytic lineage.
- Altered BMP-4 signal transduction is associated with fibrodysplasia ossificans progressive *(scenario: child with multiple areas of ossification in his body, mechanism?)*

Patterns of Transmission (Mode of Inheritance)

- Autosomal-dominant gene defects usually cause structural deformities.
- Autosomal-recessive genes defects usually cause enzymatic and biochemical defects.
- X-linked dominant: If a woman has heterozygous gene, (single allele being dominant) she will have the condition (dominant gene). If a woman has this condition, she will transmit it to 50% of her sons and daughters.

  - o If a man has X-linked dominant, he will have the condition (only one X gene), affected man transmit the condition to all of his daughters (the daughters gets his X chromosome), but to none of the sons (the sons get the Y chromosome).
- X-linked recessive
  - o Woman: An X-linked woman with the recessive allele is a carrier, but she is not affected because the allele is recessive. She can transmit the condition to 50% of her daughters (who become carriers) and 50% of her sons (the sons are affected because their only X chromosome has the recessive gene).
  - o X linked recessive man: will have disease (see above), will pass it to all his daughters (will become a carrier) and none of his sons (because the son gets the Y chromosome)

Autosomal dominant (Structure abnormality)	Achondroplasia
	Multiple Hereditary Exostosis (MHE)
	Metaphyseal dysplasia, Pseudoachondroplasia, SED congenita
	Marfan
	Cleidocranial dysplasia
	Multiple Epiphyseal Dysplasia (MED)
	Neurofibromatosis type 1 (NF1)
	Malignant hyperthermia
	Osteopetrosis Tarda
Autosomal recessive (Enzyme abnormality)	Homocystinuria
	Diastrophic dysplasia (sulfate transport protein defect)
	Hypophosphatasia
	infantile form of osteopetrosis
	Mucopolysaccharidosis (Except Hunter)
	Vitamin D dependent rickets
	Sickle cell disease (if one gene is only affected, patient will have sickle cell trait)
X-linked recessive	Hemophilia A, B
	Duchennes muscular dystrophy
	Hunter Syndrome
	SED tarda
X linked dominant	X-linked hypophosphatemia (X-linked vitamin d-resistant rickets, Hypophosphatemic rickets)
	pseudohypoparathyroidism (PHP) (Albright Hereditary Osteodystrophy (AHO)
	Leri-Weill dyschondrosteosis

- Genomic imprinting :

  o Parent Specific Gene Activation = same genetic abnormality causes different disease if inherited from different parent.
    - Example: Prader-Willi Syndrome (if the disease inherited from father) and Angleman syndrome (if it is inherited from mother)

Genetic Definitions:

- genome of a cell is the full array of genes, encoding the structure of all proteins and other genetic information.
- Plasmid are extra-chromosomal element that can replicate and be transferred independently of the host chromosome.
- Cells are completely tetraploid (4N) for the entire duration of G2 of the cell cycle.
- Apoptosis: Cell death induced by a series of programmed signaling events

- Transgene: an artificially inserted gene into a single-celled embryo.
- Recombinant technology involves the linking DNA or RNA segments into larger segments of DNA or RNA to produce specific proteins or peptides
- Transcription: first step in gene expression by formation of mRNA from DNA.
  - mRNA carries the genetic information from DNA to the ribosomes, this information is then transformed into proteins and peptides
  - Transcription is the most significant mechanism by which a cell controls its pheno-type
- Translation: second step in gene expression by formation of protein from mRNA

Genetic Tests:

- Immunocytochemical analysis: stain cells using antibody to localize a certain protein within the cells.

- ELISA (enzyme-linked immunosorbent assay): used to detect the presence of an antibody or an antigen in a sample (screening test for HIV and HCV is ELISA against their antibodies)
- Western blot (protein immunoblot): to detect **protein** by using antibodies specific against these protein.
- Northern blot and microarray expression profile analysis assess **RNA.**
- Southern blot: detect specific **DNA** sequence
- Reverse transcription polymerase chain reaction (RT-PCR): quantify the level of **messenger RNA (mRNA)** of a particular gene inside the cells.
- Cytogenetic testing (routine chromosome analysis, karyotyping): is utilized to detect numerical and/or structural chromosome abnormalities in metaphase cells.

Translocation Genes Related to Tumor (See Tumor Chapter)

Chapter 3:   Systemic Conditions

Reflex Sympathetic Dystrophy:

- Patient will display intense pain with light touch.
- Pain, allodynia (central pain sensitization (increased response of neurons)); hyperalgesia.
    - o Management: Physical therapy, anti-inflammatory drugs, and a serotonin reuptake inhibitor, if this fail: sympathetic blocks.

Charcot Arthropathy (See Foot and Ankle Chapter):

- Due to neuropathy (most commonly diabetic neuropathy, but can occur with any etiology of neuropathy). The most common etiology of neuropathy will vary with the affected area.
    - o Shoulder and elbow: cervical spine syringomyelia
    - o Knee: syphilis.
    - o Foot and ankle: diabetes mellitust.
- Patient will present with mild pain, swelling and redness.
- Investigation:
    - o Marker of infection: usually within normal.
    - o Biopsy: normal bone.
    - o XR fragmentation, subluxation, and dissolution of the joint.

Inflammatory Conditions:

Gout:

- Gout is caused by the deposition of monosodium urate crystals (purine breakdown products).
    - o Neutrophils ingest the crystals and release potent lysosomal enzymes.
    - o **Aspiration of the joint will show strongly negative birefringent needle shaped crystals.**
- Common locations of gout include the **great toe** (most common), ankle, and knee.
- Punched lesions (tophi) may be seen on radiographs in chronic cases (Fig 1 in the hand chapter).
    - o Histologically, the tophi have several features: acellular amorphous material, macrophages, foreign body giant cells.
- The treatment of gout includes
    - o Acute stage: NSAIDs and/or colchicine.
    - o Allopurinol (lowers the level of uric acid):
        - ▪ Allopurinol should be avoided in acute stages as it may increase the severity of the attacks.
        - ▪ Allopurinol is not indicated for asymptomatic hyperuricemia.

Calcium Pyrophosphate Crystals Arthropathy:

- The knee is the most affected joint.
- Clinical presentation: usually asymptomatic. Attacks of join pain (pseudo-gout) can occur due CPPC. These attacks can occur spontaneously or can be precipitated by trauma, surgery (e.g. abdominal surgery), MI, cerebrovascular accidents.
- XR: calcium deposition in the joints (e.g. chondrocalcinosis of the menisci or the TFCC (triangular fibrocartilage complex).
- Aspiration of the knee will show **weakly positive birefringent rhomboid-shaped crystals**.
- Treatment: NSAIDs, possible steroid injection. *(Scenario: 45 years old male, laparoscopic cholecystectomy 10 days ago, c/o of knee pain, XR shows chondrocalcinosis, what will the aspiration show?)*

Rheumatoid Arthritis (RA) (See Hand, Foot, Spine Chapters for Specific Rheumatoid Affection of These Areas):

- Rheumatoid arthritis is a systemic inflammatory disorder marked by erosive arthritis in multiple joints.
- Main clinical presentation is morning stiffness and joint pain.
- Pathology:
  - The main feature of rheumatoid arthritis is chronic synovitis:
    - Histologically: RA will show accumulation of lymphocytes, absence of neutrophils, intimal lining hyperplasia (no basement membrane in synovium), and increased disorganized capillaries and blood vessel proliferation
    - The pathologic lesion in rheumatoid arthritis is pannus, which is a hyperplastic synovial proliferation resulting in proteoglycan and collagen digestion (joint destruction and ligamentous instability).
  - Rheumatoid factor is present in about 80% to 90% of **adult** patients with rheumatoid arthritis.
  - Rheumatoid factor is IgM autoantibodies against the Fc fragment of immunoglobulin G (IgG).
  - Interleukin-1 and tumor necrosis factor have been implicated in the pathogenesis of rheumatoid arthritis
  - Patients with rheumatoid arthritis have impaired capacity to control infection with Epstein-Barr virus (EBV) (which may be the etiology of the increased incidence of lymphoma in patients with RA).

- o Steroid use in rheumatoid patients lead to poor bone quality, impair bony fusion, and poor wound healing. Elective orthopedic surgeries can have poor outcomes due to the above reasons.
- **Treatment of rheumatoid arthritis:**
  - o Adalimumab and etanercept, Infliximab: TNF-alpha antagonist (Infliximab and Adalimumab are monoclonal antibody that prevents the binding of TNF-α to its receptors on cells).
  - o Anakinra: IL-1 antagonist. It inhibits the action of IL-1 by binding to the IL-1 receptor
  - o Basiliximab, Daclizumab: IL-2 antagonist.
  - o Tocilizumab (Actemra): IL-6 antagonist.
- **Pre-operative evaluation of the cervical spine stability:**
  - o Flexion/extension views should be done to assess the stability of the cervical spine for RA patients before elective surgeries (e.g. THA).
    - ▪ A difference of greater than 9 to 10 mm in the atlanto-dens interval (ADI) on flexion/extension views or space available for the cord less than 14 mm is associated with an increased risk of neurologic injury and usually requires surgical treatment.
- **RA medication (DMARDs) and elective surgeries:**
  - o Methotrexate, leflunomide, hydroxychloroquine, and sulfasalazine can be continued through surgery.
  - o Biologic agents (TNF, IL1, IL2 and IL6 antagonist) should be stopped one dosing cycle (from 2-24 weeks depending on the medication) prior to surgery, then the surgery performed the following week after that (for possible increase in incidence of infection).

Ankylosing Spondylitis (See Also Spine Chapter):
- More common in young males.
- Most common initial manifestation is sacro-iliitis.
- Work up:
  - o HLA-B27 has about 90% sensitivity and specificity for AS in patients with European descents. *(Scenario: 30 years old white male with bilateral SI joint pain and stiffness of both hips, imaging shows bilateral SI joint fusion, next step? (NSAIDs and assessment of HLA-B27)).*
  - o Imaging:
    - ▪ Early in the disease process: erosion on the iliac side of the sacroiliac joint and bilateral sacroiliitis
    - ▪ Marginal thin syndesmotic osteophytes (see spine chapter).
- Patient with AS sustaining trauma to spine can develop epidural hematoma.

o Patients with AS and history of spinal trauma, should get advanced imaging studies. The condition is frequently missed on the initial radiographs.

o Patient with AS usually have a flexed posture of their neck. If they have neck trauma, they should be kept in their "normal" flexed position and do not try to extend them as this may result in neurologic injury or displacement of a non-displaced fracture.

  ▪ For non-displaced fracture: treatment is posterior column fixation. Non operative treatment can result in fracture displacement.

  ▪ Decompression may be needed if there is an epidural hematoma that is compressing the cord.

  ▪ In patients with ankylosing spondylitis, stand-alone anterior stabilization has a high failure rate. *(Scenario: 75 years old, long history of low back pain and stiffness, fell on his face, scalp laceration, XR normal, gradual development of upper and lower extremity weakness, next step? (CT), treatment? (decompression and posterior stabilization)).*

Psoriatic Arthritis:

- Clinical presentation:
  o Dactylitis and nail pitting (Radiographs will show pencil in cup deformity (very characteristics))
  o Enthesopathy (achilles tendinitis, and posterior tibial tendonitis). *(Scenario: forefoot pain, synovitis, nail pitting, diagnosis?)*

Lyme Arthritis:

- The most common tick-borne illness in the United States.
- Pathology:
  o Synovitis of the joint. Borrelia burgdorferi (the causative organism) does not produce proteolytic enzymes (in contrast to bacteria septic arthritis), this leads to less damage to the articular cartilage.
  o Usually involve large joints (the knee is involved in 90% of cases).
- Clinical Presentation:
  o History of travel to endemic areas (e.g. North-East USA).
  o Early disease: usually develops 7–14 days after a tick bite, erythema migrans is the most common presentation and is a pathognomonic skin lesion.
  o Late disease: arthritis is the hallmark of this stage, develops few months after disease onset.
    ▪ The joint is warm, swollen. The swelling is usually larger and less painful than bacterial septic arthritis.
  o Blood workup:

- ELISA for B Burgdorferi titer.
- Aspiration: positive PCR for B Burgdorferi DNA in synovial joint.
  - o **Treatment:**
    - Can be treated by oral (doxycycline or Amoxicillin) or intravenous antibiotics (Ceftriaxone or Penicillin).
    - If there is neurological affection, IV treatment is preferred.

Septic Arthritis (See Also Septic Arthritis in Pediatric Chapter):

- The antibiotic of choice for gonococcal septic arthritis of the knee is Ceftriaxone IV.

Hemochromatosis:

- Pathology: symmetrical poly arthropathy, with chronic joint pain and stiffness.
- XR shows characteristic changes in the foot and ankle: chondrocalcinosis of the ankles and bony enlargement of the midfoot and the second and third metatarsal heads.

Neurological Diseases:
Poliomyelitis:

- Anterior horn cell disease. The virus affects these cells causing lower motor neuron paralysis.
- The best method of optimizing function of muscles affected by post-polio syndrome is to exercise daily at sub-exhaustion levels.

NF (Neurofibromatosis) Type 1 (von Recklinghausen Disease) (See Also Pediatric Chapter):

- Due to mutation of NF1 gene on chromosome 17 (tumor suppressor gene).
  - o Autosomal dominant with 100% penetrance.
- Bone lesions include anterolateral bowing of tibia, pseduoarthrosis of tibia or the forearm (ulna or rarely radius), scoliosis, sphenoidal hyperplasia.
  - o Spine deformities (kypho-scoliosis):
    - Scoliosis is the most common skeletal manifestation of NF1.
    - Curves are usually dysplastic (dystrophic) with short, sharp angular angles (over 4-6 vertebrae). Dystrophic curves have "penciling" of the ribs (twisting of the ribs will make it look thinner).

- Penciling (indication of rotation) is a major risk factor of progression.
    - Modulation: the change of a spinal curve from an idiopathic-like type to a dysplastic type with rapid progression and the need for aggressive stabilization.
    - Dural ectasia (Widening of the dural sac and the spinal canal) causing erosion of the surrounding vertebral bone is a frequent manifestation of NF1. It is thought to be due to weakening of the dura which expands with the pressure of cerebrospinal fluid causing scalloping of the posterior portions of the vertebral bodies and erosion of the pedicles (CT may be needed to assess the bony elements for instrumentation planning).
    - In neurofibromatosis: circumferential fusion (combined anterior and posterior fusion) is needed to achieve correction and union (pseudoarthrosis is a common complication). *(Scenario: 14 years old with NF1, 70° dystrophic curve of upper thoracic, treatment?)*
- Other manifestations include café au lait patches (more than 5 needed for diagnosis) and axillary or inguinal freckles (>2 freckles).
    - The café au lait spots in NF has smooth border (coast of California) (in contrast to McCune Albright Syndrome with fibrous dysplasia which is ragged (coast of Maine)).
    - Patients with NF1 can develop aortic stenosis (new cardiac symptoms require urgent evaluation).

Dysplasias

Achondroplasia:

- AD (autosomal dominant), the most common skeletal dysplasia.
- Due to abnormality of Fibroblast Growth Factor Receptor 3 (FGFR3) gene (see genetic chapter).
    - The gene mutation can result in development of achondroplasia, thanatophoric dysplasia and hypoachondroplasia (but not pseudo achondroplasia).
        - Activation of the receptor limits enchondral ossification.
        - Mutation of the gene will result in phosphorylation of the tyrosine kinase domain.
        - Most cases are due to new mutation.
- Affect proliferative zone (**quantity defect not quality defect**).
- Clinical presentation:

- o Rhizomelic dwarfism (short limbs, mainly affecting proximal segments (thigh, upper arm))
  - Disproportionate dwarfism.
- o Patient with achondroplasia do NOT have spinal instability. NO C1-2 instability. NO need for assessment of upper cervical spine prior to surgeries.
- o Lumbar and cervical stenosis. Decrease inter pedicular distance (the pedicles narrow as they progress distally in the lumbar spine). This can become very disabling in adults.
- o The pelvis is low and broad with narrow sciatic notches and ping-pong paddle-shaped iliac wings. *(Scenario: short person with broad pelvis, genu varum, what genetic mutation?)*
- o Thoracolumbar kyphosis: in most cases the kyphosis will resolve with growth.
- o Can have foramen magnum stenosis, which may cause deterioration of the child neurological condition (weakness, apnea and possible sudden death). The condition can be assessed by CT or MRI. *(Scenario: 5 years achondroplasia started to have wide based gait, hypotonia, sleep apnea, diagnosis?).*

Diastrophic Dysplasia:
- Autosomal recessive affecting the sulfate transporter gene (DTDST) (proteoglycan sulfation) (see Genetics Chapter).
- Hitch hiker thumb, cauliflower ear

Cleidocranial Dysostosis.
- Autosomal-dominant condition.
- Deficiency of intramembranous ossification.
- Absence of the clavicle (which is formed by intramembranous ossification).
  - o Clinical presentation: droopy shoulders with narrow chest (absence of clavicles), short stature.
- Radiographs of the spine and chest show absent clavicles, delayed ossification of the pubis and ischium, and coxa vara.

Pseudoachondroplasia:
- Mutation of the COMP gene (see genetic chapter) (same gene as MED).
- Difference form achondroplasia:
  - o Has more normal facial appearance in contrast to achondroplasia.
  - o Commonly has C1-C2 spinal instability.

Multiple Epiphyseal Dysplasia:

- Mutation of the COMP gene (see genetic chapter).
- Affects the epiphysis. *(Scenario: Child with waddling gait. XR pelvis shows bilateral symmetrical proximal femoral epiphysis affection, diagnosis?) (NOT bilateral Perthes).*

Larsen syndrome:

- Characterized by multiple congenital joint dislocations, cervical instability and congenital cardiac defects.

Mucopolysaccharidoses

- All types are AR except Hunter (X linked recessive).
- Carpal tunnel syndrome is a characteristic finding.
- Other features: **upper cervical instability** and progressive kyphosis.

Pseudo-Hurler's Syndrome (Mucolipidosis):

- Carpal tunnel syndrome is characteristic finding.

Gaucher's disease:

- Results in the abnormal accumulation of Glucocerebrosides.
- Due to a defect in the gene responsible for β-glucocerebrosidase.
- Risk factor for AVN.

Nail-Patella Syndrome (Hereditary Onycho-Osteodysplasia):

- Abnormalities of the patellae (absent patella), elbows (radial head dislocation), and nails.
- Associated with nephropathy and possible subsequent development of renal failure.

Rickets:

- Disease of deficient bone mineralization in children.
- Common types (see table below):
  - Vit D deficiency (nutritional, deficient absorption).
  - Vit D resistant rickets (hypo phosphatemic rickets) (most common type in US).
  - Vit D dependent rickets (Type I and Type II).
- Pathology:

- o The common pathologic process that occurs in patients with rickets, regardless of the cause, is a failure to mineralize the matrix in the zone of provisional calcification.
- o Bone deformities (eg genu varum) can develop due deficient mineralization.
- XR:
  - o **Widening, cupping and fraying** (see Fig 1) of the growth plate, bone deformities (commonly, genu varum), widening of the ribs anteriorly. *(Scenario: 4 years' boy, bilateral genu varum, XR shows bowing of the distal femur and proximal tibia with widening, cupping and fraying of the proximal tibial and distal femur physes, next step?) (Obtain serum phosphorous, calcium, and alkaline phosphatase levels.))*

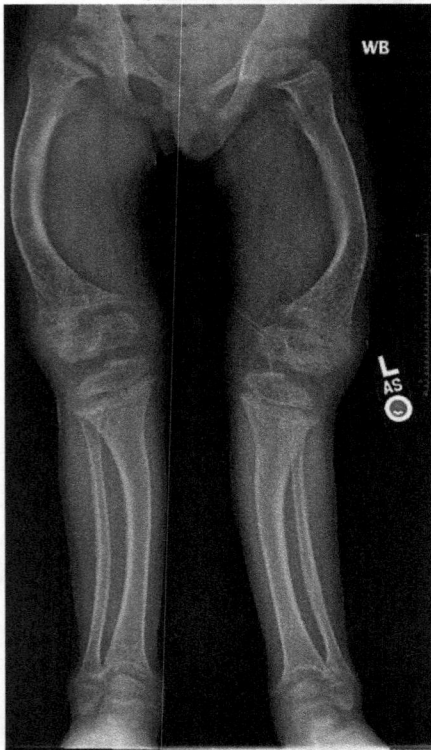

Fig 1: scangram for 4 years old patient with Vit D resistant Rickets. Notice the growth plates of the proximal and distal tibia and distal femur showing widening, cupping and fraying. Notice also the deformity of the femur and tibias.

Comparison of different types of Rickets

	Ca	Phos	Alk Phos	PTH	Vit D (total)	1,25 Di OH Vit D	Genetics
VIt D deficiency rickets	Low normal/ low	low	high	**high**	**low**	low	
Vit D resistant rickets	normal	low	High or normal	Normal/ slightly high	**normal**	normal	XD
Vit D dependent rickets Type I	low	low	high	High	normal	low	AR
Vit D dependent rickets Type II	low	low	high	High	normal	high	AR

- **Vitamin D Deficiency Rickets:**
    - Causes: nutritional (decreased Vit D intake), decrease Vitamin D absorption from the intestine (mal-absorption syndrome, steatorrhea causing loss of vit D with fat in stool).
    - Nutritional deficiency is common in developing countries, rare in United States due to use fortified food (foot with added Vit D).
    - Nutritional rickets in US is more common in African American children who are breast fed past 6 months of age without vitamin D supplementation.
    - Pathology: decreased serum Vit D, decreased calcium absorption, decreased serum calcium, secondary hyperparathyroidism.
    - Effects of increased PTH in cases of Vit D deficiency rickets:
        - Increase calcium urinary re-absorption from the kidney (decrease urinary calcium excretion).
        - Increased bone resorption (leading to increased alkaline phosphatase).
        - The two above effects will result in increased serum calcium to become normal or low normal.
        - Increased urinary phosorus excretion (low serum phosphorus).
    - **Treatment:** high dose Vit D (5000 IU per day).
- **X- Linked Hypophosphatemia Rickets (Vitamin D-Resistant Rickets) (familial hypophosphatemic rickets):**
    - X-linked dominant:
        - Caused by mutations of PH EX gene
    - Metabolic bone diseases associated with decrease phosphate in blood due impaired renal tubular reabsorption of phosphate.
    - Affected children are short in stature and have genu varum, physeal widening, and generalized osteopenia.
    - Calcium level is normal, markedly decreased serum phosphorus; Alkaline Phosphatase is often elevated, normal parathyroid hormone level (or slightly elevated).
    - Treat with phosphate replacement and high-dose vitamin D3 (Vitamin D alone will not improve clinical picture). *(Scenario: 3 years old, bilateral genu varum, physeal widening, lab studies show decreased serum phosphate levels, elevated alkaline phosphatase, but normal serum calcium, parathyroid hormone (PTH), and vitamin-D levels, diagnosis? inheritance?)*
- **Vit D dependent rickets:**
    - Type I:
        - Failure of conversion of 25-hydroxy vit D to 1,25-dihydroxy vit D.
        - 25 hydroxy Vit D will be increased with low 1,25 di OH vit D.
    - Type II:
        - End organ insensitivity to 1,25-di hydroxy vit D.

- Increase in both 25 hydroxy Vit D and 1,25 di hydroxy vit D. *(Question: what disease will result from A knock-out mouse for the Vitamin D receptor?)*

Hypophosphatasia:

- Metabolic bone diseases associated with **decreased alkaline phosphatase level and activity**.
  - o Will cause inability to mineralize osteoid.
- The chemical profile: Normal calcium, normal di-hyroxy Vit D, and low alkaline phosphatase.

Hypoparathyroidism:

- Decrease serum calcium and increase serum phosphate.
- Most common cause of hypoparathyroidism is parathyroid surgical removal during total thyroidectomy.

Pseudohypoparathyroidism (PHP):

- Sex-linked dominant condition.
- Pathology: end organ resistance to parathyroid hormone.
- Clinical presentation: short stature, short metacarpals (4th and 5th), Mental retardation, tetany

Renal Osteodystrophy:

- Pathology:
  - o Decreased hydroxylation of the 1 position of Vit D (failure to synthesize active form of Vit D), this will lead to Hypocalcemia.
  - o Hypocalcemia and possible increased phosphate (due to phosphate retention and inability to secret the phosphate by the diseased kidney) will lead to increased level parathyroid hormone (secondary hyperparathyroidism), resorption of bone by increased activity of osteoclasts due to hyperparathyroidism (brown's tumor), osteopenia and possible fractures.
  - o Metabolic acidosis (renal affection).
  - o Aluminum toxicity: due to dialysis fluid impurities which is toxic to osteoblast.
- If the condition occurs in children, it can lead to deformities of the extremities *(scenario: 8 years old, renal disease, progressive limb deformities, XR shows osteopenia, cupping widening and fraying of the physis with deformities, diagnosis?) (Scenario: end stage renal disease, hip pain, XR: bone resorption, biopsy: increase osteoclast, resorption of the bone trabeculae, what is the diagnosis? (secondary hyperparathyroidism)).*

Hyperparathyroidism:

- Can be primary or secondary to hypocalcemia (see renal osteodystrophy above).

- o Primary: increased serum calcium, decreased serum phosphate, kidney stone.
- o Secondary: in response to hypocalcemia. The calcium level can reach normal or low normal level.
- Pathology: Increase bone resorption. Brown tumor: areas of bone osteolysis can be found in the bone; histologically: giant cell (similar histologically to giant cell tumor)

Hypercalcemia:

- Causes: primary hyperparathyroidism, hypercalcemia of malignancy.
- Clinical presentation: lethargy, nausea, constipation, abdominal pains, kidney stones. EKG will show a shortened QT interval.
- Treatment: Intravenous fluid administration (first step), furesimde (lasix) diuretics.

Osteomalacia:

- Disease of deficient bone mineralization in adults (in contrast to Rickets which is a disease of children). It is due to failure to maintain adequate serum calcium and phosphate levels.
- Pathology:
    - o Disease of bone quality and not bone quantity (in contrast to osteoporosis).
    - o Blood chemistry will show low levels of Calcium (or low normal) and low phosphate levels (hemoglobin is not affected in most cases).
    - o Affect the zone of provisional calcification.

Ostporosis:

- The peak bone density is reached at the 4th decade.
- Pathology: normal mineralization of bone, decrease bone mass, abnormal micro architecture leading to enhanced bone fragility and increased fracture risk.
    - o Osteomalacia is abnormal mineralization (bone quality), osteoporosis is decrease mass (bone quantity).
    - o Most important determinant of cancellous bone strength and stiffness is bone density (the amount of bone per unit volume).
    - o Two types:
        - Post-menopausal (high turnover osteoporosis due to increased breakdown of bone): with menopause; there is a negative calcium balance with a decrease in intestinal absorption and an increase in urinary calcium loss. These changes may be directly related to decrease estrogen level. Affects about 10% of females after menopause.

- - Senile (low turnover osteoporosis due to decreased bone formation) affects males and females after the age of 70 years, associated with decrease amount of active Vit D.
- Lab study: normal blood work (CBC and BMP)
  - Elderly female with low energy fracture of the distal radius were found to have low level of Vit D.
- DEXA scan will show the decrease BMD (see below for details).
- XR: osteopenia (radiographic evidence of osteopenia and bone density loss is not apparent until 40% reduction of bone loss).
  - With increasing age, diaphyseal bone will have increased inner bone diameter and decreased cortical thickness (an attempt to increase bone strength).
- Urinary N-telopeptide (breakdown product of Type I collagen/ marker of increased bone turnover, see basic science chapter) increased with osteoporosis due to accelerated bone loss.
- Bone Mineral Density (BMD):
  - DEXA provides data on bone mineral content and soft-tissue composition (thus requiring data on cross-sectional dimension for accuracy). DEXA provides a quantitative, not qualitative, measurement of bone mineral content.
    - Osteoarthritis falsely elevates the DEXA results, especially in the AP spinal analysis.
  - The T-score: the number of standard deviations that the individual's bone mineral density (BMD) differs from the normal peak bone mass in young adults (30 years) for the gender (and ethnicity) of the patient.
    - osteoporosis is defined as BMD that is 2.5 standard deviations (SDs) or more below the peak bone mineral density (T-score lower than −2.5).
    - Osteopenia: Patients with BMD between 1 and 2.5 SDs below peak bone mineral density (T-score −1 to −2.5).
- Risk factors: **white (Caucasian) thin females**, use of steroids, anti-depressant or anti-epileptic, smoking, family history (history of hip fractures), increasing age, early menopause, lack of exercises and low protein diet, type I diabetes mellitus, malabsorption syndromes.
- Effect of fragility fracture on mortality and on getting another fragility fracture:
  - Elderly patients with vertebral compression fractures have higher mortality rate than control; this increased mortality rate is more in males than in females.

- o Previous distal radius fractures (especially in men) and previous spinal fracture (in both genders) increase the relative risk of a subsequent hip fracture
- o Proximal humerus fracture is the most consistent fracture that predicts the patient's risk for a subsequent low-energy hip fracture
- **Fracture Risk Assessment Tool (FRAX):**
  - o FRAX is a diagnostic tool used to evaluate the 10-year probability of bone fracture risk.
  - o Depends on the BMP at the femoral neck and clinical risk factors:
    - Clinical risk factors include a prior fragility fracture, parental history of hip fracture, current tobacco smoking, long-term use of glucocorticoids, rheumatoid arthritis, other causes of secondary osteoporosis and daily alcohol consumption.
    - Femoral neck BMD (it can also be pure clinical score if BMD is not known)
- **Prevention and treatment of osteoporosis**
  - o Prevention of osteoporosis:
    - Women > 50 years: should start daily supplement of Vit D and calcium (food rich in these elements is not enough).
    - Women > 65 years: recommend to have DEXA scan to assess BMD.
    - Post-menopausal women with one risk factor for fracture: recommend to have DEXA scan to assess BMD.
  - o A patient with a T-score of -1.0 to -2.5 should be considered for osteoporosis prevention therapy. This would consist of calcium (1,200 to 1,500 mg daily), vitamin D (800 to 1000 IU daily). If they have increase fracture risk (see before), then active treatment is indicated.
  - o Indication for treatment of osteoporosis:
    - T-scores lower than -2.5 (at the femoral neck or spine).
    - Age 50 and older with T-score between -1.0 and -2.5 (osteopenia) AND 10-year hip fracture probability > 3% or a 10-year major osteoporosis-related fracture probability > 20% (based on FRAX).
    - Previous fragility fracture.
      - Patient with fragility fracture: assess level of Vit D and obtain DEXA scan. If T score worse than 1.5, treatment is indicated.
  - o Pharmacologic options for osteoporosis treatment are bisphosphonates, calcitonin, Selective estrogen receptor modulators (SERMs), recombinant parathyroid hormone 1-34 (teriparatide) and RANKL inhibitor (denosumab).

- o After 3-5 years of treatment, re-assessment should be performed. Prolonged bisphosphonate treatment had been linked to sub-trochanteric and femoral shaft stress fractures.
- o Osteoporosis diagnosed after a hip fracture should have early post-operative referral to an osteoporosis clinic if possible (with orthopedic surgeon co-management).
  - Intravenous (IV) zoledronic acid within 90 days of a hip fracture, followed by annual treatment will result in reduction of vertebral and nonvertebral fractures and improvement in survival.
- **Teriparatide (recombinant form of parathyroid hormone):**
  - o Consists of 1-34 Amino-terminal residues of parathyroid hormone.
  - o Administrated as daily subcutaneous injection. yhbIntermittent PTH treatment (daily injection) increases **osteoblast** function and bone mineral density by increasing coupled remodeling between osteoclast-mediated bone resorption and osteoblast-mediated new bone formation (**anabolic effect on bone**, only FDA approved anabolic bone medication).
  - o Intermittent PTH administration mediate the anabolic bone response through receptors expressed by osteoblasts (Continuous dosing would stimulate bone resorption).
  - o Indication: severe osteoporosis (>3 SD), failure or inability to tolerate other medications. It is also used for treatment of bisphosphonate induced femoral fracture.
  - o Its use in rats was associated with an increased incidence of osteosarcoma. The medication is contra indicated in children and in patients with Paget's disease and in any patient for a period of more than two continuous years
- **Bisphosphonates:**
  - o Mechanism of action:
    - Nitrogen containing bisphosphonates (alendronarte, risedronate, ibdronate, zaledronic acid): inhibit osteoclast resorption by inhibiting the enzyme farnesyl diphosphate synthase (within the mevalonate pathway). This will result in inhibition of protein prenylation and GTPase formation (which is needed for ruffled border formation and cell survival). This results in programmed cell death (apoptosis)
    - Non–nitrogen-containing bisphosphonates (Etidronate): Metabolized into a nonfunctional adenosine triphosphate (ATP) analog (which will also cause apoptosis)
  - o Effects of bisphosphonate after orthopedic surgeries:
    - Reduced rate of spinal fusion in animal model; withholding bisphosphonate is recommended after surgery.

- No adverse effects after TKA and THA.
- Effects after fracture healing is controversial (may inhibit remodeling).
- Children with osteogenesis imperfecta (OI) on bisphosphonate treatment may have inhibition of osteotomy healing.
  o Long-term side effect for bisphosphonate treatment:
    - Osteonecrosis of the jaw: rare complication that can happens in patients with major dental intervention and in cases receiving parental bisphosphonate (e. g. cancer patients).
    - Pathological sub trochanteric and diaphyseal (insufficiency stress fractures of the femur): Occurs in the sub-trochanteric and proximal shaft region, there will be lateral cortical thickening with beaked appearance and history of thigh pain for few months prior to the fracture. *(Scenario: 80 years old with proximal femoral shaft fracture, thigh pain for months prior to the fracture, what history is related to this fracture?)*.
  o Contra-indications for bisphosphonates: pregnant females, chronic kidney disease, esophageal disorders.

Marfan's disease:

- Due mutation in the **Fibrillin-1** gene (FBN1).
- Clinical presentation:
  o Elongated limbs (dolichostenomelia), pectus excavatum, acetabular protrusion, dural ectasia, **superior** lens dislocation.
  o Positive thumb sign and collar sign (see Fig 2).
  o Cardiac anomaly (echocardiography is needed before surgery).
  o Progressive scoliosis: may require surgery to prevent progression.
    - Spinal fusion in Marfan patients has higher complication rate than regular idiopathic cases; surgeon should avoid massive correction as it may lead to cardio vascular complication.

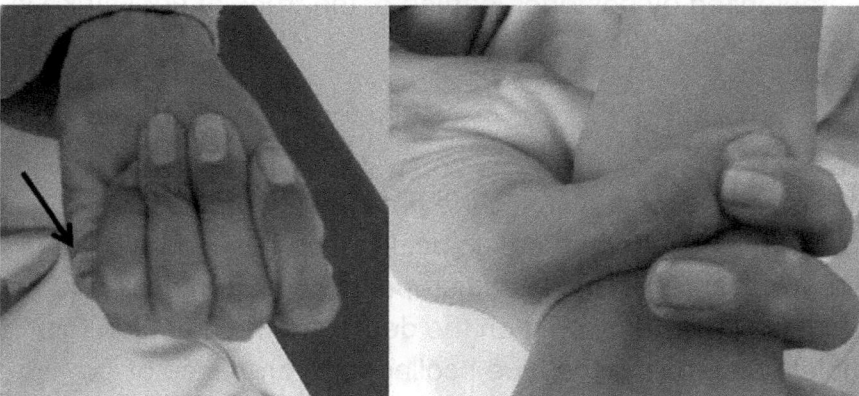

Fig 2: Thumb sign (the tip of the thumb (arrow) protrude from the ulnar side of the hand with grip) and collar sign (the thumb and small finger can encircle the wrist and overlap each other.

Hereditary Motor Sensory Neuropathies (Charcot-Marie-Tooth Disease) (Sensory Motor Demyelinating Neuropathy) (See Cavus Foot in The Pediatric Chapter):

- Pathology:
  - o Mutation of the gene of peripheral myelin protein (PMP) 22.
  - o The disease process affects myelination of the peripheral nerves (myelin sheath disease).
- The disorder can be diagnosed with DNA gene mutation test (very sensitive and specific).
- Charcot-Marie-Tooth type I (CMT I) is the most common type of CMT, affecting approximately 50%-80% of CMT patients and is autosomal-dominant.
- Peroneal nerve is the primarily affected nerve in the initial stages of CMT disease.
- The first muscles affected in the lower extremity are foot intrinsics (leading to clawing).
- Patient will present with cavus foot (more than 90% of CMT patients will develop foot deformity). Cavus will eventually progress to cavo-varus (see pediatric chapter) and 5th banionnette:
  - o This should be treated by correction of the varus deformity and not resection of the 5th metatarsal head. Fifth metatarsal head resection can lead to transfer lesion to the fourth metatarsal few years later.
- Scoliosis occurs in about 1/3 of patients with CMT.

Friedrich Ataxia:

- Spinocerebellar disorder which is characterized by ataxic gait, areflexia, muscle weakness, loss of proprioception, scoliosis, and cavo-varus foot deformity.
- Usually the gluteus maximus is the first muscle to be affected. The patient will have gluteus maximus gait characterized by posterior leaning of the trunk at heel strike in order to keep the hip extended during the stance phase.

Osteogensis Imperfect (OI):

- The main mutation in OI is glycine substitutions in the procollagen molecule.
  - o Glycine normally occurs as every third amino acid in the collagen helix. Substituting glycine for a larger amino acid disrupts the collagen helix and causes abnormal cross links (depending on the degree of the mutation this may result in complete absence of the type I collagen or presence of abnormal collagen).

- o Apophyseal avulsion fractures of the olecranon are characteristic injuries of OI.
- Treatment by bisphosphonate.
  - o It increases bone mass, cortical thickness, and the height of collapsed vertebrae.
  - o It decreases the incidence of fractures and relieve chronic bone pain.
  - o No effect on the incidence of scoliosis.
  - o Long-term use of bisphosphonate can result in appearance of radiographic bands in distal femoral and proximal tibial and fibular metaphyses parallel to the growth plates in these bones.
- If there is progression of spinal curve (>35-40°): treatment is by posterior spinal fusion with instrumentation.
- Basilar invagination can be seen in patients with osteogenesis imperfecta (will be presenting by progressive weakness) *(Scenario: 8 years old with OI, stopped walking for the last few months, no pain in the lower extremities, XR of the lower extremities does not show any fracture, there progressive weakness of all extremities, Next step? (imaging of the cervical spine))*

Apert's Syndrome:
- Affect the hand (mitten hand), feet (syndactyly). Patient will also have cranial synostosis.
- Patient may have mutation of the fibroblast growth factor receptor 2 (FGFR2) *(Scenario: a picture of new born with mitten hand, what also may this infant have? What is the genetic problem?)*

Avascular Necrosis (See AVN of Hip):
- There is complete death of all the elements inside the bone: osteoblasts, osteocytes (empty lacunae), hematopoietic cells, capillary endothelial cells, and lipocytes.
- These changes start to occur from the second week after injury.

Sickle Cell Disease:
- Point mutation of beta 2 chain hemoglobin.
- In THA, sclerosis can cause perforation of the femoral canal (see hip chapter).

Hemophilia:
- Hemophilia A: deficiency of **factor VIII**. Hemophilia B: deficiency of **factor XI**.
- Hemophylic arthopathy is due repeated hemoarthrosis causing synovitis from heme deposition.

- XR: squaring of the inferior patellar pole and femoral condyles.
- Availability of recombinant factor VIII treatment had decreased the incidence of hemophilic arthropathy.
- The knee is the most common location of spontaneous bleeding in children with hemophilia.
- 40% to 50% of normal level of factor VIII is needed to control spontaneous bleeding into the knee in children with hemophilia.
- For surgery, the replacement should be targeted to reach to 100% of the normal level of factor VIII.
  - The plasma level rises 2% for every unit/ kg body weight of factor VIII administered.
- Synovectomy:
  - Indication: recurrent hemarthrosis (especially if these attacks occurred despite optimal medical management).
  - Effective in decreasing joint bleeding. Not as effective in restoring ROM or preventing (or reversing) arthropathy.

Disseminated Intravascular Coagulation (DIC):

- Due to widespread microvascular thrombosis leading to consumption of coagulation factors and platelets, and then subsequent hemorrhage.
- Elevation in the PT and aPTT, decreased levels of fibrinogen and platelets, increased levels of fibrinogen degradation products and D-Dimer

Paget's Disease:

- Due to a defect in the process of coupling of bone formation and resorption.
- This defect in coupling is characterized by increased activity of bone resorption by the osteoclast followed by increased activity of bone formation by the osteoblast
- Three stages:
  - First stage (lytic): increase osteoclastic activity, this will be manifested by increased urinary N-telopeptide and alpha-C-telopeptide (markers of osteoclast activity).
  - Second stage (mixed lytic blastic): increased osteoblastic activity (disorganized woven bone).
  - Sclerotic.
- May be related to viral infection (paramyxovirus). The disease has increased incidence in Europe (compared to US).
- Pathology:

- o Microscopically: abnormal bony architecture. The normal trabecular appearance is distorted, with a mosaic pattern of irregular cement lines joining areas of lamellar bone.
- o Can lead to knee and hip arthritis, pathologic fracture, and rarely neurologic complications (from compression of nerves).
- o Can lead to bone deformity.
- o The bone is very vascular, can profusely bleed during surgeries (difficult THA).
- o Most common complication of TKA for Paget's knee arthritis is malalignment. Most common complication of THA for Paget's hip arthritis is excessive bleeding during surgery.
- XR: combined lytic/ blastic lesion, thickened cortices. Joint arthritis can be seen.
- Treatment:
  - o Medically: NSAIDs, bisphosphonate *(Question: Paget's disease discovered accidently in XR for patient with arthritis, treatment? (NSAIDs for the arthritis)).*
  - o Surgery may be needed for correction of deformity or arthritis.
  - o When there is a fracture or arthroplasty for arthritis with underlying severe limb deformity: restoration of mechanical alignment should be done by osteotomies to avoid early prosthetic failure in Paget's.

Osteoarthritis (OA) (See Also Cartilage in Basic Science Chapter and Knee OA in Knee Chapter):

- First stage (Early OA) (mechanical):
  - o **Decrease in the proteoglycan (decreased chain length, less aggregation) and an increase in the water content**.
    - Glucosamine supplementation act as substrate for chondroitin sulfate and hyaluronate formation.
    - It does not have anti-COX-2 inhibitory effects nor does not increase synovial fluid viscosity.
  - o Constant type II collagen content and increase in collagen type X.
  - o This results in **increased permeability and softness (less stiff)** of the cartilage.
    - A decrease of the stiffness of the cartilage makes it less able to bear loads and more susceptible for injury.
  - o Significant and progressive decrease in the tensile and shear modulus of the cartilage.
- The second stage (cellular stage):
  - o There is an increased cellular response: chondrocyte proliferation with cluster formation and increased production of extracellular matrix.

- o There is an increase in catabolic activity with removal of damaged matrix.
- Third stage:
  - o Increased inflammatory cytokines (nitric oxide and interleukin I)
    - ▪ This will increase matrix metalloproteinase activity (proteolytic enzymes) which will break down types IX and XI collagen, and affect the stability of the type II collagen structure.
    - ▪ Stromelysin and plasmin: two metalloproteinase secreted by chondrocytes and play a role in OA.
    - ▪ Tissue inhibitor of metalloproteinase (TIMPs) counteract the metalloproteinase. TIMPs can play a role in treatment of OA
    - ▪ This will cause decreases in cross-linking of collagen and increased degradation (decease content of collagen in advanced stage).
    - ▪ Loss of articular cartilage giving rise to clinical signs of degenerative joint disease
- Mice with a type IX collagen gene deletion become susceptible to early arthritis (collagen IX mutation/deletion may play a role in development of early OA).
  - o COL9A2 gene (collagen type IX alpha 2 chain) is also related to MED and Stickler syndrome (see genetics chapter).

Osteomyelitis (See Also Osteomyelitis in Pediatric Chapter):

- Pathology: Changes seen in cases of chronic osteomyelitis:
  - o Sequestrum: dead separated bone (must be excised and removed to clear infection as it has no blood supply).
  - o Involucrum: reactive periosteal new bone, does not have to be excised to clear infection.
  - o Cloaca: a defect in the bone cortex and involucrum draining purulent material.
- Antibiotics should be given for at least 6 weeks. If the organism is of low virulent that has oral antibiotics susceptibility/sensitivity, IV antibiotics can be administrated for one or two weeks, followed by 5-4 weeks of oral antibiotics.
- Malignant change can occur in the draining sinus track of patients with chronic osteomyelitis (Marjolin ulcer): occur in cases of longstanding osteomyelitis; microscopically it is squamous cell carcinoma (not sarcoma).
- The Cierny-Mader classification system:
  - o Three types of patients (host) with osteomyelitis: (A) healthy, (B) those with comorbidities, and (C) a host in whom treatment will lead to greater morbidity than the infection.

- Four types of bone affection: type I-medullary, type II-superficial, type III-localized defect with stable bone, and type IV-diffuse OM with affection of bone stability.
- Localized osteomyelitis is treated with debridement of non-viable bone (sequestrectomy), and placement of absorbable antibiotic beads (no need for application of external fixator as the integrity of the bone is not affected).

Necrotizing fasciitis
- Clinical presentation: pain in the affected extremity:
  - The pain is intense with relatively minimal initial clinical findings.
  - Progressive cellulitis despite antibiotic therapy.
  - Later in the course of disease, areas of necrosis and discoloration. Patient may develop shock, confusion and dyspnea.
- Low sodium level.
- MRI will show thickening of the subcutaneous tissues.
- Culture results are usually polymicrobial.
- Treatment is urgent aggressive debridement of skin, subcutaneous fat, and fascia *(scenario: 60 years old diabetic, presenting with leg pain, diagnosed with cellulitis, antibiotic treatment, no improvement, MRI, leg shows thickening of the subcutaneous tissues, treatment?) (Scenario: 70 years old hepatitis C positive, leg pain, antibiotic, spreading of swelling and redness, blood pressure is 80/40, treatment?)*

Gas producing infection
- Gas in the tissues suggest an infection with anaerobic bacterial infection.
- Common in farm injuries.
- This can be a life- and limb-threatening infection.
- Treatment should consist of wide debridement of all devitalized tissue, and intravenous antibiotics, wounds should be left open. *(Scenario: 30 years old, leg wound while working in farm, 48 hours later have severe pain, XR gas in tissues, treatment?)*

Vascular Disease of the Lower Extremity:
- When assessing patient with vascular condition of the lower extremity for elective surgery (e.g. atherosclerosis and TKA), start the assessment with ankle-brachial index of the affected lower extremity *(scenario: 65 years' diabetic patient, no palpable pulses in the left lower extremity wants to have TKA, next step?)*
  - If periprosthetic fracture leads to vascular injury: the treatment is urgent traction (to clear the pressure on the vessels) and management of the fracture (ORIF vs revision). If traction fails to restore flow in the femoral artery,

vascular repair will be needed (temporary shunt can be done until repair is available).

Smoking in Orthopedics (See Also the Spine Chapter):

- Smoking has been found to increase the rate of perioperative infections and wound complication rates in foot and ankle surgery.
- Smoking can cause osteoporosis, degenerative disk disease (cervical and lumbar spondylolysis), poor wound healing.
- Smoking is a risk factor for nonunion.

Tips:

- Superior lens dislocation: Marfan; inferior lens dislocation: homocystinuria.
- Dural ectasia: Marfan, neurofibromatosis.
- Achodnroplasia: mutation of FGFR3, Apert syndrome: mutation of FGFR2
- Orthopedic deformity may be associated with kidney abnormalities *(scenario: child with bone congenital condition, what else should you assess?).*

Chapter 4: Surgical Anatomy

Lower Extremity and Pelvis:

Pelvis and Hip Approaches:

- **For bone graft from iliac crest:**
  - During harvesting of anterior iliac crest bone graft, the nerve at greatest risk for injury is lateral femoral cutaneous nerve (lies within 2 cm from ASIS). *(Scenario: patient undergoes ACDF with authogenous bone graft, he has numbness of the lateral thigh, injured nerve?)*
  - Posterior iliac crest bone graft:
    - The cuneal nerve is 8 cm lateral to PSIS (at risk with **lateral** extensions)
    - The superior gluteal artery is the structure at greatest risk for injury at **distal** extensions.
- **Ilioinguinal surgical approach:**
  - Iliopectineal fascia separates the lateral muscular iliopsoas compartment (with the femoral nerve) from the medial vascular compartment. This fascia needs to be released to be able to reach to the proper pelvis.
- **Anterior intrapelvic approach (Stoppa approach):**
  - Allow best access to the quadrilateral plate of the pelvis.
  - The corona mortis is at risk at the level of the obturator foramen (about 6 cm from symphysis pubis).
  - The obturator nerve and vessels are at risk during exposure of the quadrilateral plate.
- **Smith Peterson approach:**
  - Between Sartorius (femoral nerve) and tensor fascia lata muscle (superior gluteal nerve). Deep interval is between rectus femoris (femoral nerve) and gluteus medius (superior gluteal nerve).
  - The only true inter-neural approach in the hip region.
  - It is used for the anterior approach for THA.
    - The lateral femoral cutaneus nerve (lies in lateral part of the Sartorius sheath) is at risk during this approach. *(Question: anterior approach to THA is between what muscles?) (Question: what is the structure at greatest risk during this approach?). (Question: what is the most common complication for THA done though anterior approach? (injury to lateral femoral cutaneus nerve)) (Question: what is the structure at risk with anterior approach for THA?).*
    - The Ascending branch of the lateral femoral circumflex artery (a branch of the profunda femoris artery) passes between sartoris and tensor fascia lata (needs to be ligated for adequate exposure).
- **Direct lateral (Hardinge) approach:**
  - Through the gluteus medius muscle.

- Should not split the muscle more than 5 cm (to avoid injury of the superior gluteal nerve).
  - o The anterior two thirds (or one half) of the gluteus medius is detached as a sleeve with the vastus lateralis. This will expose the gluteus minimus and iliofemoral ligament of Bigelow which both should be also detached to anteriorly dislocate the hip
- **Posterior approach to the hip:**
  - o Common approach for arthroplasty and posterior acetabular fixation.
  - o When used for arthroplasty: has higher dislocation rate.
- **Medial approach to the hip:**
  - o The superficial dissection between the gracilis and the adductor longus muscles.
  - o The deeper dissection between adductor brevis and adductor magnus.
- **Hip arthroscopy approaches:**
  - o Posterolateral portal: close to sciatic nerve (internal rotation of the hip can protect the nerve).
  - o Anterior portal: close to lateral femoral cutaneous nerve and to the ascending branch of the lateral femoral circumflex artery.
  - o Antero-lateral portal: close to the superior gluteal vessels.
- **Open surgical dislocation of the hip with trochanteric osteotomy:**
  - o Based on preserving the blood supply to the femoral head (which depends on branches from the **medial** femoral circumflex artery penetrating the capsule **posteriorly**).
  - o Digastric trochanterioc osteotomy (the mobile part of the trochanter will have both the gluteus medius and vastus lateralis attached to it) followed by anterior Z capsulotomy.
    - In the trochanteric digastric (flip) osteotomy: the posterosuperior aspect of the osteotomy should be about 2 mm anterior to the posterior insertion of the gluteus medius (the mobile piece contains the majority of the medius leaving a small cuff of muscle on the stable trochanter). This will ensure that the pyriformis muscle is not injured (which is an indication that the cut will not injure the medial femoral circumflex artery).
  - o Z capsulotomy:
    - One limb over anterosuperior neck, then proximally extend posteriorly along the acetabular rim and distally extend anteriorly towards the lesser trochanter.
    - Release of the anteroinferior capsule along the proximal femur can injure the blood supply to the femoral head if the release extends

below the level of the lesser trochanter due to possible injury to the medial femoral circumflex artery.

Pelvis and Acetabulum Anatomy

- Sacrospinous ligament separates the greater sciatic notch from the lesser sciatic notch.
    - Structures exiting the greater sciatic notch above piriformis muscle: superior gluteal nerve and artery
    - Structures exiting the greater sciatic notch below piriformis muscle: pudendal nerve, the internal pudendal artery, the nerve to the obturator internus, the posterior femoral cutaneous nerve (posterior cutaneous nerve of the thigh), the sciatic nerve, the inferior gluteal nerve, the inferior gluteal artery, the nerve to the quadratus femoris.
    - The tendon of the obturator internus (together with the two gemelli) passes through the lesser sciatic notch.
    - Superior gluteal vessels exit the pelvis by passing around the superior gluteal notch. *(Question: CT arthrogram, what is the name of the vessel turning around the superior gluteal notch.)*
    - Superior gluteal nerve passes superior to the pyriformis muscle.
- Corona mortis is formed by anastomosis between obturator vessel (internal iliac system) and inferior epigastric vessel (external iliac system). It can be arterial or venous.
- L5 nerve root lies on the anterior surface of the sacral ala. Care should be taken not to injure this structure in anterior approach to the SI joint and during IS screw insertion (see lower extremity trauma chapter).
- The iliopectineal fascia runs between the Iliopsoas muscle/femoral nerve (laterally) and the iliac vessels (medially)
- The main blood supply to the femoral head is through the **Deep branch of the medial femoral circumflex artery** *(scenario: 21 years old, fracture proximal femur, what artery injury can affect the blood supply?)*
    - The medial femoral circumflex artery passes posteriorly around the medial side of the distal part of the psoas tendon. The medial femoral circumflex artery lies medial or deep to the quadratus femoris muscle.
    - It is at risk, especially in children, during release of the psoas tendon. *(Question: anteromedial approach for DDH reduction, what vessel is at risk?).*
    - Femoral nailing through the piriformis fossa starting portal is contraindicated in adolescents with open physes because of the risk of damage to branches the medial femoral circumflex artery (see also pediatric trauma chapter).
    - Inferior gluteal artery provides the most significant secondary contribution to the blood supply of the femoral head. It anastomoses directly into the deep

branch of the medial femoral circumflex artery and in a minority of patients, it becomes the dominant blood supply into the femoral head

- o In the first 4 years of life, the main blood supply to the femoral head is both medial and lateral femoral circumflex arteries, with significant contributions also coming from the artery of the ligamentum teres.
- o Both medial and lateral femoral circumflex arise from the profunda femoris artery.
- The teardrop landmark that is used for anterior pelvic pin placement represent the column of bone running from the anterior inferior iliac spine (AIIS) to the posterior superior iliac spine (PSIS), best **visualized on the obturator outlet view.**
    - o Acetabular teardrop (XR finding):
        - Comprised of the quadrilateral surface and cotyloid fossa.
        - In absence of dyspalsia, a teardrop appear by age 18 months of age.
- The hip joint allows motion in different 3 degrees of freedom in flexion-extension, abbduction-adduction, and axial rotation (the other three degrees of freedom (translation in the medial/lateral, anterior/posterior and axial translation) are not allowed).
- Placing the hip in extension and internal rotation results in an increase in intracapsular pressure. With hip effusion, the joint lies in flexion and external rotation to decrease the pressure inside the joint.
- Ligaments of the hip joint:
    - o The iliofemoral ligament (the Y-ligament or the ligament of Bigelow) extends from the anterior inferior iliac spine to the femur (anterior inter trochanteric ridge) in front of the joint.
        - The strongest ligament of the hip joint is the ilio-femoral ligament (the strongest ligament in the body)
    - o The ischiofemoral ligament has the most significant effect in limiting hip internal rotation in both extension and flexion.
- Muscles attached to pelvic apophysis: see sports lower extremity chapter.
- To accurately determine the neck shaft angle, the XR should be taken with the leg in internal rotation in an amount similar to ante version (about 17°).
- The femoral triangle borders: inguinal ligament proximally, the sartorius muscle laterally, and the adductor longus medially. The floor triangle is made up of the iliopsoas, pectineus and adductor longus muscles

Knee:
Knee Approaches:
- **Medial parapatellar approach (See knee chapter):**

- o Can injure the 3 medial genicular arteries. If lateral release is done (in conjunction with medial parapatellar approach), it can add injury to the superior and inferior lateral genicular arteries (causing AVN of the patella).
- o Lateral menisectomy may injure inferior lateral genicular artery (see before).
- o The use of an extensile rectus snip at the proximal end of a medial parapatellar arthrotomy when needed to increase the exposure in TKA will cause no difference in outcome compared with a standard medial parapatellar arthrotomy (no change in the post-operative rehabilitation regimen). "patellar turndown" extension will delay active extension (see the knee chapter).
- o Midvastus surgical approach for TKA has the greatest potential for denervation of the quadriceps muscle (see knee chapter).
- **The postero medial approach for the knee** (eg ORIF of bi condylar tibial plateau to support the medial condyle, avulsion of the posterior cruciate ligament tibial attachment or for performing a posterior cruciate ligament tibial inlay reconstruction):
  - o Interval between medial border of the medial gastrocnemius (retracted laterally to protect the neurovascular bundle) and the posterior border of the semimembranosus tendon.
  - o With a tibial inlay-type approach for PCL reconstruction, the popliteal artery is about 20 mm from the screws used for fixation of the bone block
- **The posterolateral approach of the knee:**
  - o Intervals between the iliotibial band (anteriorly) and the biceps femoris tendon (posteriorly).
  - o Deep interval: **posterior** retraction of the gastrocnemius provides access to the posterolateral capsule.
  - o Used for the inside-out lateral meniscal repair.
  - o The inferior lateral genicular artery can be injured during this surgical approach.
- Saphenous nerve:
  - o Infrapatellar branch of the saphenous nerve (passing from medial to lateral) can be injured with mid line knee approaches (TKA or BTB for ACL) resulting in numbness of the anterolateral aspect of the knee.
  - o The saphenous nerve can be injured during harvesting the hamstring graft.
    - ▪ Knee flexion and hip external rotation relax the nerve and decrease the chance of nerve injury during harvesting the graft.

Knee Anatomy
- Structures on the lateral part of the knee:
  - o The femoral insertion of the popliteus is **anterior, distal and deep** to the femoral insertion of the lateral collateral ligament.

- The femoral insertion of the lateral collateral is proximal and posterior to the lateral epicondyle and to the femoral insertion of the popliteus.
  - The lateral collateral ligament inserts at the anterior part of the fibular head and the poplitio-fibular ligament inserts into the posterior part. The biceps tendon insertion extends into nearly all the lateral portion of the fibular head.
- The neurovascular bundle posterior to the knee has the following arrangement from lateral to medial (as well as from superficial to deep): posterior tibial nerve, popliteal vein, and popliteal artery.
  - Popliteal artery is the closest structure to the posterior knee capsule.
  - The popliteal artery lies anterior (deeper) to the popliteal vein and 9 mm posterior to the posterior aspect of the tibial plateau in 90 degrees of flexion.
- At the level of tibial bone cut in TKA, the common peroneal nerve lies superficial to the lateral head of the gastrocnemius protecting the nerve while doing the bone cut.
- **The home screw mechanism of the knee (see knee kinematics below):**
  - Unlock the knee:
    - The popliteus tendon unlocks the knee from the home screw mechanism.
    - This occurs by external rotation of the femur (or internal rotation of the tibia).
  - Locking the knee:
    - Necessary for knee stability during standing upright position
    - It occurs at the end of knee extension (between 0° and 20° knee flexion).
    - Internal rotation of the femur (external rotation of the tibia) occurs during the terminal degrees of knee extension which results in tightening of both cruciate ligaments, which locks the knee. This rotation occurs due to shape of the distal femoral condyle.
- **Blood supply:**
  - The popliteal artery gives the superior genicular, middle genicular and inferior genicular.
    - The superior genicular splits into medial and lateral branches supplying the patellar cartilage and the posterior cruciate ligament.
    - The middle genicular artery supplies the ACL, PCL, and collateral ligaments.
    - The inferior genicular splits into medial and lateral branches and supplies the menisci
- Knee kinematics:
  - The radius of curvature of the lateral femoral condyle is greater than of the medial femoral condyle.
  - During normal knee flexion:

- With the beginning of knee flexion, the tibia rotates internally in relation to the femur and then keeps this rotational position until flexion past 90° when more internal rotation occurs.
- With beginning of flexion, the lateral tibiofemoral contact point translates posteriorly greater than the medial side direction resulting in more rollback, and medial pivoting.
- **Medial pivot:** during knee flexion, the lateral femoral condyle will roll back on the tibia while the medial femoral condyle remains relatively stationary in its position. This movement is related to the larger diameter of the lateral femoral condyle. ACL, and to a lesser degree PCL, also play a role in this rotational movement.
- Screw home: see before.
- The meniscofemoral ligaments:
  - Connect the posterior horn of the **lateral** meniscus to the intercondylar wall of the medial femoral condyle.
  - The ligament of Humphrey passes anterior and the ligament of Wrisberg passes posterior to the PCL.
    - The ligament of Humphrey (anterior meniscofemoral ligament) and ligament of Wrisberg (posterior meniscofemoral ligament) are delineated by their anatomic relationship to the posterior cruciate.
    - Only about 50% of the knees have both anterior and posterior meniscofemoral ligament
- The average orientation of the knee joint line relative to the mechanical axis of the limb is 3° of varus.
- Anterior Cruciate Ligament (ACL) (see also the lower extremity sport chapter):
  - The ACL is an intra-articular and intrasynovial structure, innervated by posterior articular branches from the tibial nerve.
    - This contributes to proprioceptive function of the knee.
  - The middle genicular artery is the primary blood supply of the ACL. *(Scenario: knee injury, hemoarthrosis, MRI shows ACL injury, what artery is responsible for hematoma?)*
  - Tension force in the ACL (native and reconstructed) is highest at full extension.
  - The ACL plays a primary role in anterior-posterior stability and secondary role to limit internal rotation of the tibia.
  - The anterior cruciate ligament is composed of the anteromedial and posterolateral bundles.
    - The lateral bifurcate ridge separates the anteromedial and posterolateral bundles from one another.

- The anteromedial bundle originates (from the lateral femoral condyle) anterior and proximal to the posterolateral bundle and inserts in the anterior and medial part of the ACL footprint on the tibia.
- The two bundles are parallel with the knee extended. With knee flexion, the anteromedial bundle rotates in relation to the posterolateral bundle.
- The anteromedial bundle is tight in flexion while posterolateral bundle relaxes in flexion.
- Posterolateral bundle provides more rotational control than the anteromedial bundle (see lower extremity sport chapter).
- Posterior Cruciate Ligament (PCL):
  - PCL has two bundles: anterolateral and posteromedial.
  - In PCL: The anterolateral bundle is shorter, thicker, and stronger than the posteromedial bundle.
- Menisci:
  - Menisci move anteriorly with extension and posteriorly with flexion.
    - The lateral meniscus is more mobile than the medial meniscus because of less soft-tissue attachments.
  - Collagen type I is the predominant collagen in the menisci.
- The superficial portion of the MCL is the primary constraint against valgus loading (especially in flexion).
  - Secondary stabilizers include: the deep MCL and posteromedial capsule (and to lesser degrees The ACL and PCL).
- Baker cyst: the stalk is between the semimembranosus (medially) and medial head of the gastrocnemius muscles (laterally).

Lower Leg:

Lower Leg Approaches:
- The anterolateral approach to the distal tibia and ankle for open reduction and internal fixation of pilon fractures can injure the deep peroneal nerve (course over the plate)
- Posterior approach to the lower leg (eg performing a gastrocnemius recession):
  - Sural nerve is at risk as it crosses over the lateral border of the Achilles tendon at an average of 9.8 cm above its insertion.

Lower Leg Anatomy:
- The peroneus brevis (evert the foot and subtalar joint) is the primary antagonist to posterior tibialis (primary invertor) (see below).
- Peroneus brevis is closer to bone (anterior) than peroneus longus.

- The plantaris muscle originate from the posterolateral aspect of the distal femur
  - The tendon courses between the soleus and the medial head of the gastrocnemius.
- The neurovascular bundle in the leg is located between the soleus and posterior tibialis muscle (see nerve section below).

Ankle and Foot
Ankle and Foot Approaches:
- **Postero lateral approach:**
  - Between peroneal tendons laterally and flexor hallucis longus medially.
  - The sural nerve is at risk in this approach and should be identified. *(Scenario: posterior malleolus fracture, surgery for ORIF by postero-lateral approach, neuroma of which nerve?)*
- **Lateral approach to the fibula**
  - The superficial peroneal nerve is at risk during the lateral approach to the fibula.
    - It exits the fascial hiatus approximately 12 (10-14) cm proximal to the tip of the distal fibula anterior to the mid-lateral plane of the fibula.
- **Anterior exposure to the ankle:**
  - The nerve at greatest risk for injury during an anterior surgical exposure of the ankle is the dorsal medial branch of the superficial peroneal nerve.
- **Talus approach (see talus anatomy):**
  - In cases of double incision for ORIF of talus neck fracture dislocation the only remaining blood supply to the talus is the deltoid branch of the artery of the tarsal canal originating from the posterior tibial artery. This remaining blood supply must be preserved to avoid AVN of the talus.
- **Extensile lateral approaches for calcaneus fracture:**
  - Arterial blood supply to the raised flap consisted of three arteries: **the lateral calcaneal artery**, the lateral malleolar artery, and the lateral tarsal artery.
    - The lateral calcaneal artery is the one responsible for most of the blood supply to the corner of the flap.
    - This artery is about 1.5 cm anterior to the Achilles tendon. The vertical incision should be 0.5 cm anterior to the Achilles tendon, and horizontal incision should be at the junction of the lateral skin and the plantar glabrous skin.
    - This approach gives best exposure to obtain anatomic reduction.
- The plantar medial cutaneous nerve is at risk during surgical approach to the medial sesamoid.

- o This nerve lies at the junction of the glabrous skin of the big toe, injury can cause painful neuroma during shoe wear.
- Incision for bunion surgery: see foot chapter.
- **Ankle Arthroscopy Portal:**
  - o Antero-lateral: lateral to the peroneus tertius tendon, can injure superficial peroneal nerve (or its intermediate dorsal cutaneous branch).
  - o Antero-medial: medial to the tibialis anterior tendon, can injure saphenous nerve.
  - o Postero lateral: lateral to the Achilles tendon, can injure sural nerve (or its branch "lateral calcaneal nerve" that innervate the lateral heel pad) and the lesser saphenous vein. *(Scenario: 9 months after ankle arthroscopy, the patient has shooting pain to the medial foot when his lateral portal is tapped, what nerve was entrapped? what is the treatment? (If the nerve is in good condition, release of the nerve. If the nerve is cut or severely thinned, excise and bury it.))*
  - o The most common injured nerve during ankle arthroscopy in general is the intermediate dorsal cutaneous branch of the superficial peroneal nerve.
- The superficial peroneal nerve (after existing from the crural fascia) can be injured during approaches for distal fibula fractures and during arthroscopy (anterolateral ankle portal).

Ankle and Foot Anatomy:

- At the distal part of the lower leg level, the anterior tibial artery lies medial to the extensor hallucis longus tendon. The artery passes beneath the Y-shaped inferior extensor retinaculum deep to the muscle to reach the dorsum of the foot as the dorsalis pedis artery lateral to the tendon of extensor hallucis longus muscle (so it starts medial to the muscle then becomes lateral). The artery lies medial to anterior tibial nerve.
- Intrinsic muscles of the foot flex the metatarsophalangeal joints and extend the interphalangeal joints (similar to the hand).
- The five major compartments of the foot are medial, lateral, central, calcaneal and interosseous (4 interosseous compartments). There is no dorsal compartment in the foot.
- Syndesomsis ligamnents (see ankle fracture in lower extremity trauma chapter):
  - o Anterior tibio-fibular ligament between the fibula and the antereo lateral part of the tibia. Avulsion of this bony attachment in the tibia will result in the "Tillaux fracture".
  - o Posterior tibio-fibular ligament between fibula and postero lateral part of the tibial is smaller than the anterior one.
- Muscles:

- o The FHL (Flexor hallucis longus) tendon run lateral to the posteromedial tubercle of the talus then turn around the sustentaculum tali (can be irritated with long screws (e.g during fracture fixation) below sustentaculum tali going from lateral to medial below the subtalar joint). Then it crosses the flexor digitorum at the knot of Henry to insert into the base of the distal phalanx of the big toe.
- o In the peroneal groove behind the fibula, the peroneus brevis lies anterior and medial (closer to bone, deeper) to the peroneus longus. The peroneal (fibular) tubercle of the lateral surface of the calcaneus separates between the peroneus brevis (anterior/superior to the tubercle) and peroneus longus (underneath/inferior the tubercle).
- o Peroneus longus and brevis everts the subtalar joint. In addition, peroneus longus plantar flexes (pronates) the first ray (helping to create the foot arch).
- o The function of the peroneus tertius is ankle dorsiflexion and eversion of the subtalar joint.
- o Posterior tibial muscle (inverts and plantar flex) and peroneus brevis (everts) muscles are antagonists.
- o Gastrocnemius-soleus is the main ankle plantar flexor. Calcaneus deformity of the ankle (dorsi-flexion of the ankle and foot) is the result of weakness of gastrocnemius-soleus.
  - ▪ The Achilles tendon is the conjoint tendon of gastrocnemius-soleus. Its fibers rotate 90° before their insertion (the superficial fibers becomes lateral).
- • Ligaments:
  - o The Lisfranc ligament connects **medial** cuneiform and **second** metatarsal.
  - o The **spring ligament** connects between the calcaneus and navicular bones. It supports the talonavicular articulation (maintaining the position of the talar head) and prevents the collapse of the arch.
    - ▪ It is composed of the superomedial calcaneonavicular ligament and the inferior calcaneonavicular ligaments.
  - o Lateral ankle ligaments:
    - ▪ Anterior talo fibula ligament (ATFL) is under maximum stress in inversion and plantar flexion.
    - ▪ Calcaneo fibular ligament (CFL) is under maximum stress in inversion and dorsiflexion.
- • Hallux sesamoids (see foot and ankle chapter):
  - o Each hallux sesamoid sits within its respective head of the flexor hallucis **brevis** tendon. It increases the mechanical force of the muscle.
  - o Excision of one sesamoid can result in weakness in its flexor hallucis brevis tendon head.

- Removing the medial sesamoid can lead to hallux valgus. Removing the lateral one can lead to hallux varus. Repair the respective head of flexor hallucis brevis tendon is important to avoid this complication. *(Question: what structure you have to repair with excision of medial sesamoid?)*
    - The two hallux sesamoids are held together by the inter-sesamoid ligament and plantar plate (which inserts into the base of the proximal phalanx of the hallux).
    - The tibial sesamoid is bipartite in about 10% of individuals (25% of these are bilateral).
    - The conjoined tendon (inserts along the lateral base of the proximal phalanx of the great toe and the lateral sesamoid) is made up of two muscles: flexor hallucis brevis and adductor hallucis.
    - The flexor hallucis longus tendon passes between the two sesamoids.
- Contents of the anterior tarsal tunnel:
    - Extensor hallucis longus, tibialis anterior, extensor digitorum longus, dorsalis pedis artery, deep peroneal nerve (NOT the superficial).
- Blood supply to the talus:
    - The artery of the tarsal canal (branch of the posterior tibial artery), and the artery of the sinus tarsi (branch of the peroneal artery with its anastomosis with anterior tibial artery).
    - Artery of the tarsal canal: main blood supply to the lateral two thirds of the talar body) and deltoid ligament.Injury to this vessel can cause osteonecrosis of the talus
    - Artery of the tarsal sinus: main blood supply of the intrasinus of the talus.
    - The talar body receives most of its blood supply by retrograde flow from the talar neck. Displaced fracture of the talar neck can cause osteonecrosis.
- Blood supply to the heel pad:
    - The medial calcaneal branch of the posterior tibial artery. Heel avulsion can lead to necrosis of heel pad.
- Foot position during gait:
    - Early stance (first rocker): subtalar joint in everted (pronated), this will unlock the mid tarsal joint, and will allow the foot to absorb the shock of ground hitting (first rocker)
    - Mid and late (second rocker) subtalar joint in inverted, this will lock the transverse tarsal joint (talonavicular and calcaneocuboid joint (Chopart)), and will allow rigid platform for push off in the gait cycle.
- "Bassett's ligament":
    - Accessory anterior inferior fascicle of the tibiofibular ligament which is present in most ankles.
    - Rarely, it may get inflamed causing of anterolateral ankle impingement.

- o Treatment: Resection of fascicle.
- In Tarso-metatarsal articulations: the second TMT joint has the least motion while the fourth and fifth have the most motion.

Nerves of the lower extremity:

- **Femoral nerve (L2-4):**
  - o Supplies: quadriceps femoris, iliacus, pectineus, sartorius.
  - o To differentiate femoral nerve palsy from L3 radiculopathy
    - Assess the function of the adductor muscles (supplied by L3 through the adductor nerve not femoral nerve).
  - o The femoral nerve runs within the fascial sheath of the iliopsoas muscle (lateral to the vessels and separated from them by the ilio-pectenial fascia).
    - A bleed into the muscle will compress the nerve causing pain and weakness. *(Scenario: 14 years, hemophilic, pain in the thigh, weakness of the quadriceps, diagnosis?)*
- **Sciatic nerve (L4-5, S1-3):**
  - o In most individual: sciatic nerve passes deep (anterior) to piriformis muscle, then it exits the pelvis through the **greater sciatic notch** between piriformis and superior gemellus.
    - Less frequently, it pierces the piriformis muscle.
  - o It then passes posterior (superficial) to the short external rotators (superior gemellus, obturator internus, inferior gemellus), quadratus femoris before it passes deep to the biceps femoris.
  - o Will divide into tibial nerve and common peroneal nerve.
- **Lateral femoral cutaneous nerve:**
  - o Passes under the inguinal ligament before piercing the fascia lata.
  - o Lies in the interval between tensor fascia lata (TFL) and sartorius (within the lateral part of the sartorius sheath).
- Genitofemoral nerve lies on the antero-medial surface of the psoas muscle (see spine chapter).
- **Tibial nerve:**
  - o Innervates:
    - The posterior compartment of the thigh (all hamstring muscle except short head of biceps) (the adductor magnus muscle has dual innervation by tibial nerve and posterior division of the oburator nerve).
    - The posterior compartments of the lower leg (superficial and deep) (gastrocnemius, popliteus, soleus, tibialis posterior, plantaris, FHL, FDL).

- o Divides to medial and lateral plantar nerves which supply the muscles of the feet.
- **Common peroneal nerve:**
  - o Will end by dividing into superficial and deep peroneal nerves.
  - o Stretched by knee extension.
    - In case of post-operative palsy, first maneuver is flexion the knee (see Knee chapter)
  - o Innervates:
    - The only thigh muscle innervated by peroneal nerve is the short head of biceps femoris. *(Question: tibial nerve supplies all hamstring muscles except?)*
    - Deep peroneal nerve (anterior tibial nerve): EHL, EDL, Tibialis anterior, peroneus tersius and EDB (dorsiflexor of the ankle and toes).
    - Superficial peroneal nerve: see below.
  - o **Superficial peroneal nerve:**
    - It innervates the muscles of the lateral compartment of the lower leg (peroneal longus and brevis).
    - It ends as the intermediate and medial dorsal cutaneous nerves of the foot.
    - Supplies the skin of the dorsum of the foot and toes except for the first web space.
    - At risk during the lateral approach to the ankle (10-14 cm from the tip of the fibula) (see approach section).
- **Sural nerve:**
  - o Formed by contributions from both the tibial and common peroneal nerves.
  - o Provides sensation to the dorso-lateral aspect of the foot
  - o The small saphenous vein lies medial to the sural nerve in the mid-calf and can be used to identify the nerve.
- **Baxter's nerve (nerve to abductor digiti quinti muscle, 1st lateral plantar nerve):**
  - o The first branch off the lateral plantar nerve, it innervates the abductor digiti quinti (see Fig 1).
  - o Impingement of this nerve can occur deep to the abductor hallucis muscle.
    - Will cause heel pain that can be confused with plantar fasciitis.
    - Tapping on the nerve will produces a Tinel's sign along the nerve
- **Saphenous nerve:**
  - o **Sartorial branch of the saphenous nerve:**
    - At risk during medial meniscus repair
    - Lies posterior to the sartorius; dissection should remain anterior to the muscle. The nerve is anterior to the semitendinosus with the knee in extension.

- - The branch becomes extra-fascial (superficial) between the gracilis and the sartorius.
  - o **The infrapatellar branch of the saphenous nerve**
    - - Exits the adductor canal and travels to the anteromedial aspect of the knee.
  - o The saphenous nerve lies on the posterior border of the sartorius muscle at the level of the knee.

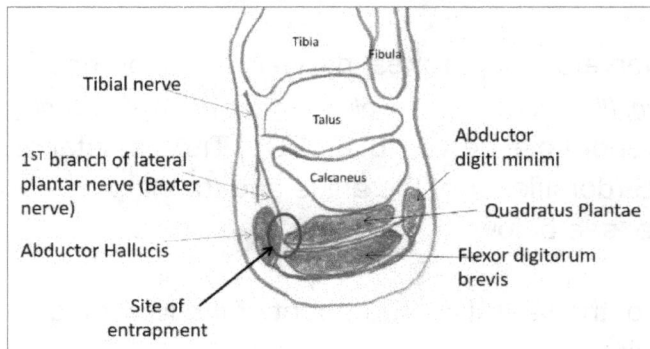

Fig 1: Anatomy of Baxter nerve (1st branch of lateral plantar nerve). The nerve changes direction and passes under the deep fascia of the abductor hallucis.

Root anatomy (see spine chapter for more details):
- o S1 nerve root innervates:
  - - Peroneus longus and brevis muscles, Gastrocnemius-soleus complex, Gluteus maximus muscle.
- o L5 nerve root innervates:
  - - **Extensor hallucis longus,** extensor digitorum longus and extensor digitorum brevis, **Gluteus medius.**
- o Tibilias anterior muscle: supplied primary by L4.
- o To test for S2 function: peri-anal sensation.
- o L4: supplies the medial aspect of the lower leg, foot, and great toe
- o L5: supplies the lateral aspect of the lower leg, dorsum foot and toes 2 through 4.
- o S1: supplies the lateral aspect of the foot and the fifth toe.
- o Reflexes and associated nerve roots:
  - - Patellar tendon reflex: L4; Achilles tendon reflex :S1 (NO clinically used reflex for L5)

Shoulder and Arm:
Shoulder and Arm Approaches:
- posterior approach to the glenoid neck is between infraspinatus muscle proximally (suprascapular nerve) and teres minor distally (axillary nerve).
  - o The Axillary nerve is at risk during this approach.

- Using an infraspinatus-splitting incision allows for better exposure of the posterior capsule and minimizes the risk of injury to the axillary nerve which lies inferior to the teres minor in the quadrilateral space.
    - o Excessive superior retraction on the infraspinatus can cause injury to the suprascapular nerve and/or artery.
- Acromial branch of the thoracoacromial artery:
    - o Crosses at the superior extent of the deltopectoral interval (anterior to distal the edge of the clavicle).
    - o Can be injured during anterior shoulder or acromial approaches. *(Scenario: bleeding during distal clavicle excision or RC surgery. What artery responsible?)*
- Delto pectoral approach (see shoulder arthroplasty):
    - o Require cutting the subscapularis muscle to be able to reach the shoulder joint. Repair of the tendon must be done at the end of the procedure.
    - o Post operatively: restriction of both active internal rotation and passive external rotation more than 90 should be done (to avoid failure of the repair).
- Lateral deltoid-splitting approach:
    - o Can cause injury to the axillary nerve.
    - o The distance between the nerve and the lateral margin of the acromion is about 5 cm and decreases with shoulder abduction.
- The modified posterior approach: elevation of the medial and lateral heads of the triceps can expose about 95% of the humeral shaft.
- The traditional posterior triceps-splitting approach (with radial nerve dissection) exposes about 60-65% of the humeral shaft (the distal part of the humerus).

Shoulder/ Brachial plexus/ Axilla/ Humerus Anatomy:
- Anatomy of the brachial plexus: (see Fig 2).
    - o Roots, trunks, divisions and cords.
    - o Some nerves come directly from the roots or the trunks (see Fig 2).
    - o *Scenarios: endless number of scenario can be presented, you must know the anatomy by heart and be able to know where is lesion (Scenario: stab wound to the axilla, exam shows weak shoulder abduction, weak shoulder internal rotation, weak wrist extension, weak thumb IP extension, what structure affected? (posterior cord)) (Scenario: stab wound to the axilla, on exam, weak wrist and thumb extension, what structure affected? (posterior division of the lower cord))*

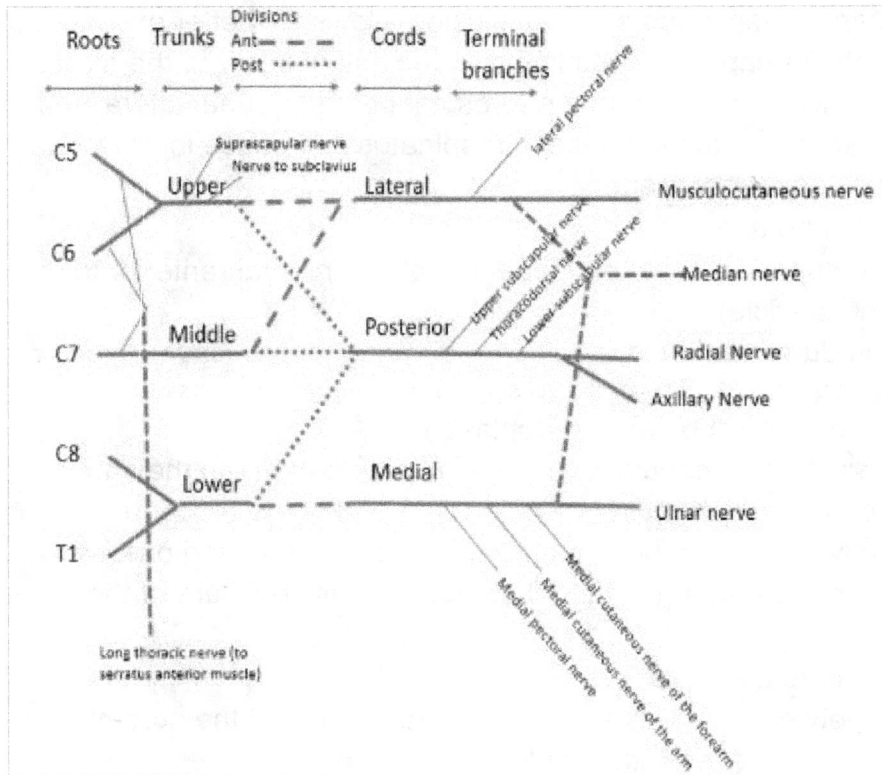

Fig 2: Anatomy of the brachial plexus. There are 5 components of the plexus: roots, trucks, divisions, cords and terminal branches. Long thoracic nerve comes off from roots C5-7.

- Pectoralis major is supplied by medial and lateral pectoral nerves (all root of brachial plexus C5-T1).
- Long thoracic nerve (nerve supply of serratus anterior muscle) arises from C5,6,7.
- Thoracodorsal nerve arises from posterior cord of the brachial plexus. It innervates latissimus dorsi muscle.
- C5 and C6 nerve roots will form the **upper trunk of the brachial plexus**; injury to it will give the classic Erb's palsy (obstetric brachial plexus birth palsy or traumatic):
    - Weakness of the deltoid muscle (weak shoulder abduction), weakness of supra spinatus and infra spinatus (weak shoulder external rotation), weakness of brachilis (weak elbow flexion) and weakness of biceps (weak supination) and weak wrist extension. This will cause waiter's tip position deformity (see also the pediatric chapter). _(scenario: MVC, patient has weakness of the deltoid and infraspinatus muscles, where is the anatomical lesion?)_
- Axillary artery in divided into 3 parts depending on it relation to pectoralis minor.
- Quadrangular space (see Fig 3):
    - Contents: axillary nerve and posterior humeral circumflex vessels.
    - Borders: medial: long head of triceps; lateral: humeral shaft; superior: teres minor; inferior: teres major.
    - Quadrilateral space syndrome (see shoulder chapter):

- ▪ Axillary nerve palsy: weakness of the deltoid and teres minor muscles.
- ▪ Teres minor action: external rotation with the arm abduction 90°
- Triangular space:
  - ○ Contents: scapular circumflex artery.
  - ○ Borders: superior: teres minor; inferior: teres major; lateral: long head of triceps.
- Triangular interval:
  - ○ Contents: radial nerve and profunda brachii vessels.
  - ○ Borders: superior: teres major; medial: long head of biceps, lateral: lateral head of triceps.

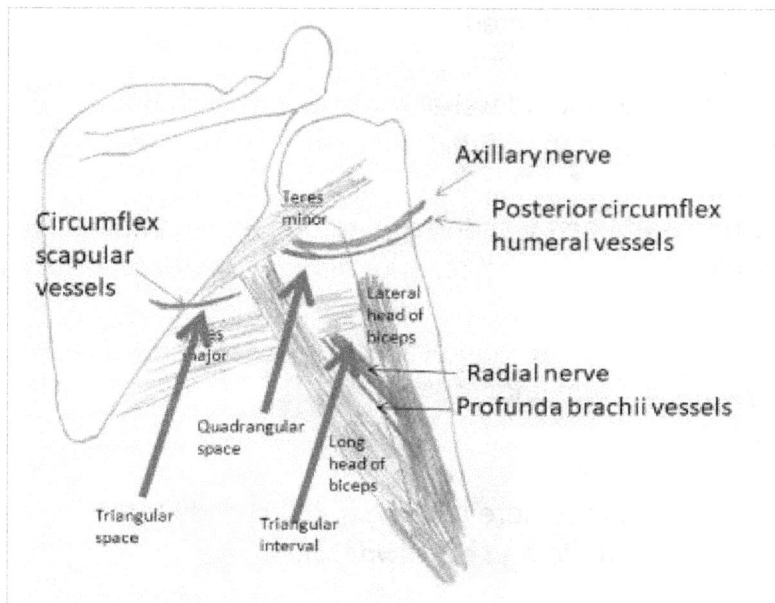

Fig 3: Contents and borders of the quadrangular space, triangular space and triangular interval.

- The rotator interval:
  - ○ Contents: coracohumeral ligament, the superior glenohumeral ligament (NOT middle), the glenohumeral capsule, and the biceps tendon.
  - ○ Boundaries: medial (base): coracoid process; lateral (apex): the transverse humeral ligament at the biceps intertubercular sulcus, superior border: anterior border of the supraspinatus; inferior border: superior border of the subscapularis.
  - ○ Closure of rotator interval results in reduction in posteroinferior translation of the humerus in relation to the glenoid.
- Coracohumeral ligament (one of the rotator internal structures) is the primary restraint to inferior translation of the shoulder.
- The superior glenohumeral ligament primarily restrains inferior translation of the humeral head with the arm in adduction.

- o Both coraco-humeral ligament and SGH ligament prevent inferior translation of adducted arm and both are components of the rotator interval.
- The middle glenohumeral ligament (MGHL) prevent anterior and posterior translation in the midrange of abduction (45°).
- The IGHL: anterior band prevent anterior translation at 90° of shoulder abduction (cooking position), posterior band to limit posterior translation
- The three gleno humeral ligaments: provide the primary ligamentous restraint to anterior glenohumeral translation in different arm positions:
  - o Inferior glenohumeral ligament (anterior band): arm abducted 90° and externally rotated (the position of apprehension).
  - o Middle glenohumeral ligament: arm abducted 45°.
  - o Superior glenohumeral ligament: arm adducted.
- The MGHL (present in about two-thirds of shoulders) arise from the labrum and glenoid immediately below the superior glenohumeral ligament.
- The blood supply for humeral head:
  - o In previous literature, the humeral head was thought to be supplied primarily by the anterolateral ascending branch of the anterior circumflex artery.
  - o More recently the posterior humeral circumflex artery was found to provide more than 60% of the blood supply to the humeral head, whereas the anterior humeral circumflex artery supplied less than 40%.
- **Muscles action around the scapula:**
  - o Serratus anterior: protracts the shoulder.
  - o Trapezius: rotate the scapula to obtain more global shoulder abduction (upward movement of the inferior angle and downward movement of the medial border)
- **Nerve supply to muscles around the shoulder:**
  - o Axillary nerve: deltoid and teres minor muscles
  - o Suprascapular nerve: supraspinatus and infraspinatus muscles.
  - o Upper and lower Subscapular nerves: subscapularis muscle.
  - o Teres major: lower Subscapular nerve.
- **Stability:**
  - o Sternoclavicular (SC) joint: the posterior part of the capsule is the main stabilizer for the SC joint.
  - o The superior acromioclavicluar ligament (thickening of the capsule) is the primary restrain against anteroposterior translation of the AC joint. The thickest part of the superior capsule is its posterior aspect (**postero-superior part**).
  - o Vertical stability of AC joint is mainly by the conoid part of the CC ligament.

- CC ligament: the conoid part is stronger and posteromedial to trapezoid part.
    - Concavity compression (controlled by RC muscles) is the most important stabilizing mechanism in the midrange of motion of the glenohumeral joint.
    - In the position of 90° forward flexion and internal rotation, the most important static stabilizer of the glenohumeral joint is the posterior band of the inferior glenohumeral ligament (in this position the posterior band is under tension in an anterior-posterior direction)
- **Rotator cuff (see shoulder chapter):**
    - The average maximum insertional length (anterior to posterior distance), and width (medial to lateral distance) of the supraspinatus insertion was 23 x **16mm** respectively.
    - 7 mm of exposed bone lateral to the articular margin (Arthroscopic measurement) represent about 50% of the tendon substance.
    - Rotator cuff muscles provide dynamic glenohumeral stability by compressing the humeral head against the glenoid.
- The long head of biceps tendon attaches to the labrum at variable positions. Most common form of attachment of biceps tendon to labrum is "predominantly posterior", followed by entirely posteriorly followed by equal anterior and posterior.
    - The long head of biceps tendon is controlled in the biceps groove by the insertion of the subscapularis and the biceps pulley (CH and SGHL ligaments) to prevent medial subluxation.
- The biceps groove:
    - Laterally: pectoralis major; medially: teres major; floor: latissimus dorsi.
    - Biceps tendon runs in the groove (lateral to teres major and latissimus muscles and medial to pectoralis major).
- The acromial branch of the thoracoacromial trunk (see before, approach section):
    - Can cause bleeding in surgery around the acromion.
    - Courses along the coracoacromial ligament starting about 5 mm from its acromion insertion.
        - To avoid injury of the artery, division of the AC ligament should be done at its insertion on the acromion.
- Humerus growth: 80% of the growth from proximal end and 20% of the growth from distal end.

Elbow:

Elbow Approaches:

- Anterior approach to the biceps tubercle and neck of the radius: the lateral antebrachial cutaneous nerve is the most commonly injured nerve (NOT PIN).

- Kocher approach (postero lateral approach to the elbow):
  - The forearm should be kept pronated to lessen the chance of injury to PIN.
  - Care should be taken to avoid injury to the lateral ulnar collateral ligament which lies posteriorly under the anconeus.
- **Portal for elbow arthroscopy:**
  - **Posterior portal:** 3 cm proximal to the tip of the olecranon
  - **Postero lateral portal:** 3 cm proximal from the tip of the olecranon and lateral to the triceps.
  - **Anterolateral portal:** risk of injury to the radial nerve (assessed by extension of the metacarpophalangeal joints)
  - **Anteromedial portal:** risk of injury to median nerve
  - Least safe elbow arthroscopy portals regarding ulnar nerve proximity is posteromedial portal (not used anymore).

Elbow Anatomy:

- See elbow dislocation in elbow chapter.
- The medial collateral ligament complex of the elbow consists of three portions: the anterior band, the posterior band, and the transverse component. The origin of the ligament is from the anteroinferior undersurface of the medial epicondyle.
  - The anterior band is the primary stabilizer of the elbow to a valgus stress in flexion and extension. It originates from the anteroinferior medial humeral epicondyle and inserts on the medial portion of the coronoid (the sublime tubercle).
  - The posterior band is tight in flexion and resists stress between 60° and full flexion.
- The biceps muscle is mainly responsible for supination of the forearm. The brachialis muscle is mainly responsible for elbow flexion strength.
- Cubital tunnel:
  - Boundaries (Fig 4):
    - Roof: cubital tunnel retinaculum (Osborne's ligament) which extends from the medial epicondyle to olecranon.
    - Floor: medial collateral ligament (posterior band).
    - laterally: olecranon process

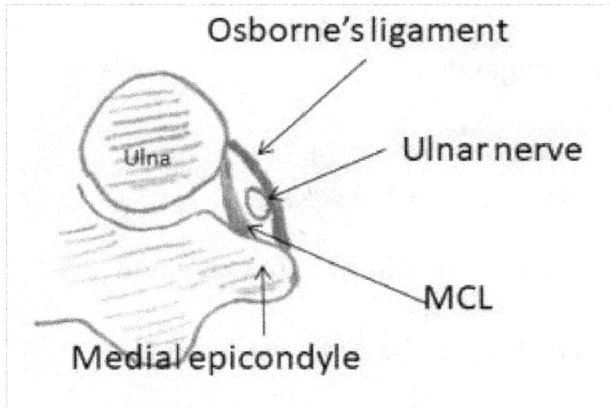

Fig 4: Roof and floor of the cubital tunnel.

- About 1/3 of the radial head (about a 100° arc) does not articulate with ulna at any position of supination-pronation. This part corresponds to the part from radial tuberosity to Lister's tubercle.
- The sequence of the growth plate **appearance** is
  - C-R-I-T-O-E: Capitellum, Radial head, Internal (medial) epicondyle, Trochlea, Olecranon, External (lateral) epicondyle. The age of appearance is 1,3,5,7,9, 10 in girls (two years later in boys (except for capitelum which also appears at the age of 1 year).
- The last growth plate to **fuse** is the medial epicondyle epiphysis, around the age 16-19 years old in boys (1-2 years earlier in females).

Forearm:
Forearm Approaches:
- Anterior approach for the radial shaft (Henry):
  - The internervous plane: laterally: the brachioradialis (radial nerve); medially: flexor carpi radialis distally, and pronator teres proximally (median nerve).
  - The radial artery lies in the interval between the tendons of the flexor carpi radialis and the brachioradialis.
  - Proximally, the posterior interosseous nerve (PIN) is the structure at most risk. The arm should be kept in supination to avoid injury to the PIN.
- The posterior approach to the radial shaft (Thompson):
  - The internervous plane: radially: extensor carpi radialis brevis muscle (ECRB) (radial nerve); ulnarly: extensor digitorum communis (EDC) muscle (PIN). Retraction between ERCP and EDC will expose supinator proximally and abductor polices longus distally.
- In both approaches, the arm should be kept in supination during disection of the proximal radius to protect the PIN nerve.

Forearm Anatomy:

- The axis of forearm rotation occurs around a longitudinal forearm axis between radial head proximally and ulnar head distally.
- Anterior and posterior interosseous arteries are branches of the common interosseous artery off the ulnar artery. *(Question: arthrogram, identify artery in the forearm which gives most of the branches? (Ulnar)).*
- The main function of biceps is supination (flexion of the elbow is mainly achieved by the brachialis).
    - With biceps rupture or injury to its nerve supply; the main weakness is supination (not elbow flexion). *(Scenario: biceps rupture, what movement affected?).*
- FCR is supplied by median nerve (see nerve section below).
- FDS:
    - The tendon for ring and middle are volar to those of small and index at the level of carpal tunnel.
    - Innervated by median nerve; flexes PIP (inserts in P2)
- FDP: Innervated by ulnar (ulnar two digits) and anterior interosseus nerve (branch of median) (radial two digits); flexes DIP and PIP (inserts on P3).
- Flexion of MCP is by mainly achieved by intrinsics (lumbricals and interossei).

Hand and Wrist

Hand and Wrist Approaches:

- The palmar cutaneous branch of the median nerve (PCBMN) arises from the median nerve on the radial side approximately 4 to 6 cm (range 3-20 cm) proximal to the wrist crease then passes between FCR (radially) and median nerve and palmaris (ulnarly). It supplies the skin of the thenar region. This nerve is at risk for injury in distal radius approaches.
- Wirst arthoroscopy portals are named according to the extensor compartment:
    - The 1-2 portal can injure the superficial branch of the radial nerve.
    - The 6U portal can inure the dorsal sensory branch of the ulnar nerve.

Wrist and Hand Anatomy:

- Most of the radio-ulnar deviation occurs through the mid-carpal joint, most of the flexion extension occurs through the radiocarpal joint.
- Stresses across the wrist joint:
    - Neutral alignment of the radius/ ulna: 80% through the radio-carpal and 20% through the ulna.
    - For ulna positive articulation: 1mm positive (30/70), 2mm positive (40/60).
    - For ulna negative articulation: 1mm negative (10/90).

- Vascular anatomy of the hand:
  - Superficial arch (mainly from ulnar artery): will give the common digital arteries, these will give the proper digital arteries.
  - The radial artery passes dorsally by curving around the wrist at the level of the anatomic snuff box then it enters the palm between the two head of the 1st dorsal interosseus muscle, and then it passes between the transverse and oblique heads of adductor pollicis to become the deep palmar arch.
    - Princeps pollicis artery origniates from the radial artery just distal to the location of the deep palmar arch then passes on the palmar aspect of the adductor pollicis and then becomes subcutaneous at the thumb metacarpophalangeal flexion crease. It lies beneath the flexor pollicis longus tendon muscle and divides into two branches.
- 6 dorsal compartments of the wrist (1st and 3rd moves the thumb):
  - First: Abductor pollicis longus and extensor pollicis brevis (APL may have multiple slips)
  - Second: Extensor carpi radialis longus and brevis (ECRL and ECRB).
  - Third: extensor pollicis longus (EPL) (lies ulnar to Lister's tubercle, then turn radially to insert in the distal phalanx of the thumb).
  - Fourth: Extensor digitorum communis (EDC), extensor indicis proprius (EIP), posterior interosseus nerve (PIN) (the only compartment which has a nerve).
    - The extensor indicis proprius tendon has the most distal muscle belly, and it lies deep and **ulnar** to the extensor digitorum communis branch to index finger (help in identification of correct tendon repair in cases of laceration of the tendon and in cases of tendon transfer).
  - Fifth: Extensor digit mini (EDM). EDM usually has two slips. EDM is ulnar to digital slip of the EDC.
  - Sixth: Extensor carpi ulnaris (ECU).
- Flexor tendons receive their nutritional supply from the synovial fluid; distal parts of the tendons receive nutrition from vinculae vessels.
- **Interossei:**
  - 4 dorsal (abduct), and 3 palmar (adduct).
  - All supplied by ulnar nerve,
- **Lumbrical**
  - Origin from the radial side of tendon of FDP.
  - Nerve supply: ulnar 2 supplied by ulnar nerve; radial 2 supplied by median nerve (through its anterior interosseous branch).
  - Insertion on the lateral extensor hood.
- The interossei muscles pass dorsal to the deep transverse inter-metacarpal ligament, the lumbrical muscles pass palmar to the ligament.

- - Force vector of both interossei and lumbical is volar to the joint axis at the MCP (flexion of the MCP) and dorsal to IP joints (extension of the IP joints).
- The extensor mechanism of the fingers:
  - 2 lateral bands and 1 central slip.
  - The central slip extends the PIP, the lateral band extend the DIP
- **Sagittal bands:**
  - Act to centralize the tendons of EDC at the MCP.
  - Attached to the tendon on one side and the volar plate on the other side.
  - Rupture will cause subluxation of the tendon away from the affected side(see later).
- **The triangular ligament (Fig 5):**
  - Located on the dorsal aspect at the base of the middle phalanx just distal to the central slip. It keeps the lateral bands at the dorsal aspect of the digit.
  - **Disruption** of the triangular ligament will lead to volar subluxation of the lateral band causing flexion of the PIP (boutonniere deformity).
  - **Contracture** or tightness of the triangular ligament will lead to hyperextension of the PIP (Swan-neck deformity)
- *Transverse* **retinacular ligament (Fig 5):**
  - Extends from the edge of flexor tendon sheath at PIP to the lateral edges of the lateral bands. It prevents dorsal subluxation of the lateral bands (opposite of triangular ligament).
  - **Disruption** of transverse retinacular ligament will lead to excessive dorsal subluxation of lateral bands, hyperextension of the PIP and secondary Swan-neck Deformity.
  - **Contraction** of transverse retinacular ligament will lead to volar subluxation of the lateral bands and boutonniere deformity.
- *Oblique* **retinacular ligament (Fig 5):**
  - Originates from the flexor tendon sheath and volar aspect of proximal phalanx and extends distally and dorsally to inserts into the distal aspect of the lateral band close to the distal phalanx.
  - It coordinates the movement of the PIP and DIP (coordinated flexion and extension).
- **Carpal tunnel:**
  - Carpal tunnel has 9 tendons (4 FDS, 4 FDP and FPL) and median nerve (FCR is NOT).
  - It has an hourglass shape which is narrowest at the level of the hook of the hamate.

- o The transverse carpal ligament is the volar boundary of the carpal tunnel. It attaches to the scaphoid and trapezium radially and the pisiform and the hook of the hamate ulnarly.

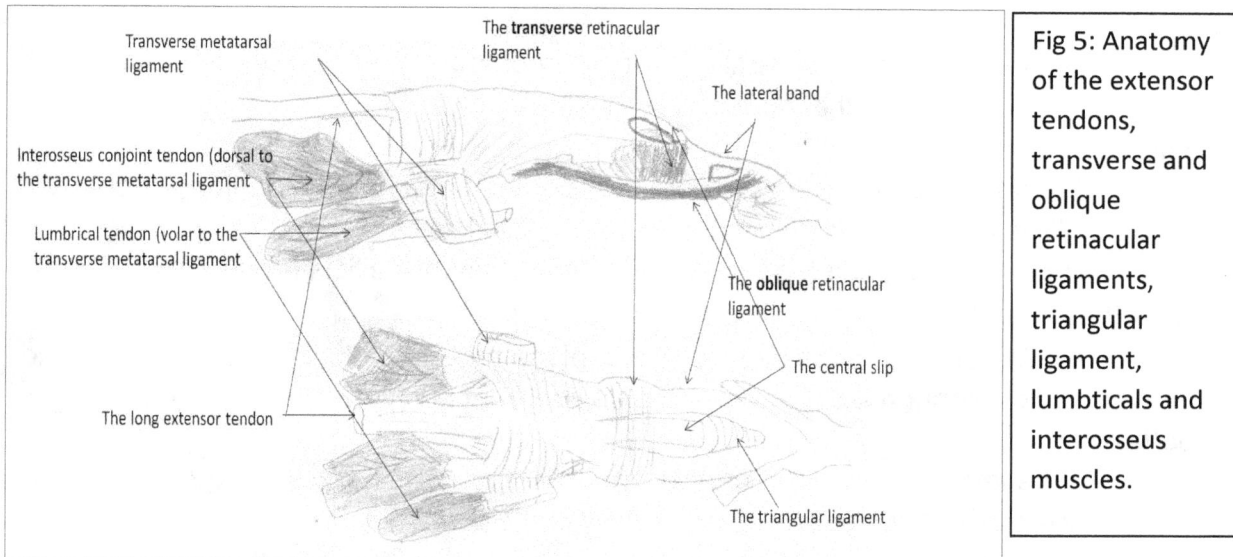

Transverse metatarsal ligament

The **transverse** retinacular ligament

The lateral band

Interosseus conjoint tendon (dorsal to the transverse metatarsal ligament

Lumbrical tendon (volar to the transverse metatarsal ligament

The **oblique** retinacular ligament

The central slip

The long extensor tendon

The triangular ligament

Fig 5: Anatomy of the extensor tendons, transverse and oblique retinacular ligaments, triangular ligament, lumbticals and interosseus muscles.

- **Guyon's canal (see also the hand chapter):**
  - o 4cm longitudinal tunnel.
  - o Borders: the pisiform (ulnar) and hook of hamate (radial); roof is formed by palmar carpal ligament and pisohamate ligament; floor: transverse carpal ligament.
  - o Contains the ulnar artery and ulnar nerve.
- **Pulley mechanism:**
  - o Annular and cruciform pulley in the digits proceed from proximal to distal as A1, A2, C1, A3, C2, A4, C3.
    - ▪ A2, A4 annular pulleys of the flexor tendon originate from the phalanges. These are the ones who prevent "bow stringing" (more important clinically).
- The A2 and A4 pulleys are the most important parts of the pulley system. They prevent "bow-string" and allow full finger IP flexion.
  - o A2 pulley is over the proximal phalanx and the A4 pulley is over the middle phalanx.
- The flexor tendon sheath of the small finger and thumb communicate with ulnar and radial bursa respectively through the Parona's space (between the pronator quadrates fascia and FDP conjoined tendon sheath)
- **Ligaments:**

- o The radioscaphocapitate ligament is a volar structure running obliquely from the radial styloid to the scaphoid waist, then inserting on the proximal radial aspect of the capitate.
- o Dorsal scapho-lunate ligament is the strongest part of the scapho-lunate intercarpal ligament.
- Luno-triquetral bony coalition is the most common bony coalition of the hand. It is asymptomatic condition that is discovered accidently in XR.
- **Thenar muscles:**
  - o Median nerve: supplies the abductor pollicis brevis (APB) and opponens pollicis and superficial head of flexor pollicis brevis.
  - o Ulnar nerve: supplies adductor pollicis and flexor pollicis brevis (deep head)
- Hypothenar muscles: all supplied by ulnar
- Neurovascular bundle in the digit is held in place by Cleland's ligament (dorsal) and Grayson's ligament (volar) (only Grayson's ligament is involved in Dupyutern pathology).
  - o At the level of digits: the nerves are volar to arteries. *(Scenario: volar laceration of the digit with arterial injury, what other structure affected?).*
- **DRUJ:**
  - o Articular disc: meniscal-like structure, about 20% of the load across the wrist (between the ulnar carpal bones and the ulnar head) passes through the disc, it has almost no stabilizing function.
  - o The radioulnar ligaments: the dorsal and volar thickened margins of the articular disc (origin from the foveal area of the ulnar head and styloid and insert into the dorsal and volar margins of the sigmoid notch), primary restraints to dorsal and palmar translation of the radius on the ulna.

Nerves of Upper Extremity:

- **Axillary nerve:**
  - o Divides into anterior and posterior branches: anterior branch: supplies the deltoid; posterior branch: supplies the teres minor and continues as the upper lateral cutaneous nerve of the arm (superior-lateral brachial cutaneous):
    - The posterior branch of the axillary nerve travels within 1-3 mm of the inferior capsule of the glenohumeral joint and can be injured during posterior-inferior labral repairs. The nerve can also be injured in cases of plication or thermal shrinkage procedures of the inferior capsule (see shoulder chapter).
    - Injury to the posterior branch will lead to teres minor weakness (weak external rotation with the arm abducted) and sensory symptoms in the lateral upper arm (over the lateral aspect of shoulder).

- **Suprascapular nerve:**
  - See shoulder chapter (compression areas).
- **Long thoracic nerve (nerve to serratus anterior):**
  - Injury to the long thoracic nerve will cause medial scapular winging (see shoulder chapter).
- **Spinal accessory nerve**
  - Supplies the trapezius muscle. Injury to the spinal accessory will cause lateral scapular winging (see shoulder chapter).
- **The musculocutaneous nerve:**
  - Supplies the coracobrachialis, biceps brachii, and the medial part of the brachialis.
  - Enters the conjoint tendon 1 cm to 5 cm distal to the coracoid process.
  - Can be injured by proximal humeral fractures or dislocations; also at risk during surgical exposure of proximal humerus if excessive lateral retraction is placed on the conjoint tendon.
  - If the nerve is affected by traction, the antebrachial cutaneous nerve (which is the terminal branch of the musculocutaneous nerve) will cause numbness over the anterolateral aspect of the forearm). *(Scenario: biceps rupture, what is the part of the upper extremity sensation affected by the nerve supplying this muscle?)*
- **Ulnar nerve:**
  - Supply the FDP to the 4th and 5th digit, FCU, most intrensics (all interossei, ulnar two lumbericals, all hypothenars, thumb adductor, deep head of FPB).
  - Ulnar nerve injury: will cause loss of thumb adduction, Froment's sign and Wartenberg sign (see below), inability to extend 4th and 5th IP joints
  - Froment's sign: when the patient is asked to adduct the thumb to hold a paper between the thumb and palm, the patient will flex the thumb IP. *(Scenario: patient is able to flex DIP of the fingers with positive Froment's sign, what is the injury? (ulnar nerve at wrist)).*
  - Wartenberg's sign: the little finger held in an abducted position; it is due to accessory slip of the extensor digiti minimi (supplied by radial) attached to the **abductor digiti minimi** tendon and to the ulnar side of the proximal phalanx of the 5th digit (not being counteracted by the dorsal interosseous muscle).
  - Ulnar nerve is the most common nerve to demonstrate increased signal intensity about the elbow in asymptomatic patients.
  - The ulnar nerve is ulnar (outer) and dorsal (deeper) to the ulnar artery at the level of the wrist
- **Median nerve:**
  - Give two motor branches: the anterior interosseous nerve (AIN), and the recurrent motor branch.

- o Median Nerve supplies the FDS, pronator teres, FCR. AIN supplies FPL, FDP to the index and middle finger, pronator quadratus. The recurrent motor branch of the median nerve innervates the thenar muscles (except the adductor pollicis and the deep head of FPB which are supplied by the ulnar nerve).
- o At the level of elbow: the structures from lateral to medial are: biceps tendon, brachial artery and median nerve. Then the brachial artery divides to radial and ulnar arteries. The ulnar artery will pass deep to the medican nerve (from lateral to medial) with the deep head of the pronator teres separating the nerve (superficial to it) from the ulnar artery (deep to it).
- o The nerve will pass deep to the fibrous arch of the superficialis muscle, and deep to the superficial head of the pronator teres muscle (the nerve passes in-between the two heads of pronator teres). Then the nerve travels in the interval between the flexor digitorum superficialis muscle and the flexor digitorium profundus muscle.
- o At the level of the wrist, the median nerve is dorsal and ulnar to the FCR.
- o Anterior interosseous nerve (off median nerve) supplies the flexor pollicis longus and flexor digitorum profundus to the index finger and middle finger. It is tested by "OK" sign (flexion of the IP of the thumb and DIP of the index). It also supplies the pronator quadratus.

- **The radial nerve**
  - o The radial nerve pierces the lateral intermuscular septum (from posterior to anterior) at the junction of the middle and distal thirds of the humerus, then passes anterior to the elbow joint at radiocapitellar joint.
  - o Supplies the triceps, lateral part of brachialis, anconeus, brachioradialis (first muscle to be innervated after reaching the anterior compartment of the arm), ECRL and ECRB (ERCB may get dual nerve supply from both radial nerve and PIN).
  - o Branches into the superficial branch and deep branch (posterior interosseous nerve) at the level of radio-capitellar joint.
    - ▪ Radial nerve supplies more muscles through its PIN branch.
  - o The superficial branch continues deep to the brachioradilis muscle, then exits the muscular fascia to become subcutaneous between the brachioradialis tendon and the extensor carpi radialis longus tendon (dorsal side of brachioradialis muscle) 8 cm proximal to the radial styloid.
    - ▪ Wartenberg's syndrome: compression of the sensory branch of the radial nerve. *(Scenario: burning pain at the dorsum of the thumb with positive Tinnel sign with percussion 8 cm proximal to radial styloid, after failure of non-operative treatment, decompression should be done for radial nerve at which interval?)*

- o Posterior interosseous nerve: supply EDC, EDM, EIP, APL, EBP, EBL, ECU and supinator.
- o Injury to the PIN: finger drop (inability to extend the fingers and thumb). Patient will be able to extend the wrist (ECRL and ECRB are supplied by radial nerve) but, the wrist will go into radial deviation (ECU not functioning). No sensory loss. The nerve can be injured during most elbow and proximal forearm approaches (see approaches section) or surgeries on the radial head and neck.
- o The return of function (or the re-enervation) usually occurs in the following pattern: brachioradialis, extensor carpi radialis longus, extensor carpi radialis brevis; then the PIN recovery: extensor digitorum comminus, extensor carpi ulnaris, extensor pollicis longus (last easily testable muscle to recover), **extensor indicis proprious** (variations may occur) *(Scenario: PIN injury, what is the last muscle to recover? (EIP causing hyperextension of the index MCP joint)).*
- Brachialis muscle has dual innervation (mainly by musculocutaneous nerve, lateral part gets nerve supply from radial nerve)
- Martin Gruber connection: motor neural communication between median and ulnar nerves in forearm.
  - o Most common neural anomaly (about 25%).
  - o Can result in abnormal clinical presentation in cases of nerve laceration proximal to the connection. *(Scenario: ulnar nerve laceration at the wrist, patient can adduct and abduct finger, explanation?)*
- Spinal accessory nerve (cranial XI): can be injured in posterior neck procedures.
  - o Patient will have pain in the shoulder girdle and will be unable to elevate his shoulder
- Root anatomy (see spine chapter):

C5	Shoulder abduction	Biceps reflex
C6	Elbow flexion wrist extension	Brachioradialis reflex
C7	Elbow extension wrist flexion	Triceps reflex

Spine
Cervical Spine Approaches (See Also Spine Chapter):
- **The Anterior Cervical Spine Approach:**
  - o Complications include: Horner syndrome, dysphasia, injury to recurrent laryngeal nerve, injury to hypoglossal nerve and/or injury to superior laryngeal nerve.
  - o Carotid sheath (containing carotid artery (common and interna), internal jugular vein, and the vagus nerve) lies lateral to the dissection.

- o During cervical spine approaches, injury to the sympathetic chain (inferior ganglion) can lead to "Horner syndrome" (pre-ganglion injury to the inferior symptathetic ganglion).
  - The patient will report a drooping of the upper eyelid and dryness on the affected side of the face.
- o Hypoglossal nerve can be injured nerve during the anterior exposure of C2-3 (upper cervical spine approach)
- o Omohyoid can be encountered during surgical approaches to C5-6. The posterior digastrics can be encountered during surgical approaches to C3-4. These two muscles run horizontally.
- o In revision anterior cervical spine surgery, before deciding to do the approach on the contra lateral side from the one used in the first surgery, assessment of the vocal cord function should be done (by formal ENT or pulmonologist consult).
  - If the vocal cord on the side of the first surgery is found to be paralyzed, second surgery must be done on the same side.
- o Vocal cord paralysis occurs with equal incidence in right-sided or a left-sided approach.
- **The Posterior Cervical Spine Approach:**
  - o The vertebral artery lies close to the posterior midline.
    - On the superior aspect, the groove for the vertebral artery lies about 1 cm (8-12 mm) from the midline. On the posterior aspect of the vertebral body, the vertebral artery lies about 2 cm (12-23 mm) from the midline.

Cervical Spine Anatomy (See Spine Chapter):

- C1-C2 ligaments (Fig 6):
  - o The transverse atlantal ligament (main stabilizer) runs horizontally behind the dens.
  - o Apical ligament, 2 alar ligaments and one transverse atlantal ligament (transverse cruciate apical alar ligament complex).
- The cervical root exits the spine in the space above the same numbered vertebrae (e.g. C4 root exits between C3-C4 vertebrae)
- Surgical land mark

Hyoid	C3
The upper border of the thyroid cartilage	C4
The lower border of the thyroid cartilage	C5
Cricoid cartilage	A midline structure at the level of C6

	(external landmark that is easily palpable).
Carotid tubercle	Anterolateral aspect of C6 (internal landmark after superficial dissection).

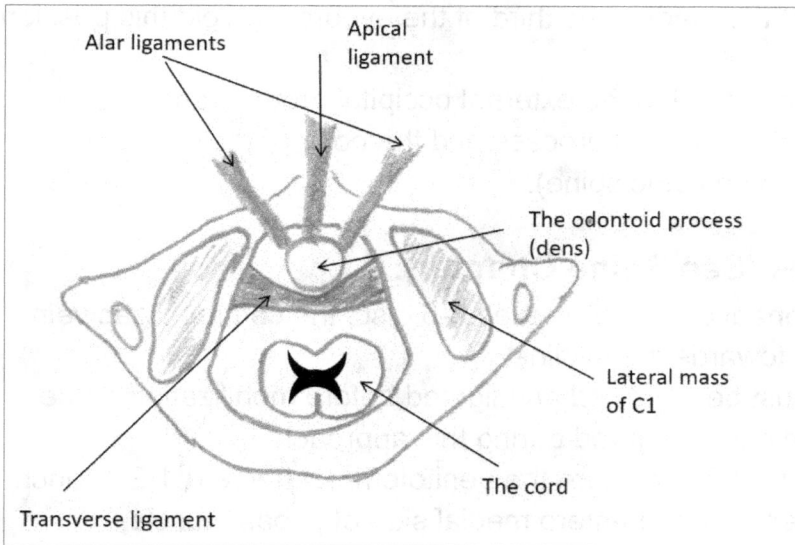

Fig 6: C1 vertebra with the dens (odontoid process) kept in place with the transverse ligament and ligaments connect the dens to the craniums

- Greater occipital nerve:
  - C2 nerve root.
  - It exits the cervical spine posteriorly between C1 and C2 vertebrae.
- Structures from anterior to posterior (Fig 7):
  - Sympathetic chain, Longus coli (on the anterior wall of the vertebra), vertebral artery (in the foramen), cervical root (in the lateral recess), then lateral mass. (note that artery is anterior to nerve root). _(Question: what is the relation of the lateral mass screw starting point to vertebral artery? (posterior))_

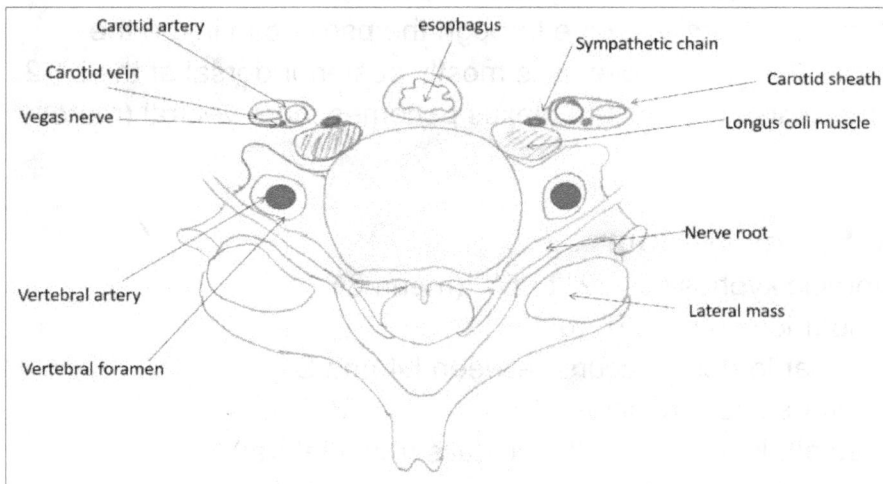

Fig 7 showing the relationship for different structures at the level of the cervical vertebra.

- The vertebral artery is contained within the vertebral foramen and thus tethered alongside the vertebral body, making it vulnerable to injury if a drill penetrates the lateral wall *(Scenario: burr into the lateral wall, what structure can be affected)*.
- Supraorbital nerve, passes at the medial one third of the eyebrow (avoid this position in halo application)
- The occiput is thickest at 5 cm lateral to the external occipital protuberance.
- The synchondrosis bewteen the odontoid process and the body of the axis fuses around the age of 6 years (see pediatric spine).

Lumbar Spine Approaches (See Spine Chapter):
- During an anterior retroperitoneal approach to the L4-5 disc, the common iliac vein should be retracted medially towards the midline.
    - The Iliolumbar vein must be identified and ligated before mobilization of the iliac vessels. This vein can be injured during this approach.
- Retro-peritoneal approach for L2-3 can injure the genitofemoral nerve (L1-2, branch of the lumbar plexus, emerges from the antero medial side of psoas muscle, innervates cremaster muscle and the skin over the anterior thigh).
- The iliohypogastric nerve innervates the external and internal oblique muscles, transversus abduminus muscle, and skin over the lower anterior abdomen.
- Anterior transperitoneal approach to L5-S1 can lead to retrograde ejaculation due to injury to superior hypogastric plexus (sympathetic).
- The most commonly injured vascular structure during lower levels lumbar disc surgery is the common iliac artery.
- Direct lateral approach:
    - Thigh pain and psoas weakness after direct lateral approach to the lumbar spine are common to occur, but usually they are transient.
    - Approaches to the lateral lumbar spine through the psoas can injure the lumbosacral plexus. The lumbar plexus is mostly posterior/dorsal at the L1-2 disc spaces. At more distal levels, the plexus becomes more ventral (more prone to injury).

Lumbar and Thoracic Spine Anatomy:
- The normal range of thoracic kyphosis is 20° to 50° (mean 35°).
- The normal range of lumbar lordosis is 40° to 80° (mean 60°).
    - The majority of lumbar lordosis occurs between L4 and S1
- Paraspinal muscles (erector spinae muscles):
    - Spinalis (most medial), longissimus, Ilio-costalis (most lateral)
- Vascular anatomy:

- o Segmental arteries lie directly related to the vertebra.
  - o The main feeder for the lower thoracic spine cord is the greater medullary artery or artery of Adamkiewicz.
    - It arises from left lower thoracic segmental arteries (T9-T11).
    - In lower thoracic spine: the right-sided approach is preferred to avoid the aorta and segmental artery of Adamkiewicz.
  - o The aorta lies anterior to the L4 vertebral body.
  - o The bifurcation of the aorta into the left and right common iliac arteries occurs over the L4-5 disc or L5 verterbal body.
  - o The vena cava bifurcates just distal to L4.
  - o Right and left common iliac vessels lie in front of L5.
- The ureters lie to both sides of the anterior spine.
- Sympathetic chain descends along the anterolateral aspect of the lumbar spine into the pelvis close to the vertebral column
- The sensory supply at the:
  - o Nipple line is by T4.
  - o Umbilicus is by T10.
- Pedicle anatomy:
  - o The diameter of the pedicle is lowest at the mid thoracic and highest in the lower lumbar.
  - o L1 has smallest diameter in lumbar spine.
  - o T4-T5 has smallest diameter overall.
  - o S1 has average diameter of about 19mm.
  - o In the thoracolumbar area (T12,L1): the L1 pedicle is smaller than T12.
  - o The axial plane transverse angulation of the thoracic pedicles is about 25° medial at T1; 15° at T2; and 10° medial from T3 to T10.
- The superior articular facet (of the vertebra below) is anterior to the inferior articular facet (of the vertebra above).
  - o In the lateral recess, the superior articular facet will be closer to the root (as it is more anterior).
- Thoracic duct:
  - o Lies on the left side, lateral to the esophagus.
  - o Loops around the subclavian artery, and drains into the subclavian vein.
  - o With exposure of upper thoracic segments, consider a right sided approach (to avoid the thoracic duct).

Anatomy of The Cord/Intra-Thecal Roots (Fig 8):
- Spinal tracts:

- o Main descending motor pathway in the spinal cord is the lateral corticospinal track.
- o Posterior column tracts (gracilis and cuneate) transmits deep sensations (sense of position, sense of vibration, sense of movement).
- o The spinothalamic tract transmits sensory sensation from the body to the brain. It is further divided into two:
  - ▪ The lateral tract transmits pain and temperature.
  - ▪ The anterior tract transmits crude touch and pressure sensation.
- Roots relation: the more proximal roots will be lateral to the more distal roots (so it can exit from the foramen). *(Question: what is the relation of L4 root to L5 root in the vertebral canal?)*
- All the somatic sensory innervations have their cell body in the dorsal root ganglion.

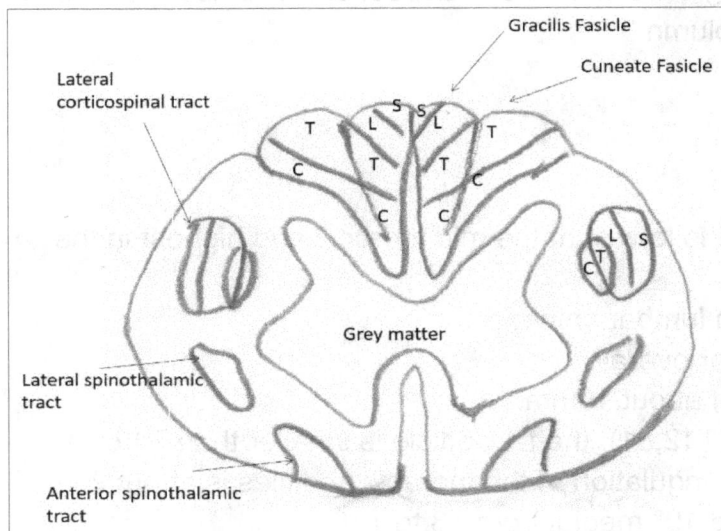

Fig 8: anatomy of the ascending and descending tracts. Notice that in the posterior column tracts, the sacral roots are more medial while in the lateral corticospinal tract, the sacral roots are more lateral.

Intervertebral Disc (See Basic Science Chapter):

- Composed of nucleus pulposus, annulus fibrosus and vertebral end plate
  - o The nucleus pulposus mainly resists compressive loads.
    - ▪ The nucleus pulposus is composed primarily of type II collagen. The nucleus pulposus is rich in aggregating proteoglycans (aggrecan). This attracts water and help maintain disc height.
    - ▪ The nucleus pulposus consists of chondrocyte-like cells that have a limited vascular supply and generate energy through anaerobic glycolysis
  - o The annulus fibrosus mainly resists tensile/ torsion loads.
    - ▪ The annulus fibrosus is composed primarily of type I collagen. The annulus fibrosis has a multilayer architecture; each layer is oriented at

30° to the horizontal in an opposite direction to the adjacent layers. This composition allows the annulus to resist torsional and tensile loads.
- The anulus fibrosus is innervated by the sinuvertebral nerve.
  - With increasing age, the disc cells produce less aggrecan and type II collagen, leading to decrease in proteoglycan and water content.
    - The nucleus pulposus desiccates, disc height is decreased and the annulus fibrosus develops fissures.
- Disc nutrition occurs via diffusion through pores in the end plates. The disc has no direct blood supply
- Ninety percent of asymptomatic individuals older than 60 years have MRI evidence of disc degeneration.
- BMP 2 and TGF Beta increase stimulate the cells to produce disc matrix (without increasing cell proliferation). ILGF-1 and FGF increase cell proliferation.

Tips:
- Wartenberg sign (ulnar nerve palsy), Wartenberg syndrome (compression of radial sensory nerve)
- Sciatic L4-S2, femoral L2-4 (L4 has contribution to both)

Chapter 5:   Pediatric Orthopedics

Normal growth and development

- Age of rolling:
    - From front (tummy) to back at the age of 4 months.
    - From back to front 6 months *(Scenario: 4 months old boy, on his back, rolled over and broke his femur, next step? (contact CPS, the story in not convincing as he cannot roll)).*
- Sitting unsupported: at the age of 6-9 months.
- Walking is usually by 12 months. If not walking by the age 18 months, underlying developmental or neurological condition should be suspected.
    - Clubfoot, DDH, rotational deformity, cleft foot, foot deformity, rotational deformity of the extremity should not significantly delay walking. *(Scenario: 15 months old boy, not walking, next step? (wait if no obvious pathology))*
- Infants and toddlers are normally ambidextrous (can use both hands). Most children develop hand dominance during their third year.
    - Strong hand preference in a child younger than age 2 may indicate a neurological deficit while persistence of ambidexterity is not pathological. *(Scenario: 18 months old girl, right hand dominant, next step? (Neurological evaluation, not supposed to have dominance at 18 months)).*
- Abnormal pathological reflexes/ findings:
    - Moro's reflex after 6 months.
    - Asymmetric tonic neck reflex, extensor thrust, absent foot placement.
- Parachute reflex: normal findings. It starts around the age of 6 months and persists after that.
- Onset of menarche is most reliable method to predict the amount of growth remaining in girls.
    - Females continue to grow for about 2-3 years after menarche. *(Scenario: female with idiopathic scoliosis requiring bracing or athletic female needing ACL surgery, what is the best method to detect growth remaining?)*
- Peak growth velocity occurs prior to menarche and prior to Risser 1

Normal Knee Alignment

- The knee joint is in varus until 2 years of age.
- The alignment of the knee changes to valgus which reach maximum around the age of 3-4 years.
- The normal adult alignment (7 degrees of valgus) is usually reached by the age 8 years. *(Question: Physiologic bowing of the lower extremities should spontaneously correct by what age? (24-36 months)). (Scenario: twin brothers, 18 months, bilateral genu varum, treatment? observation)) (Scenario: bilateral genu varum in 16 months' boy, mother concerned, treatment?)*

Lower extremity rotation:

- Etiology of intoeing: excess femoral anteversion, internal tibial torsion, or metatarsus adductus.
- Excess femoral anteversion:
  - Normal version: at birth the femoral version is about 40°. Then it decreases gradually to reach about 20° at the age of 8 years.
  - With excess femoral anteversion: hip internal rotation will be more than external rotation.
  - Treatment: observe until the age of 8. If it persists after age of 8: possible surgical interventionK.
- Tibial Torsion:
  - Normal version: at birth the tibial torsion is about -10° (internal). Then it, change gradually to about 10° (external) by the age of 3 years.
  - In toddlers, the thigh foot angle (which represents tibial torsion) will be negative (foot pointing inward in relation to the thigh with the child lying prone with flexed knee).
  - Treatment: observe until the age of 8 years. *(Question: what do you tell families of kids with internal tibial torsion? (Resolution by age 8 years with observation in most patients.)) (Scenario: 18 months, tripping, exam shows negative thigh foot angle, treatment? prognosis?)*
    - "Orthopedic" shoes and/ or orthoses are ineffective treatments for treatment of tibial torsion or femoral version.
- Metatarsus adductus:
  - Most cases of metatarsus adductus will resolve spontaneously in the first year.
  - Patients with persistent rigid metatarsus adductus after one year can be treated by serial casting or bracing.

General Considerations About Pediatric Patients:

- Healthy child has about 75 milliliters (mL) of blood volume per kilogram of body weight. *(Scenario: 4 years old, 16KG, how much blood does she have?)*
- **Amputation in children:**
  - Syme's amputation:
    - Ankle disarticulation.
    - Can accommodate a prosthesis to equalize the LLD.
  - Boyd amputation:
    - Talectomy and fusion between distal tibia and calcaneus (to prevent the problems associated with heel pad migration).
    - May provide better end bearing.
    - Excessive length can interfere with prosthetic foot options.

- o Amputation through bones in children (femur, tibia, humerus) is commonly complicated by continuation of bone growth resulting in protrusion of the bone through the end of the stump (common in humerus >fibula >tibia >femur).
  - o Age of fitting of prosthesis:
    - Upper extremity: sitting age (6 months); lower extremity: walking age (12 months).
- Intraosseous (IO) access is recommended in all children after 2 failed attempts of intravenous access or during circulatory collapse.
  - o Blood products and medications can be administrated through IO. It should not be left in place for more than 72 hours.

General Conditions Affection Musculoskeletal Systems (See Also the General Chapter and Genetic Chapter)

- **Streeter's dysplasia (constriction band or amniotic band syndrome):**
  - o Congenital condition, in which the child will have an obvious constriction band with swelling of the distal part.
  - o Can be associated with club foot or syndactyly, cleft palate, renal and cardiac anomalies.
  - o Treatment is circumferential band excision and z-plasty (single or two stages). If there is a need for skin grafting, full thickness skin graft should be used.
  - o Tight bands around the peroneal nerve can lead to nerve damage. Patient will have neuropathy with insensate foot that may lead to ulcers and osteomyelitis.
- **Juvenile Rheumatoid Arthritis (Juvenile Idiopathic Arthritis (JIA)):**
  - o Diagnostic criteria: arthritis in any joint for greater than 6 weeks before the age of 16 years.
  - o Clinical diagnosis: the diagnosis depends on thorough history and physical exam.
  - o Clinical presentation: **Joint stiffness, soft tissue swelling**. One or more joints involved with swelling of **6 weeks or longer**.
    - Radiographic and serological evaluation may be unremarkable.
  - o Subtypes: pauciarticular, polyarticular, and systemic-onset:
    - Pauciarticular form (affection of fewer than five joints) is the most common form, usually presents early in life (before the age of 4 years).
  - o Systemic symptoms are frequent in children including rash, lymphadenopathy, uveitis, and intermittent fevers.
    - Uveitis occurs in about 25% of cases may lead to blindness. Referral to ophthalmologist is needed (the condition can start asymptomatic).

- The cervical spine may be involved in a child with polyarticular or systemic JRA which may lead to cervical instability and spinal cord injury during intubation or positioning in the presence of an unstable cervical spine. Radiographic assessment of the cervical spine should include lateral flexion-extension views *(Question: what is the most important preoperative evaluation test for children with juvenile arthritis?)*
    - o Rheumatoid factor is present in only 20% of patients with JRA (compared with 80% of adults with RA). Rheumatoid factor is seen only in patients 8 years or older at the time of presentation.
    - o Screening test is **antinuclear antibody** (positive in 70% of children with pauciarticular JIA) *(Scenario: 4 years old girl, knee swelling and decrease ROM for 2 months, XR negative, what test order?)*
- **Sickle cell disease.**
    - o Children with Sickle cell disease are more prone to sustain osteomyelitis.
    - o Most common organism for osteomyelitis is staph aureus.
    - o Most specific organism is Salmonella.
- **Arthrogryposis**
    - o Congenital disease characterized by stiffness of the joints.
    - o It may be a primary pathology (arthrogryposis multiplex congenital (AMC)) or can be secondary to many other condition.
        - AMC has normal mentality.
    - o Clinical presentation: stiffness of the joints with loss of skin creases over the joints:
        - Elbows and knees flexion contracture.
        - Shoulders: internal rotation contracture.
        - Clubfeet.
    - o Can be associated with hip dislocation (teratologic hip dislocation):
        - Negative Ortolani (irreducible dislocation).
        - Treatment is open reduction around the age of 6 moths.
        - In early age (<12 months), this can be done bilateral in the same stage through medial approach. Later in life, anterior approach (Smith Peterson) approach is needed (one side at a time). *(Scenario: 9 months' girl, elbow and knee contracture, XR broken Shenton line, treatment? (Bilateral open reduction performed through a medial approach.)) (Scenario: neonate with athorgyposis with clubfeet and left hip dislocation, treatment? (Management of clubfoot, and wait until the child is about 6 months for hip.))*

Non Accidental Trauma (Child Abuse) (NAT):

- When suspecting NAT or child abuse: Inform the child health and protective services and admit the child to the hospital.

- o If a child tells you that he is mistreated or being abuse (eg. sexually) by a teacher or a couch: Inform the child health and protective services.
- Bone (skeletal) survey should be done to assess if there is other bony lesion (other fracture in different stage of healing).
- Although physical abuse may potentially have the highest morbidity and mortality for the child, neglect is the most common form of child abuse.
- Fractures are the second most common injuries in NAT after soft tissue lesions (bruising, burns).
- Fractures with high suspicion for NAD: fracture shaft femur in non-ambulatory child, trans physeal elbow fracture (distal humerus physeal separation) (Fig 1), both bones forearm in child less than zone-year-old, fracture with abundant callus at the time of presentation. *(Scenario: 9 months old with fracture shaft femur, next step? (skeletal survey and child protective service involvement, bone scan is only used when no fracture can be detected in skeletal survey and there is high suspicious of bony injury.)) (Scenario: 9 months coming with step father, shaft humerus fracture, skeletal survey: possible distal tibial corner fracture, next step? Admit the child).*
- Most common fracture (not most specific) is single long bone transverse fracture (transverse fractures are more common than spiral fractures).
- Most common non accidental bone fractures are humerus, femur and skull.
- **Shaken baby syndrome (SBS) (abusive head trauma)**: subset of the of child abuse, often fatal and can cause severe brain damage, resulting in lifelong disability. Can be associated with chest ecchymosis and head trauma. Classically was described as a triad subdural hematoma, retinal bleeding, and brain swelling (retinal hemorrhages are often found, but are not pathognomonic).

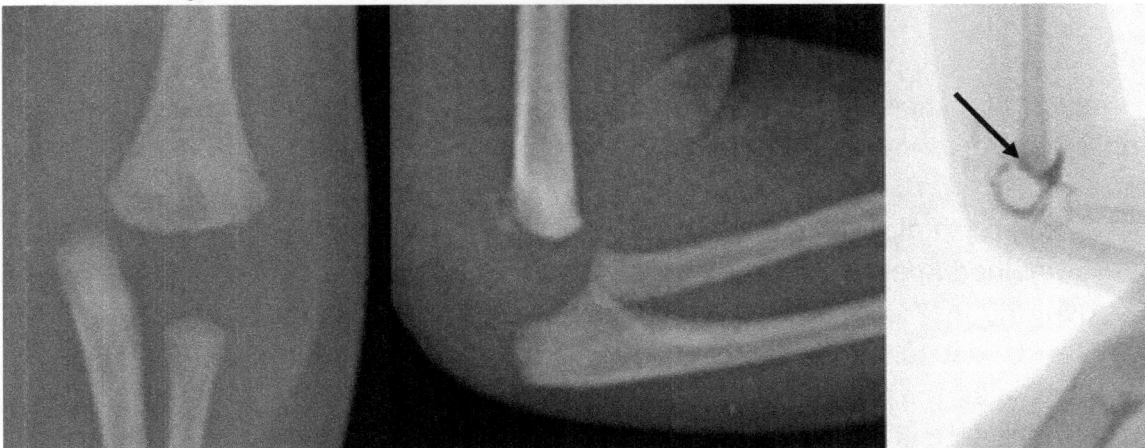

Fig 1: Trans-physeal elbow fracture. Notice that the fracture line cannot be seen as it passes in the physis. There is obvious displacement of the axis of the forearm in relation to the humerus axis. Arthrogram was done to better delineate the anatomy; the dye can be seen in between the epiphysis and the shaft indicating the presence of a fracture.

Neurologic diseases:

Cerebral Palsy (CP):

- Definition: non progressive injury to growing brain (prenatal, natal or early post-natal) resulting in motor affection.
- requirement of diagnosis:
  - Non progressive insult to the growing brain (the musculoskeletal manifestations can be progressive, but the injury to the brain should not be).
  - Presence of musculoskeletal manifestations for the brain injury.
- Periventricular leukomalcia: related to intra uterine brain ischemia (common pathology for prenatal CP)
- Types of cerebral palsy:
  - According to muscle tone: Spastic, athetoid, hypotonic, combined.
    - In general: tendon transfers are non-predictable in athetoid cerebral palsy.
  - According to part of body affected: diplegic, hemiplegic, quadriplegic:
    - Diplegic: affection of four limbs with lower extremities affected more than upper extremities.
      - Spastic diplegia: usually related to pre maturity (low birth weight) and ischemia.
    - Hemiplegic: affection of one side of the body (usually upper extremity is involved more the lower extremity).
      - The unaffected side can be in mild equines as an accommodation for the affected side (no need to address the unaffected side).
    - Quadriplegic: affection of the four extremities.
- The most prognostic sign for the ability of a young child with cerebral palsy to walk is the ability to sit independently by age 2 years.
- Crouch gait:
  - Common in diplegic CP.
  - Combined knee and hip flexion position to maintain the center of body mass over the feet for stability, resulting in the characteristic crouched posture.
  - Can be associated with either equines or calcaneus deformity of the ankle.
- Braces (see also the rehabilitation chapter):
  - Ground reaction AFO: helps to push the tibia backward (extending the knee) to decrease the crouch gait.
  - Posterior leaf spring AFO: used for mild cases of equines (spasticity has to be minimal to use this brace) in which there is loss of the heel strike (1st rocker) with normal mid and late stance and increase plantar flexion during swing phase.

- It helps to clear the toes in the swing phase and prevent foot slap at initial contact.
- **Management of spasticity**
  - Local treatment: muscle stretching, therapy, bracing, and Botox injection (see basic science chapter for mechanism of action).
  - Baclofen: oral or intra-thecal (by intra-thecal pump).
  - Surgical: selective dorsal rhizotomy (SDR). SDR is best suited for young children with spastic diplegia, limited community ambulation and crouched gait. SDR will result in permanent decrease in lower extremity muscle tone.
- **Hip affection with CP:**
  - The deformity usually starts with adduction/ flexion contracture (the flexion contracture is assessed by Thomas test).
  - In quadriplegic CP (and to less extent diplegic CP), the natural history will include subluxation and dislocation of the hips with coxa valga deformity of the proximal femur.
  - Imaging: subluxation can be assessed by the percentage of uncovered femoral head (migration index) (Fig 2)
  - Treatment:
    - Early: stretching, Botox injection and adductors/flexor release.
    - For older children (6 years and older): Varus derotation osteotomy. *(Scenario: 2 years diplegic CP, limited abduction, increase migration index, treatment?) (Same previous scenario but 8 years?)*
- **Knee:**
  - Knee flexion contracture can be commonly treated by hamstring lengthening +/- posterior capsular release (other options include distal femoral osteotomy or guided growth of the anterior distal femoral physis).

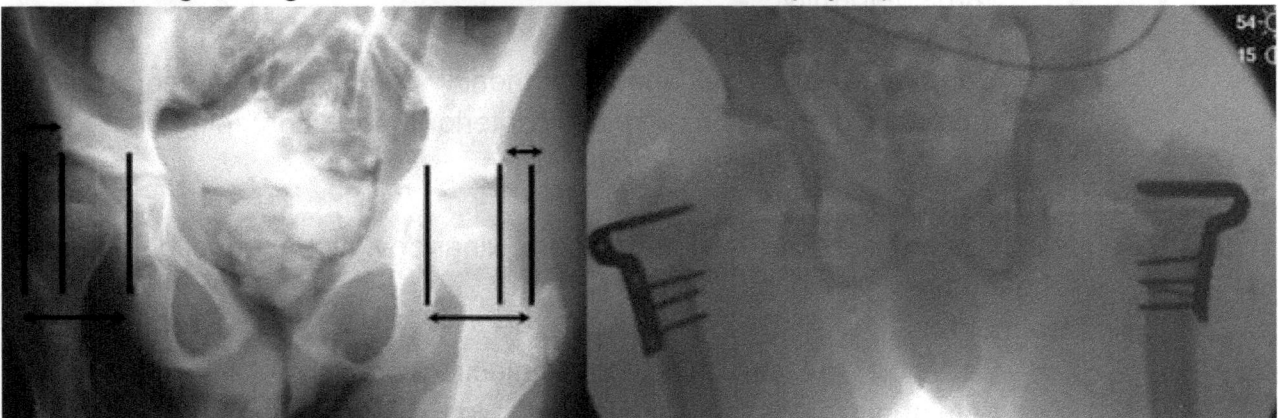

Fig 2: Pelvis AP for 9 years old CP showing bilateral hip dysplasia. The migration index is the ratio of the uncovered part of the femoral head to the whole width of the femoral head. Bilateral proximal varus femoral osteotomy was done to treat the dysplasia, note that both femoral head became covered in the acetabulum after the osteotomy.

- **Foot deformity in CP:**
  - General rule: Rigid deformities typically require bony reconstruction procedures.
  - Bunion: if it is causing symptoms and could be not be treated by shoe modification, surgical treatment by first MTP joint arthrodesis has the highest overall success rate compared to other surgeries in ambulatory and non ambulatory children with cerebral palsy.
  - Equines deformity:
    - Young children with mild equines: serial casting can bring the ankle to normal then application of AFO can be done to maintain correction. This can be facilitated by Botox injection prior to casting (to relax the gastrocnemius muscle).
    - Failure of non surgical treatment: Achilles tendon lengthening. Avoid over lengthening to prevent the development of calcaneus deformity (recession of the musculo-tendinous junction (eg Vulpius or Strayer) is preferred over Z lengthening of the tendon which can result in over lengthening).
    - AFO Brace cannot be applied to equines deformity before obtaining correction (can be used to maintain correction not obtaining it).
  - Flexible equino varus deformity: can be treated by release or split transfer of posterior tibial tendon (after failure of non-surgical treatment).
  - Varus deformity:
    - Can be due to over activity of either tibialis anterior or tibialis posterior muscle.
    - Dynamic EMG can help to identify which muscle is responsible for the varus deformity.
  - Valgus deformity:
    - Can be treated by calcaneal lengthening combined with medial column (talo-navicular) fusion or tibialis posterior tendon tightening or peroneus brevis lengthening.
- **Hand deformity in CP:**
  - Flexion deformity of the wrist and fingers, ulnar deviation, adduction deformity of the thumb.
  - Treatment:
    - Early: therapy, stretching, Botox injection, bracing.
    - Late: muscle release, transfer (FCU to ECRB) or wrist fusion. Combining wrist fusion with proximal row carpectomy can improve finger flexion deformity.
- **Spine deformity in CP:**
  - See neuromuscular scoliosis in Spine chapter.

- **Fractures:**
    - Non-ambulatory patients are at higher risk for fracture due to osteoporosis (non weight bearing and anti-seizure medications).
    - Think in non accidental trauma (developmental delay is a risk factor).

Duchenne's Muscular Dystrophy (DMD):
- Progressive muscular weakness.
- Cardiomyopathy (common cause of death in DMD): comprehensive cardiac evaluation, including an EKG and an echocardiogram should be done as preoperative assessment before major surgery (eg posterior spinal fusion).
- X linked recessive disorder (dystrophin gene):
    - The disease is transmitted from the mother (carrier), who will have mildly elevated levels of CPK (no clinical affection), to their male children (affected).
- Calf pseudo-hypertrophy occurs in about 85% of patients (characteristic finding).
- Lab: Elevated CPK. Confirm the diagnosis with DNA analysis
- Patients develop scoliosis after being wheel chair bound; treatment is by posterior fusion from upper thorax to pelvis.
    - Indication of fusion of the spine: when the curve starts to progress (>20) (which starts soon after being wheel chair bound).
- Steroid treatment helped to increase survival, increase walking period, decrease scoliosis development.
- Patients with DMD are at higher risk for malignant hyperthermia when undergoing surgery under inhalational anesthesia (treatment by dantrolene).

Myelodysplasia (Spina Bifida):
- Pathology: Neural tube defect.
- Neural axis lesions may be associated with visible midline abnormalities such as a hairy patch or nevus.
- Related to pre-conception maternal deficiency of folic acid *(question: what foot supplement can decrease incidence of neural tube defect?)*
- The higher the level of affection, the worst the condition.
- High percentage of latex allergy. Latex precautions should be done for all patients with this condition. *(Scenario: spina bifida patient, undergoing surgery, developed hypotension, why?)*
- Fractures in patients with myelodysplasia can present with picture similar to infection (red, swollen and hot). XR will show the fracture. The treatment is usually non-surgical.

- The functional motor level (lowest (most caudal) anatomical level of functional motor unit) of the patient is of most important factor in determining prognosis and outcome:
  - o Thoracic level and high lumbar: non ambulatory
  - o Mid lumbar: early in life: ambulatory with assistive device, then later in life will be mostly wheel chair (the child will become hevier).
  - o Low lumbar: ambulatory.
  - o Sacral level: minimal affection, usually have cavus foot.
- Myelodysplasia patient who starts to show rapid deterioration of their neurological condition may be developing tethering of their spinal cord. *(Scenario: 3 years old, spina bifida, walker with crutches, for last 2 months cannot ambulate, next step? (MRI of the lumbar spine for possible tethered cord))*
- **Foot and ankle:**
  - o The most common **congenital** foot deformity associated with myelomeningocele is equinovarus (clubfoot).
  - o Valgus ankle (due to distal tibia deformity):
    - In children with open growth plate: treatment by medial epiphysiodesis (mostly by screw from tip of medial malleolus).
    - In children with closed growth plate: treatment by supra malleolar osteotomy.
  - o L5 spina bifida will have working ankle dorsiflexor and nonfunctioning ankle plantar flexor resulting in **calcaneus deformity** (dorsiflexion of the ankle).
    - This can be treated by transfer of tibialis anterior muscle to posterior calcaneus. *(Scenario: picture of child with calcaneus deformity, what is the level of affection?)*
- **Knee:**
  - o See CP knee flexion deformity.
- **Hip dysplasia in myelodysplasia:**
  - o Hip dislocation is commonly seen especially with higher level of affection.
    - Thoracic and upper lumbar level: no treatment (Observation with range-of-motion exercises to minimize contractures).
    - Mid lumbar level: Unilateral dislocation: surgical reduction. Bilateral dislocation: observation.
    - Low lumbar and sacral level: surgical reduction.

Spinal Muscular Atrophy (SMA):

- Autosomal-recessive disorders characterized by progressive weakness of the lower motor neurons (congenital disease of anterior horn cell) (SMN1 and SMN2 genes).
- Affected children will have progressive weakness and muscle fasciculation.
- Can be associated with hip dislocation: no treatment (observation). *(Scenario: 6 years with unilateral hip dislocation, painless, management?).*

- Types (according to severity and age of presentation):
    - Acute infantile (type I or Werdnig-Hoffman disease): patients present before 6 months of age, severe, progressive muscle weakness with flaccid or reduced muscle tone (hypotonia).
    - Chronic infantile (type II): most children present between the ages of 6 and 18 months with developmental motor delay (failure to stand by 1 year of age).
    - Juvenile form (type III or Kugelberg-Welander disease): present around the age of 2 years and longevity can extend well into middle adult life.
- All types of SMA will have functional loss of both SMN1 genes, but disease severity depends on the number of copies of SMN2 that remain functioning.

Pediatric Musculoskeletal Infections:

Septic Arthritis:
- See septic arthritis of the hip in the hip section.
- Clinical presentation: general signs of infection, pain and rigidity of the joint, inability to bear weight on the affected extremity.
- Septic arthritis is most common in children in the first two years of life.
- **Confirmation of the diagnosis**: by aspiration of affected joint (image guided aspiration). Septic arthritis diagnosed by positive cultures or WBC count > 50,000-75,000/ml. *(Scenario: 3 years old, hip pain, flexed position, fever, increase CRP, normal WBCs, next step? (Hip aspiration)).*
- Organisms:
    - Most common organism for septic arthritis: Staph aureus.
    - Kingella Kingae:
        - A common cause of pediatric musculoskeletal infection.
        - Slowly-growing gram-negative coccobacillus.
        - It should be suspected with culture negative cases. It requires certain aerobic blood culture medium.
        - Kingella kingae is the **most common bacterial cause of osteoarticular infection in children younger than 4 years.**
        - It causes more cases of septic arthritis than osteomyelitis.
        - Susceptible to penicillins and cephalosporins, trimethoprim-sulfamethoxazole. Clindamycin does not cover about 40% of Kingella isolates.
        - For suspected septic arthritis in young children, joint aspirate should be cultured on blood culture bottle to evaluate for Kingella infection.
- Septic arthritis in neonate:
    - Multiple-joints affection is common.

o Aspiration of the joint (image guided) will confirm the diagnosis. Ultra sound is a quick test that can show the effusion. Bone scan will detect if there are other areas of involvement.
o Septic hip arthritis in a neonate:
  ▪ The hip will be kept in flexed, abducted, and externally rotated position.
  ▪ Passive movement of the hip will cause discomfort. *(Scenario: child in neonatal ICU, fever, shoulder swelling, hip limited range of motion, next step? (US), what other studies can be done? (Bone scan))*.
- Joint with intra articular metaphyseal bone: hip, shoulder, elbow, and ankle.
  o Septic arthritis of these joints can develop as sequelae of nearby osteomyelitis.

Acute Osteomyelitis

- Clinical presentation: pain, swelling, redness.
  o Refusal to walk (for lower extremity osteomyelitis).
- Labs: increased markers of infection (WBCs, CRP, ESR).
  o CRP reflect the response to treatment more rapidly than CBC and ESR (it starts to decline 48 after successful treatment and returns to normal at about 1 week).
  o ESR return to normal 2 to 4 weeks after the infection has been appropriately treated.
- Culture: Blood culture, culture from area of infection (for antibiotic selection).
- Imaging: periosteal reaction requires about 10-14 days to show up in XR. MRI and bone scan becomes positive early in the disease process.
- If clinical picture is suggestive of osteomyelitis: MRI then needle biopsy (from bone) to obtain tissue culture. *(Scenario: 5 years old, leg pain, elevated ESR, CRP, MRI distal femur osteomyelitis, blood culture taken, what is next step? (Bone aspiration for culture))*.
- MRSA osteomyelitis (see MRSA in the Basic Science):
  o 4 independent predictors (temperature > 38.0 C, white blood-cell count > 12000 cells/L, hematocrit < 34%, and C-reactive protein > 13 mg/L) to reliably differentiate between MRSA and MSSA osteomyelitis. (92% if the 4 parameters are met).
  o If suspecting MRSA: start with vancomycin or clindamycin.
  o MRSA osteomyelitis has a higher incidence of DVT (than other causes of osteomyelitis). Older children, with MRSA osteomyelitis and C-PR > 6mg/dl have 40% incidence of DVT on presentation. (The presence of the Panton-Valentine leukocidin gene encoded in strains of MRSA bacteria may explain the deep venous thrombosis).
- **Treatment:**
  o **Osteomyelitis is a primary medical problem.**

- o Treatment is mainly by antibiotics (appropriate duration, dose, and route) according to culture results.
- o The usual regimen is 2 weeks IV follow 4-6 oral (if cultures shows possible effective oral therapy).
- o Indication for surgical intervention: sub-periosteal abscess (on MRI), no improvement after 36-48 hours of appropriate antibiotic treatment, associated septic arthritis. _(Scenario: child with osteomyelitis, MRI shows abscess, treatment is? (antibiotic and debridement))_

Chronic Osteomyelitis:

- XR will show signs of bone destruction.
  - o The classic sign on radiograph is "bone-in-bone". This often signifies new bone (involucrum) surrounding the necrotic "trapped" separated sequestrum (Fig 3).
- Treatment surgical debridement of all necrotic sequestrated bone and open biopsy (to exclude malignancy and obtain appropriate culture), followed by intravenous antibiotics according to the culture. _(Scenario: 8 year old, one month of knee pain, XR bone destruction of the upper tibia, with elevated markers of infection, treatment?)_

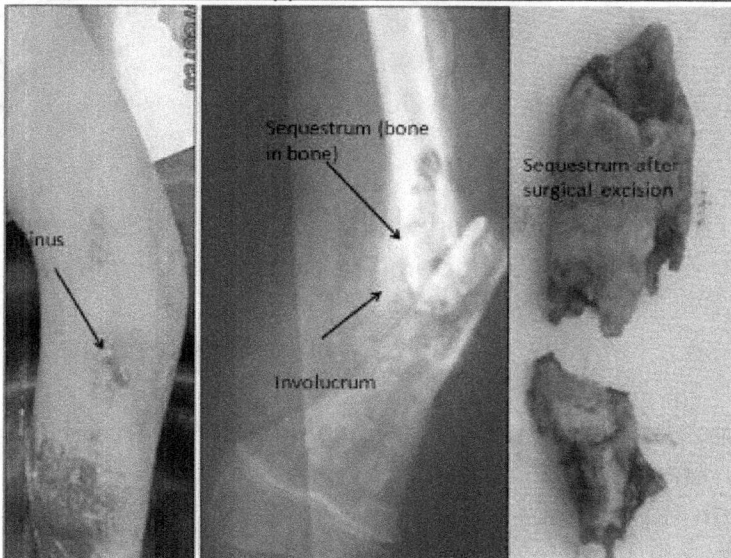

Fig 3: 12 years old male with left femur chronic osteomyelitis complicated with pathological fracture. The clinical picture shows the purulent discharge from anterior sinus of the mid thing. XR shows the pathological fracture, the sequestrum bone that lies inside the involucrum (the periosteal reaction) given the "bone in bone" appearance. Surgical debridement was done to excise the sequestered bone which is seen to the right of the picture.

Musculoskeletal Infections After Varicella

- Varicella (Chicken Box) Can be complicated by musculoskeletal infections (including osteomyelitis, septic arthritis, necrotizing fasciitis and deep soft tissue abscess).
- The most common organism causing bacterial musculoskeletal infections following varicella is group A beta-hemolytic streptococcus

Lyme Disease (see general disease chapter).

Hip:

Developmental Dysplasia of the Hip (DDH):

- Risk factors: **breech presentation** (most important), first born birth order, female, family history, condition associated with tight uterus (eg metatarsus adductus and congenital knee dislocation, and torticollis) (clubfoot is not a risk factor).
- Clinical presentation:
  - Screening at birth -6 months: by Barlow and Ortolani tests.
    - Positive Ortolani means dislocated hip. Positive Barlow means dislocatable hip.
    - If the exam shows positive test (clunk): apply the Pavlik harness.
    - If there is click, or US shows dynamic instability with normal exam: repeat the exam after 2 weeks
  - After 6 months:
    - Child will have negative Ortolani and Barlow tests (cannot elicit them after 6 months' age).
    - Limited hip abduction.
    - LLD (positive Galeazzi sign) in unilateral DDH.
    - Limping gait.
- Imaging assessment:
  - Ultra sound is used in the first 4 months (the proximal femoral is cartilaginous and cannot be seen in XR). Early ultrasound (before 4 weeks) has high false positive results.
    - Alpha angle should be more than 60° and beta angle should be more than 55°.
    - Ultrasound can assess dynamic stability (assessment of the hip stability with hip movement of adduction).
  - XR can be done after **6 months of age.**
    - Sings of instability (see Fig 4)

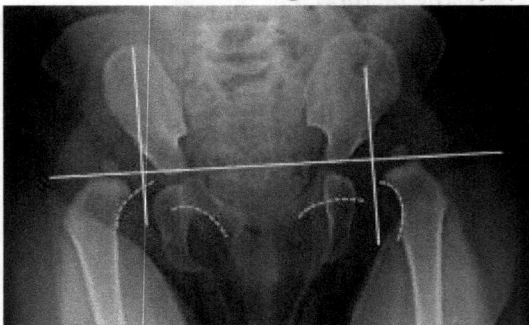

Fig 4: 10 months old girl with bilateral hip dislocation. The ossific center lies in the superior lateral quadrant in crossing made by Hilgenreiner line (horizontal line across the tri radiate) and Perkin line (perpendicular line to the horizontal line). The Shenton's line is "broken" (imaginary line from the superior edge of the obturator foramen to the inferior neck of the proximal femur.

- Treatment:
  - 0-6 months of age: Pavlik harness, re assess after 2 weeks, if hip is still out, assess that the family are applying it correctly and are compliant, and possible application for another 1-2 weeks. If not reduced after 3 weeks of appropriate application, discontinue the harness to avoid "harness disease" (displaced hip pushing on the acetabular wall causing posterolateral acetabular dysplasia).
    - Pavlik harness works by keeping the hips flexed and abducted. The hips should be flexed between 90 and 100 degrees (avoid excessive flexion to decrease the incidence of femoral nerve palsy) (controlled by anterior straps). The hips should be abducted so that with distance between the two knees cannot be less than 3–4 finger breadths (avoid excessive abduction to decrease the incidence of AVN) (controlled by posterior straps).
    - If the hips are reduced by Pavlik harness, the harness is left for (age at application + 2 months (e.g., if the Pavlik harness was applied at the age of 1 month, it should be left for 3 months).
    - If there is failure of Pavlik harness, **trial of hip abduction brace can be done.**
    - Failure of the Pavlik Harness and abduction brace: closed reduction, arthrogram and casting is the next line of treatment
  - From 6-18 months: Treatment by arthrogram, closed reduction and casting.
    - After closed reduction: the reduction is assessed either by a CT or MRI. If reduction is adequate, the child can return to operating room after 6 weeks for repeat arthrogram, spica cast for another 6 weeks
    - If closed reduction fails, open reduction through medial approach can be attempted.
  - More than 18 months: open reduction (by anterior approach which allows capsuloraphy. *(Question: advantage of anterior approach over medial approach for treatment of hip dislocation?)*
    - Obstacles to reduction: iliopsoas tendon, capsule constriction (hour glass capsule), hypertrophy of pulvinar fat, hypertrophy of ligamantom teres, inverted limbus, tight transverse ligament.
  - For late presentation (older than 24 months):
    - Femoral shortening/de-rotation osteotomy and/or pelvic osteotomy may be needed.
  - Complication of treatment of hip dysplasia: **Residual dysplasia (most common),** AVN, re-dislocation.

Hip dysplasia in adolescent:

- Adolescent with symptomatic hip dysplasia and closed tri radiate cartilage: surgical intervention is by peri- acetabular (Bernese, Ganz) osteotomy (see below). *(Scenario: 16 years old, rugby player, hip pain, cannot play due to pain, XR: hip dysplasia with closed tri-radiate cartilage, failed non operative treatment, what is the surgical option?)*
    - o The false profile view of the hip: best view to assess anterior coverage of the femoral head.

Pelvic Osteotomies

- Types:
    - o Reshaping (change the shape of the acetabulum): eg. Dega osteotomy, Pemberton osteotomy (the hinge of these types of osteotomy is the tri-radiate cartilage).
    - o Redirecting (change the position of the acetabulum): triple, periacetabular osteotomy, dial osteotomy, Salter osteotomy (hinges on symphysis pubis).
    - o Salvage (the articulation will be through fibrous cartilage by metaplasia of the hip capsule (not hyaline cartilage)): Chiari osteotomy, shelf osteotomy.
      (Scenario: 14 years old, severe dysplasia with mismatch between femoral head and acetabulum and non-reducible hip joint, what type of osteotomy needed?) (Question: what osteotomy does not require concentric reduction?)
- Salter osteotomy: pelvic osteotomy running from the notch to AIIS, hinge on the symphysis pubis, the distal fragment is pulled anteriorly, laterally and inferior (to give more anterior coverage).
- PAO (periacetabular osteotomy):
    - o Indication: hip dysplasia without arthritis in a young skeletal mature patient (closed tri-radiate cartilage).
    - o The posterior column in left intact. It does not affect the blood supply to the acetabulum. It can produce correction of the acetabular position in multiple planes.
    - o Avoid retroversion the acetabulum (both retroversion and overcorrection can lead to pincer impingement). *(Scenario: 23 years' female, left hip pain, XR dysplasia with no arthritis, NSAID and therapy failed to control symptoms, treatment?) (Scenario: 35 years old, pain with activity, full ROM, no impingement, XR deceased center edge angle, no arthritis, failed non operative treatment, what surgery can be done?)*

Coxa Vara

- XR: inverted Y sign (Fig 5) (see also Fig 2 in the basic science chapter for an XR example of case of bilateral coxa vara).
- Indication for surgery: Hilgenreiner's physeal angle > 60°, or neck shaft angle <90°.
- Valgus overcorrection of the proximal femoral deformity is the goal of surgery.

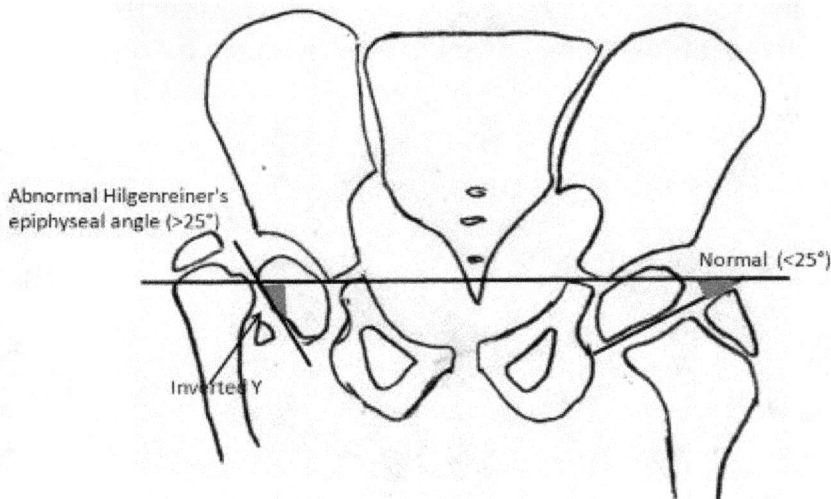

Fig 5: drawings for the pelvis AP. left side is a normal side with small Hilgenreiner's epiphyseal angle. On the right side, the Hilgenreiner's epiphyseal angle is markedly increased due to the cox vara deformity.

Slipped Capital Femoral Epiphysis SCFE:

- Clinical presentation: patients may present with knee pain (referred from the hip though the anterior branch of obturator nerve), this may lead to delay in diagnosis. *(Scenario: 13 years old boy, knee pain for one month with limping, XR knee is normal, next step? (Hip XR)).*
    - SCFE leads to decrease in the following hip movements: internal rotation, abduction, and flexion. Osteotomy to correct chronic deformity will include these three components.
    - About half of patient with SCFE have bilateral involvement: simultaneous or subsequent.
- Imaging:
    - SCFE is better detected in lateral view of the hip (Fig 6):
        - Cross table lateral can be used in both stable and unstable SCFE.
        - Frog leg lateral only in stable cases as it may cause more displacement in unstable cases.
    - Radiological severity is assessed by Southwick method (difference in the angle formed by the axis of the shaft and the perpendicular of the physis between the affected side and the normal side using the lateral hip XR (Fig 7)).
- Classified to **stable** (able to bear weight with or without crutches) and **unstable** (unable to bear weight with or without crutches)
- The incidence of avascular necrosis is much higher is unstable SCFE (around 20%-40%) compared to stable SCFE (around 0%). *(Question: what is the most important prognostic factor for development of osteonecrosis in SCFE?)*
- Chondrolysis:

- o Rapid loss of joint space.
- o Can be a consequence of unrecognized screw penetration. Transient screw penetration at the time of surgery does no increase risk of chondrolysis.

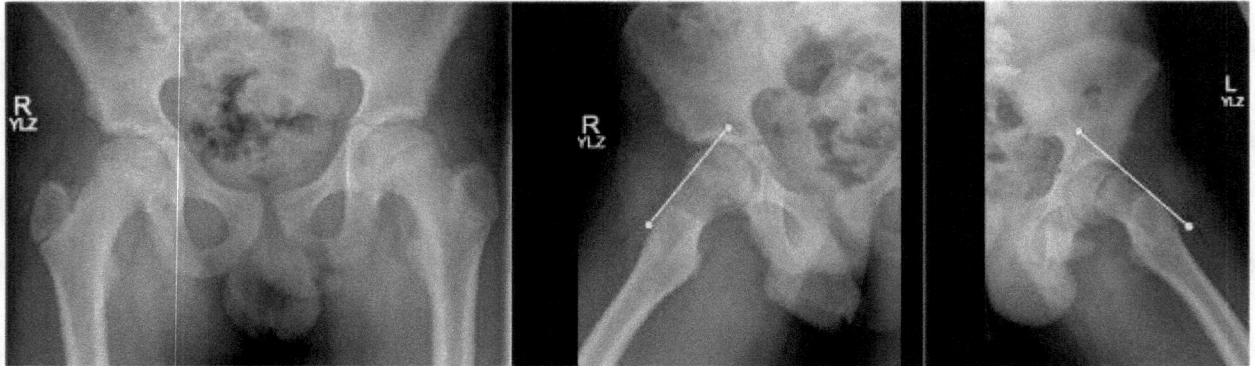

Fig 6: 13 years old boy with left hip/knee pain. Pelvis AP does not show obvious deformity (subtle changes can be seen in the left hip), however the lateral view of the left hip shows SCFE with Klein's line not bisecting the capital epiphysis. Comparison to the right side shows the difference.

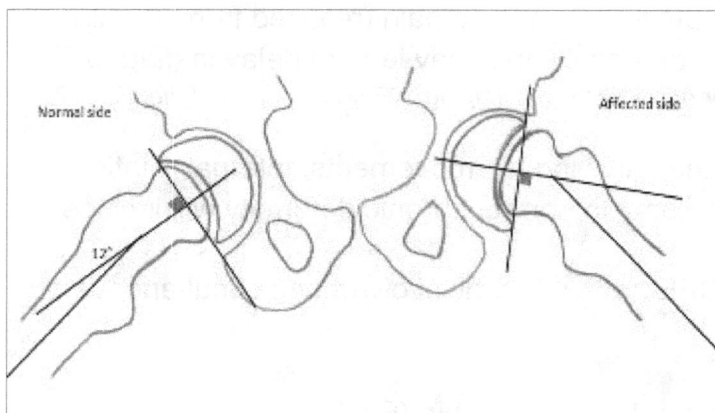

Fig 7: Assessment of severity of the SCFE by measurement of the Southwick angle. The angle is formed by the intersection of the perpendicular line to the capital epiphysis and the axis of the shaft. The Southwick angle is the difference between the affected side and the normal side. In case of bilateral affection, you can use 12° as the normal value

- **Treatment**:
  - o In-situ pinning (standard of care). *(Scenario: 13 years, knee pain for 3 months with external rotation, limping, XR shows left SCFE moderate, treatment?) (12 years, hip pain, 5 months' hip pain, lack of internal rotation and abduction, and external rotation with hip flexion, XR moderate to severe SCFE, treatment? (Still Same treatment)).*
  - o Acute unstable SCFE:
    - ▪ Gently positioning can reduce the acute element of the deformity.
    - ▪ Capsulotomy to relieve hematoma may be added (to relive pressure).
  - o About half of patient with SCFE have bilateral involvement: simultaneous or subsequent.
    - ▪ Simultaneous affection: always assess the other hip for possible SCFE. If the other hip has radiological evidence of SCFE (even if not

symptomatic): in situ pinning. *(Scenario: 13 years old boy, right hip pain, XR pelvis moderate right SCFE, mild left SCFE, treatment? (bilateral in situ pinning)).*

- Subsequent involvement: patient should be instructed if he/she started to have pain in the other side, XR should be done urgently to assess affection of the other hip. If the XR is normal, MRI can be done to assess the physis.
- Pre-SCFE: normal XR with MRI picture of edema around the physis, treatment is in situ pinning. *(Scenario: 13 years old, Right hip pinning one year ago, now left hip pain, XR normal, MRI shows increased signal around the physis in the left, diagnosis? Treatment?)*

- o Prophylactic pinning: indications include endocrine etiology (eg hypothyroidism), children less than 10 years old at the time of presentation.
- o If screw head on the anteroposterior view is medial to the intertrochanteric line, it can cause impingement at the edge of the acetabulum.
- o Avoid screw insertion in the posterior superior quadrant of the femoral head.

Hip/Pelvic Infections:
- See pediatric infection section.
- **Septic Arthritis Vs Transient Synovitis of the Hip Joint:**
  - o **Septic Arthritis:**
    - Kocher's criteria for **prediction** of septic arthritis of the hip: fever >38.5°, inability to bear weight, ESR>40 mm/h, and WBC count>12,000/ml. Modification of the original criteria includes adding CRP more than 20 mg/L. The more criteria present, the more likely to have septic arthritis.
    - **Final confirmation for the diagnosis**: by aspiration of hip joint (image guided aspiration). Septic arthritis diagnosed by positive cultures or WBC count > 50,000-75,000/ml. *(Scenario: 3 years old, hip pain, flexed position, fever, increase CRP, normal WBCs, next step? (Hip aspiration)).*
    - In equivocal cases, lean towards open drainage (to avoid the dreadful consequence of missed septic hip arthritis).
    - Untreated septic arthritis (especially in very young age) can lead to complete destruction of the femoral head or femoral head dislocation. Femoral head dislocation due to septic arthritis differs from the those due to DDH by absence of dysplasia on the acetabular side.
  - o **Transient synovitis:**
    - Unknown etiology (may be related to viral infection or trauma).
    - Treatment: NSAIDs, rest and observation.
    - Occasionally the differentiation between hip septic arthritis and transient synovitis is difficult.

- If you are not able to differential between transient synovitis and septic arthritis based on clinical exam and lab, aspiration of the joint for cell count and culture (transient synovitis will have negative culture and less than 50,000 WBC/ml). *(Scenario: 3 years old, hip pain, flexed position, fever, increase CRP, normal WBCs, next step? (Hip aspiration)).*
- **Other causes of infection of the pelvic area (other than hip septic arthritis):**
  - Pelvic pyogenic myositis, proximal femoral osteomyleitis, iliac osteomyelitis, sacro-iliac joint pyogenic arthritis.
    - Less common causes of hip pain with fever.
    - Imaging studies (**MRI** and bone scan) will show the exact pathology.
    - Treatment of all them is blood culture and antibiotics (medical treatment).

Legg Calve Perthes (LCP):

- AVN of the head of the femur in a skeletally immature child. The disease is a self-limiting condition.
- The pathological stages are: Necrosis; Revascularization; Fragmentation, Re-Ossification and remodeling.
- Classification:
  - Lateral pillar classification at the end of fragmentation stage (not at the time of presentation).
    - Depends on the height of the lateral pillar of the femoral head.
    - Classified to: A (maintaining the lateral height), B (maintaining more than 50% of the height), BC (maintaining around 50%), C (height less than 50%).
- Prognosis depends on: age at presentation, extent of head involvement (lateral pillar classification) and range of motion of the hip.
  - The most important prognostic factor is the age at presentation.
    - Children with disease process starting before the ages of six years have a good chance of achieving favorable outcome.
    - Children with presentation at an age older than 9 years old will have bad prognosis in the majority of cases.
  - Loosing adequate hip abduction is an indication for intervention (aggressive therapy, casting, or tenotomy).
  - Poor prognostic signs: hip subluxation, total head involvement, older age at time of presentation.
  - The shape of the femoral head at the age of skeletal maturity and its congruency with the acetabulum (Stulberg classification) will correlate with the long term function.

- o Lateral subluxation of the femoral head is an important radiological sign indicative of poor prognosis.
- The pathology can be bilateral (10 % of cases). In bilateral cases, the two hips are usually at different pathological stages (the disease starts in one hip and later on affects the other hip). If there is a child with bilateral symmetrical hip affection, consider different diagnosis (for example multiple epiphyseal dysplasia or spino-epiphyseal dysplasia). *(Scenario: 4 years old child, 3 weeks' history of right hip pain, XR bilateral symmetrical collapse of both hips, next step? (XR of the knees and spine to assess multiple epiphyseal dysplasia or spino-epiphyseal dysplasia)).*
- LCP before 6 years of age: symptomatic treatment: no physical education or sport participation, NSAIDs for pain, therapy to maintain abduction.
- Sequelae of old Perthes:
  - o Hinged abduction: the femoral head has a groove in its contour that causes hinge abduction (rather than rotating in the acetabulum). Treatment is with valgus osteotomy.
  - o Deformed mushroom shaped head: treatment by osteochondroplasty, and/ or increase acetabular coverage (shelf osteotomy or PAO).

Knee:

Knee coronal deformity (genu varus and genu valgus):

- See normal development section for normal knee alignment in different ages.
- Mechanical axis of the limb: from the center of the femoral head to the center of the ankle joint.
  - o Should pass in the center of the knee.
- For children with open growth plate: treatment is by **guided growth (temporary hemi-epiphysiodesis):**
  - o Follows Hueter-Volkmann principle (see later).
  - o At the apex of the deformity on the affected bone:
    - If there is knee varus deformity arising from the tibia, the treatment is by a plate applied to the lateral proximal tibial physis.
    - Valgus deformity of the knee in a growing child: guided growth of the medial proximal tibial physis (in most cases the pathology is from the proximal tibia).
  - o It is left in place until the deformity is corrected, then removed.
  - o Usually used for children with at least two years of growth remaining (12 years' old girl and 14 years' old boy).
  - o Cannot be used if the deformity is due to growth arrest (e.g. cannot be used to correct varus deformity that developed due to complete arrest of the medial

proximal tibial growth as there is no growth potential to correct the deformity); less effective in cases of bone dysplasia (needs longer times).

- For children with closed growth plate: osteotomy of the affected bone (either closing or opening wedge osteotomy depending on the side). (*Scenario: girl with genu valgum, mDFLA 75, MPTA 88 (deformity from femur) (fig 8): if she is skeletal immature (eg 14 years), treatment? (guided growth (temporary hemi ephiphysiodesis of the medial part of the distal femoral growth plate))). (Same scenario but she is skeletal mature (eg 18 years), treatment? (distal femoral osteotomy (medial closing or lateral opening)))*

- Rachitic deformity (e.g. genu varum) should be initially treated with medical treatment (Vit D) before proceeding to osteotomy.

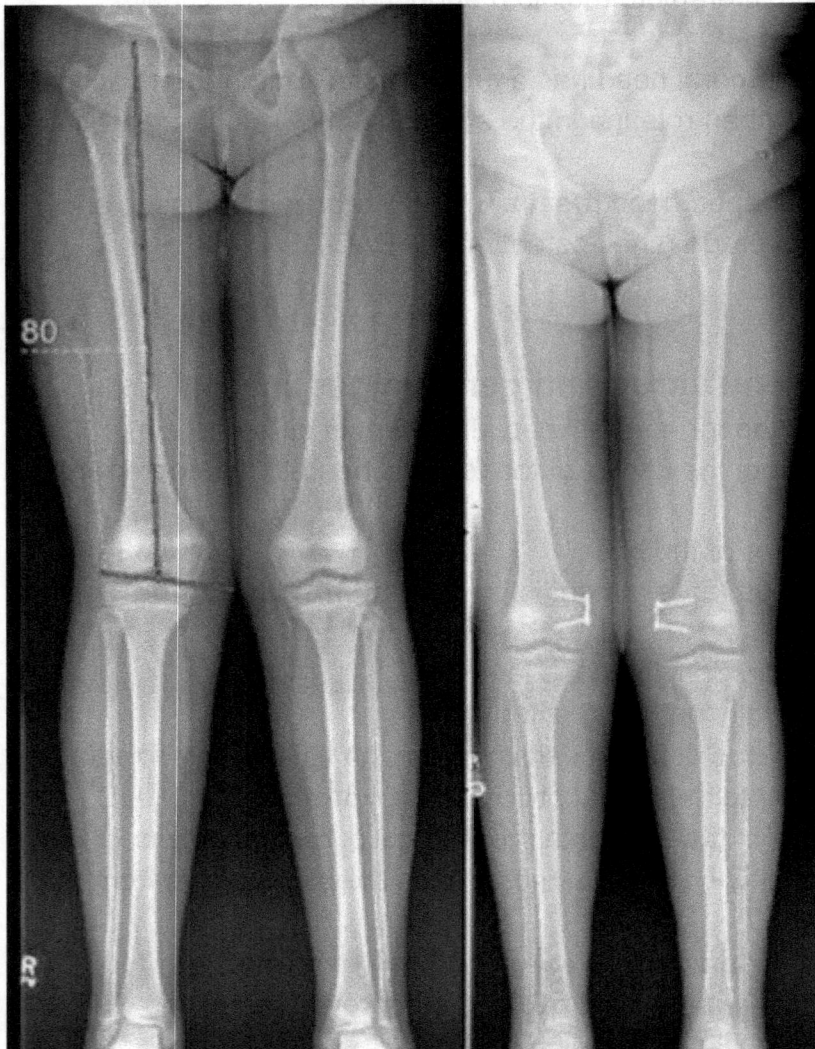

Fig 8: 11 years old female with valgus knee. Her tibial mechanical axis is normal, however, her mLDFA is 80° indicating that the valgus deformity is originating from the femur. Treatment by guided growth plate was performed resulting in correction of the deformity.

Knee sport injury:
- **See sport chapter.**

Discoid meniscus:

- Much more common in the lateral meniscus.
- On exam: clunk with each time the knee flexed at about 10°.
- Watanabe classification
    - Type I (stable, complete), the lateral meniscus covers the entire lateral tibial plateau
    - Type II (stable, partial), the lateral meniscus covers 80% of the tibial plateau. Type III (Wrisberg variant) (unstable, hypermobile) lack posterior meniscal attachments except the meniscofemoral ligament of Wrisberg.
        - On knee extension, the meniscus is pulled posteromedially into the intercondylar notch (instead of gliding forward), resulting in "snapping knee" syndrome.
- MRI: will show at least three consecutive sagittal cuts with continuous meniscal signal.
- Treatment:
    - Asymptomatic: No treatment needed.
    - If symptomatic: by saucerization of the meniscus. If there is a tear in the mid portion of a stable discoid meniscus: partial meniscectomoy with saucerization.

Blount's disease:

- Varus deformity due to medial proximal tibia growth plate disturbance.
- Two main categories: infantile and adolescent.
- **Infantile:**
    - Starts early before the age of three years.
    - Common in obese, black boys.
    - Commonly associated with internal tibial torsion and can also be associated with distal femoral **valgus** deformity.
    - XR:
        - Changes of the medial side of the proximal tibial physis.
        - Metaphysio-diaphyseal angle (angle between line connecting metaphyseal beaks and a line perpendicular to the longitudinal axis of the tibia):
            - More than 16°: diagnostic of Blount's disease.
            - Less than 11°: normal.
    - Treatment:
        - If the child is less than 3 years old, initial management can be with knee bracing.

- Surgical treatment: Failure of brace or children 3 years and older:
  - Early stages: guided growth plate hemiepiphyiodesis (reversible hemiepiphyiodesis) (Fig 9) or proximal tibial osteotomy.
  - With advanced stage (Langenskiold type IV and V), the hemiepiphysiodesis becomes less effective and tibial osteotomy is the preferred treatment for the advanced lesions. *(Scenario: 5 years old, advanced Blount's, treatment?).*
  - Proximal tibial osteotomy can be complicated by compartment syndrome. Some surgeon would advocate prophylactic fasciotomy with the osteotomy.

- **Adolescent:**
  - Around the age 12 years old, common in obese boys.
  - Can be associated with distal femoral **varus** deformity that should be addressed.
  - Management: surgical treatment (guided growth plate hemiepiphyiodesis or proximal tibial osteotomy). For guided growth, at least 2 years of remaining growth potential is needed.

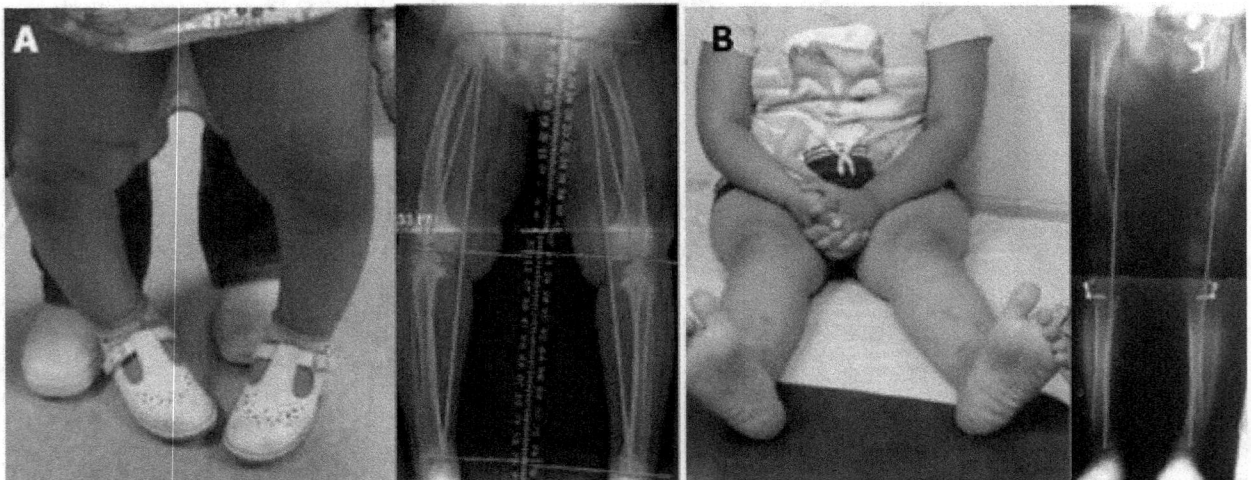

Fig 9: A) 4 years old girl with bilateral Blount's disease. B) Patient was treated by guided growth on the lateral proximal tibial physis (together with distal tibial external rotation osteotomy); the deformity was corrected gradually.

Osteochondritis dissecans (OCD):
- Most common side is the postero-lateral aspect of the medial femoral condyle.
- On exam: pain during knee extension with internal rotation of the tibia, and relief of pain with tibial external rotation (Wilson's test) (Fig 10).
- XR: the lesion is best seen in tunnel view (AP with knee flexion).

- Treatment:
    - Initial treatment for stable (non separated) lesion in skeletally immature children is non operative (**non weight bearing for 6-8 weeks and activity modification until healing occurs**)

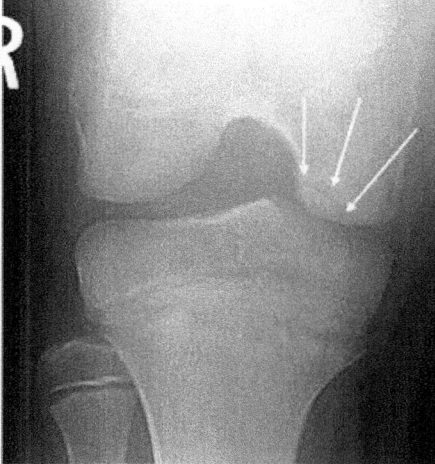

Fig 10: 14 years old boy with 6 months history of right knee pain. AP XR of the knee did not show obvious anomaly, however, tunnel view (notch view) showed OCD lesion of the medial condyle (arrows).

    - Indication for surgical treatment: failure of trial of non operative treatment (6 months), or separated (unstable) lesions.
        - Surgical treatment: drilling for stable injury, fixation or excision of separated lesion (based on the size and/or fragmentation). If excision is done, management of the condral defect should be done (see cartilage repair section in sports lower extremity chapter).
- Good prognosis (possibility of healing of the lesion by non operative treatment) is most related to the presence of **open physis** (skeletal immaturity).
    - Presence of edema behind the lesion in the MRI scan is associated with poor prognosis for healing

Osgood-Schlatter:

- Osteochondritis of the tibial tubercle, with pain and tenderness over the tibial tubercle.
- Treatment is by activity modification and NSAIDs

Pediatric ACL (See ACL injury in the sport lower extremity chapter):

- Difference from adult ACL:
    - ACL collagen fibers extend to the epiphyseal cartilage.
    - More ACL injuries occur at the tibial insertion.
    - Tibial eminence avulsion fractures can accompany ACL injury.
    - Associated meniscal injuries are common.
    - Partial tear can be managed non operatively.

○ Surgery (if crossing the physis) can lead to physeal arrest (especially in patient with more than 2 years from skeletal maturity)

Congenital Knee Dislocation:

- Can be Associated with hip dysplasia and congenital hip dislocation.
- Treatment: closed reduction then application of a splint or Pavlic harness.
- If associated with hip dislocation: treat the knee dislocation first (to be able to apply the Pavlik harness).

Patellar Dislocation in Children

- Can be associated with osteochondral fragment from the **medial** patellar facet or the **lateral** femoral condyle.
  - ○ If suspecting osteochondral fragment (flake of bone in XR or persistence of swelling and pain): MRI should be obtained.
    - ▪ The treatment should consist of arthroscopy or arthrotomy and attempted internal fixation of this fragment. If fixation is not possible, the loose body should be excised.
- Surgery is not indicated after the first traumatic dislocation.
  - ○ Acute surgical treatment of MPFL in children is not indicated.

Tibial Bowing

- Three types (according to the apex of the deformity):
- **Antero-lateral:**
  - ○ This is the one that needs special attention, has the risk of developing congenital pseudo arthrosis of the tibia (Spontaneous fracture in the area of the bowing).
  - ○ 50% of cases associated with neurofibromatosis (10% of NF patients have antero-lateral bowing).
  - ○ Treatment by fulltime bracing with a clamshell ankle-foot orthosis until maturity (osteotomy is contra indicated).
- **Postero-medial:**
  - ○ Associated with calcaneovalgus deformity of the foot.
  - ○ Resolves spontaneously, but can be associated with shortening of the extremity and LLD (around 4 cm of final LLD). *(Scenario: newborn, pictures and XR showing posteromedial deformity and calcaneovalgus foot, management? (Observation); what is the prognosis?)*
- **Antero-medial:**
  - ○ Associated with fibular hemimelia (see fibular hemimelia)

Limb Length Discrepancy (LLD):

- About 70% of population has up to 1 cm LLD.
- Common etiologies are congenital; growth plate affection by trauma, infection or tumor; post traumatic.
  - In congenital cases: a gradually progressive limb length discrepancy will occur at a relatively constant ratio (the long and short limbs will have relatively constant ratio).
- On average: growth ceases at a chronological age of 15-16 years in boys and 13-14 years in girls:
  - Children continue to grow for 3 years after the onset of puberty.
- Growth of distal femur is approximately **0.9-1 cm/year**; proximal tibia is 0.6 cm/year; distal tibia 0.4-0.5 cm/year; proximal femur 0.3-0.4 cm/year.
- To assess the final LLD (LLD at the end of skeletal growth) for a child presenting with LLD before skeletal maturity:
  - Paley's multiplication method (current difference multiplied by age-specific and gender-specific multiplier).
  - Moseley graph method: requires at least two measurements of both limbs that are plotted in a graph. This graph is used to predict the final LLD.
  - Arithmetic method (simplest, least accurate, most popular in exams)
    - 0.9 cm/year for distal femur, 0.6 cm/year proximal tibia; 14 end of growth in girls, 16 end of growth in boy (see above). _(Scenario: 10 years old girl, fracture distal femur one year ago, now completes closure of the physis and 1 cm LLD, what is the final LLD?)._
- Assessment: CT scanogram (to detect LLD) and left hand AP XR (to detect skeletal age).
  - The most accurate way to measure a limb-length discrepancy in a patient with a knee flexion contracture is a lateral CT scanogram.
- Treatment outlines (variations exist):
  - 2 cm is usually well tolerated (can use shoe lift).
  - 2-5 shortening of the long extremity (or lengthening of the short extremity if family wants).
    - Epiphysiodesis to stop the growth of the long extremity is simple alternative to shortening. It requires growth potential equal to the amount of required shortening. _(Scenario: 15 years old, female, 4 cm LLD from old injury to distal femur physis, treatment? (lengthening) (cannot stop the growth of the other side as the growth potential for 15 years old girl is minimal))._
  - More than 5 cm LLD: lengthening of the short side.
  - More than 15 cm LLD: discuss amputation and prosthetic option (debatable as some families will still choose to lengthen big LLD).

- o Limb equalization interventions should account for the final expected LLD at the time of skeletal maturity, and not only the LLD present at the time of surgery.
- To assess the time of surgical physeal arrest (epiphysiodesis) for treatment of LLD:
  - o White-Menelaus Formula:
    - 0.9 cm/year for distal femur, 0.6 cm/year proximal tibia, 1.5 cm/year for both; 14 years: end of growth in girls, 16 years: end of growth in boy. Allows rough calculation of impact of epiphysiodesis (commonest in exams). *(Scenario: 12 years old girl, LLD 1.5 cm with right side shorter due to fracture distal femur 18 months ago, XR complete closure of the right distal femur physis, treatment and at what time? (Left distal femur and proximal tibia epiphysiodesis at the current time (distal femur to prevent increase in discrepancy and proximal tibia to obtain correction))).*
    - Other methods: Anderson and Green graph method, Paley's method, Moseley graph method.
- LLD can lead to pelvic obliquity and scoliosis (lumbar curve will be larger). *(Scenario: 12 years old girl with XR showing small lumbar curve, minimal thoracic curve, pelvic obliquity (one iliac bone is higher than the other) (Fig 11), next step? (Assessment of LLD)).*
- In cases of proximal tibial epiphysiodesis, proximal fibula epiphysiodesis does not have to be added as the proximal fibula will follow the growth of the tibia.

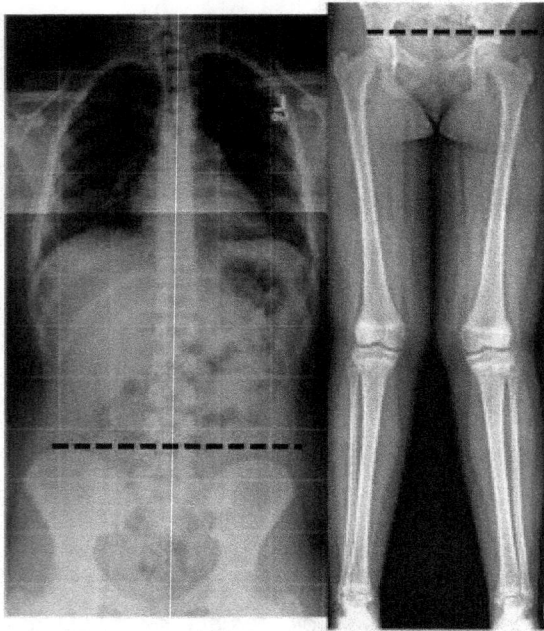

Fig 11: 12 years old girl with small lumbar curve referred to orthopedic surgeon for evaluation. There is obvious pelvic tile. Scanogram radiographs were taken showing limb length discrepancy (LLD) with right side being longer than the left; this is the reason for the lumbar curve (secondary to LLD).

Congenital Femoral Deficiency (Proximal Femoral Focal Deficiency):

- Broad spectrum of pathology (from complete absence of femur to mild shortening of the femur compared to the other side.

- Can be associated with deficient lateral femoral condyle, fibular hemimelia, coxa vara, and ACL deficiency.
- Treatment: according the extent of pathology (see treatment of LLD before).

Fibular Hemimelia

- Longitudinal limb deficiency associated short or absent fibula and short extremity.
- More common cause for LLD than tibial hemimelia
- Can be associated with short femur, valgus knee (distal femoral condyle deficiency), unstable knee (deficient cruciate ligaments), valgus ankle, deficient lateral foot rays, anteromedial tibial bowing (see tibial bowing).
- Treatment: see treatment of LLD before.
  - If ankle is severely unstable with large LLD: consider Syme's amputation.

Tibial Hemimelia:

- Associated with short or absent tibial and short extremity.
- Much less common than fibular hemimelia.
- The condition has genetic transmission (unlike fibular hemimelia): mostly autosomal dominant.
- Treatment depends with extensor mechanism (quadriceps function)
  - If there is no extensor mechanism: knee disarticulation
  - If there is extensor mechanism: lengthening and reconstruction.
    - Tibiofibular synostosis: fusing the short tibia with the longer fibula to act as a single bone.
    - Brown procedure (fibular centralization): higher failure rate.

Hemihypertrophy:

- Congenital disorder characterized by overgrowth of one side of the body in comparison with the other.
- It can affect the whole hemi body or part of it (e.g. one extremity, half of face, **tongue**)
- Can be isolated disorder or part of Beckwith-Wiedemann Syndrome (BWS) (macroglossia, gigantism, and neonatal hypoglycemi, hemihypertrophy).
- Increased risk of developing certain cancers during childhood (eg. Wilm's tumor, tumors of the liver).
  - Ultrasound is recommended every 3-6 month until the age of 8 years (this recommendation is constantly changing). *(Scenario: 2 years old with large tongue and 2 cm LLD, what other studies needed?)*

Lengthening / Deformity correction:

- Distraction osteogenesis:
  - ○ This is achieved by corticotomy followed by period of rest (5-7 days in children and 10-14 days in adults) to allow formation of soft callus, then gradual distraction of about 0.75 to 1 mm/day until achieving the required length.
  - ○ The regenerate is then left for consolidation (about double the time of distraction).
- Complication during lengthening:
  - ○ Incomplete corticotomy: When the patient starts distraction, tension develops in the frame, with increasing difficulty in distraction and limb pain. With continued frame distraction, sudden spontaneous completion of the osteotomy may occur and patient will have severe pain followed by pain rellief.
  - ○ Premature consolidation, after a period of successful distraction, lengthening will become more difficult due to consolidation of the regenerate. *(Scenario: fibular hemimelia: frame applied for lengthening, lengthening started day 5 which is very hard, in day 11 sudden popping and pain, reason?) (Same scenario but 1 month after lengthening, patient started to have difficulty lengthening, reason?)*
- There are 6 direction/ types of deformities:
  - ○ 3 angulations (sagittal, coronal, axial (rotation)
  - ○ 3 translations (medio-lateral, anterior-posterior, shortening-lengthening)
- CORA:
  - ○ Center of rotation and angulation, bisector of the deformity (see fig 12).
  - ○ If correction of the deformity is done of the concave side of the deformity, correction of the deformity will be associated with shortening; if it is done on the convex side of the deformity, correction of the deformity will be associated with lengthening.

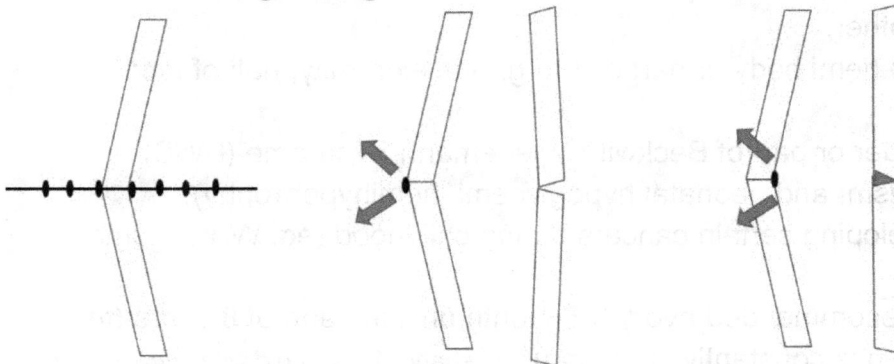

Fig 12 The concept of CORA. If correction was done on the convex side, lengthening will follow the correction of the deformity (open wedge). For correction on the concave side, a wedge of bone must be removed (the colored triangle) to correct the deformity (shortening wil follow).

OBPP (Obstetric Brachial Plexus Palsy)

- **Erb's palsy:**
  - C5 and C6 palsy.
  - Most common type of OBPP.
  - Mainly affecting the shoulder and elbow joint.
    - Shoulder: internal rotation and adduction
    - Elbow: extended pronated
    - Wrist: flexed (waiter's tip position)
  - Carries best prognosis for recovery
    - Most cases are due to neurapraxia.
    - About 85% will have complete recovery.
- **Klumpke's palsy:**
  - Rare type of OBPP, distal brachial palsy affection leading to affection of the hand function mainly.
  - Bad prognosis (usually due to avulsion of the roots)
- **Total flail limb:**
  - Worst prognosis.
- Good prognostic signs in children with OBPP:
  - Return of elbow flexion against gravity (biceps function) by 3 months of age.
  - Preservation of shoulder ROM (indicates absence of shoulder dislocation)
- Bad prognostic signs (indicates pre synaptic injury/avulsion injury):
  - Associated Horner's syndrome (ptosis, myosis, and anhydrosis).
  - Paralysis of the dorsal scapular nerve (rhomboids).
- Indication of early surgery (micor surgery for neurological repair):
  - No return of biceps movement by the age of 4 months.
  - There is total limb affection with Horner's syndrome.
- Rapid loss of ROM of the affected shoulder in young infants with Erb's palsy is an indication of early dislocation of the gleno-humeral joint.
  - MRI or ultrasound to assess the shoulder joint. *(Scenario: 1 year old with Erb's palsy, last visit he had 25° of external rotation, lack of any active or passive shoulder external rotation in this visit, failure of therapy, next step?)*
- Shoulder deformity in older patients with Erb's palsy:
  - Posterior subluxation of the humeral head in relation to the glenoid.
  - Retroversion of the glenoid surface.
  - Development of "pseudo" glenoid (posterior to the original glenoid).
  - Dislocation of the gleno-humeral joint.
- Shoulder XR in older children with Erb's play (Fig 13):
  - Prominent elongated coracoid, deficient glenoid.

- Shoulder reconstruction in cases of Erb's palsy (late intervention):
  - The condition of the glenohumeral joint should be assessed by CT (if the child is older than 5 years old) or shoulder MRI (if the child is younger than 5 years)
    - If there marked deformity of the shoulder (pseudo glenoid) or chronic posterior shoulder subluxation or dislocation: humeral osteotomy.
    - If the shoulder deformity is mild with no chronic dislocation: soft tissue releases and muscle transfer (teres major/latissimus dorsi to the posterior humerus to act as external rotator).

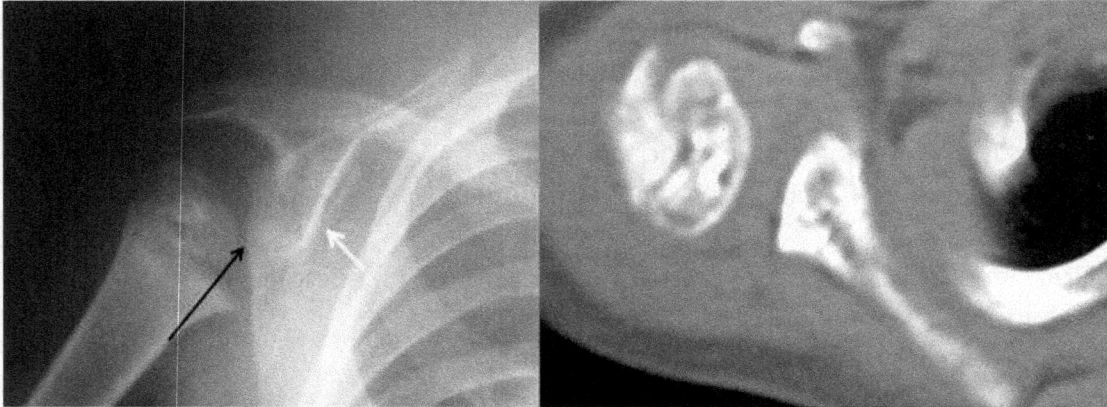

Fig 13: Right shoulder XR and CT of a 6 years old boy with Erb's palsy. XR shows deficient glenoid (black arrow) and prominent elongated coracoid (white arrow). CT shows the retroverted convex glenoid.

Foot:
Clubfoot:

- Pathology:
  - Main pathology: ankle and hind foot equines, hind foot varus, forefoot adduction, cavus foot (pronation of the forefoot in relation to the hindfoot).
  - Some cases are associated with internal tibial torsion, small lower calf muscles size, shorter lower leg (intrinsic hypoplasia) and small foot size.
- Treatment:
  - Serial casting by Ponseti technique.
    - Never pronate/evert the foot (the forefoot is already pronated).
    - Never touch the heel (manipulation is through the leg and forefoot).
    - Above knee cast in 90 flexion°, weekly change of cast.
    - First casting: supinate the first (elevate/ dorsi-flex the first ray) to correct the cavus component.
    - Following casts (after the first one): gradual external rotation of the forefoot (until you can reach about 60-70°)
      - Will correct forefoot adduction and hindfoot varus.

- - The hinge of the rotation (the position of the thumb of the physician) is laterally over the talar neck.
  - Equines:
    - Last component of the deformity to be addressed. Corrected after reaching the desired degree of external rotation (60-70°)
    - If adequate dorsiflexion (20-30°) cannot be achieved by manipulation, Achilles tenotomy (percutaneous) with casting in external rotation and dorsiflexion for three weeks (the final casting session lasts 3 weeks).
    - Percutaneous tenotomy in required in about 70% to 90% of cases.
  - The sequence of correction is cavus, forefoot adduction, hindfoot varus and finally equines.
  - After correction of the deformity, the affected foot is held in 60-70° external rotation in foot-abduction brace (eg Dennis Brown Bar) (in unilateral cases, the unaffected foot is put in about 30-45° of external rotation).
  - Most important factor determining the risk of recurrence of clubfoot (after successful treatment by Ponseti casting) is family's compliance with bracing.
  - Relapse after Ponseti casting in young child (up to age of 3 years): repeated session of serial casting.
  - Relapse after Ponseti in child 3-4 years old (dynamic supination/ forefoot adduction during gait and normal hindfoot on exam): treatment by ATTT (anterior tibial tendon transfer).
    - Needed in about 30% of patients.

Metatarsus Adductus:

- Pathology: forefoot adduction.
  - May be related to tight uterine space (may be associated with DDH).
  - There is absence of equines and hind foot varus (different than clubfoot).
  - Severity is assessed by a line bisecting the heel (this line should normally be in line with the second toe).
- Treatment:
  - For children less than one year: observation.
  - If older than one year with rigid deformity: serial casting or braces.
  - Surgery is indicated only after failure of serial casting. Surgery can be soft tissue release (capsulotomy) for young children (2-4 years) or osteotomies (older than 4 years). *(Scenario: 3 years old with severe metatarsus adductus, treatment? (serial casting))*

Tarsal coalition:

- Common to present in children around 11-14 years old.
- Clinical presentation:
  - Most cases are asymptomatic and discovered accidentally during radiographs taken for other reasons.
  - Commonly associated with fixed valgus deformity (pes planus).
  - Hindfoot pain (the origin of pain in not fully understood).
  - Decrease subtalar motion
  - Spastic peroneal muscles
  - Repeated ankle sprain.
- Two common types:
  - Talocalcaneal (subtalar) coalition:
    - Radiographs: talar beaking and a positive C sign (see Fig 14)

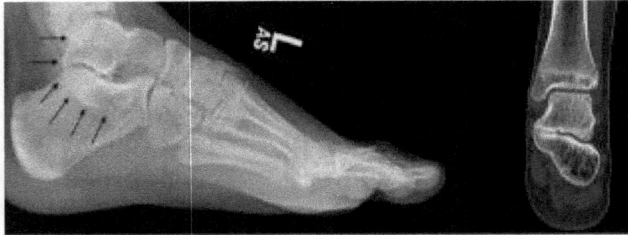

Fig 14: lateral foot XR and coronal CT of 12 years old boy with foot pain. The lateral foot XR shows the C sign of the talus. CT shows cartilaginous fusion of the medial subtalar joint.

    - CT/ MRI: bony bar fusion between the talus and calcaneus (bony coalition) or narrowing of the subtalar joint and edema in the MRI (fibrous coalition).
  - Calcaneo-navicular type:
    - Most common type.
    - lateral view will show ant eater sign (long anterior process of the calcaneus), oblique view will show narrowing (or bony bridge) between the calcaneus and navicular (Fig 15).

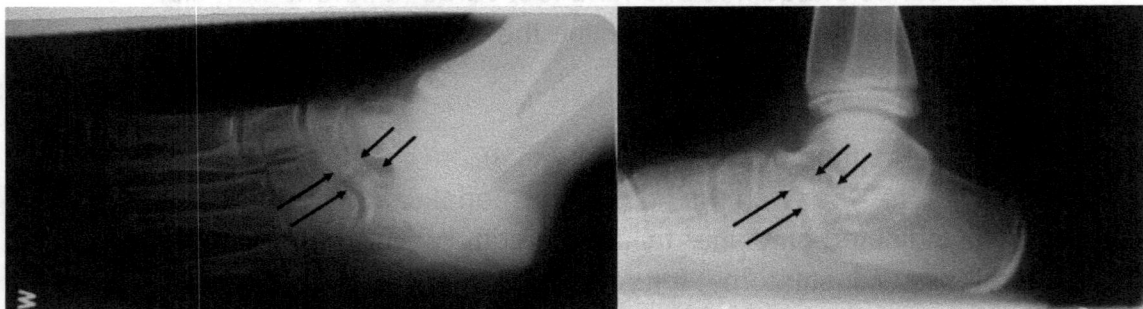

Fig 15 showing of 14 years old boy with foot pain: Left (oblique) showing the bony bridge between calcaneus and navicular; right (lateral) showing elongated anterior process of calcaneus (ant eater sign)

- Treatment:
  - ○ Initial treatment is by casting for few weeks. *(Scenario: 18 years, tarsal coalition, therapy made him worse, CT shows coalition, next step? (Immobilization)).*
  - ○ If non operative treatment fails: surgery.
    - ▪ CT scan to assess the presence of multiple tarsal coalition (present in about 15% of cases).
    - ▪ For cancaneo-navicualr coalition: excision of coalition.
    - ▪ For subtalar coalition: CT to assess the exact extend of the coalition coronal CT view (this typically shows the entire of the middle facet of the subtalar joint):
      - ▪ Excision of the coalition if < 50% of the joint surface or fusion of the joint if the coalition is >50%.
      - ▪ For patient presenting at adult age >20 years, fusion is better option). *(Scenario: 13 years old boy, 6 months' history of foot pain, casting helped for few weeks, now pain has recurred and he cannot play basketball, XR shows calcaneo-naviculur coalition, treatment?) (Same scenario with CT showing small area of talo-calcaneal fusion, treatment? (excision of the fustion mass)) (Same Scenario: CT shows 60% bony fusion of the talocalcaneal middle facet, treatment?)*
  - ○ If there is significant valgus of the hind foot, the resection of the coalition should be combined with lateral lengthening osteotomy or calcaneal medial displacement osteotomy.

Flexible Flat Foot:

- Medial longitudinal arch develops at the age of 4 years and reaches adult level at the age of 8 years. *(Scenario: mother of 3 years old complain the child has flat foot, treatment? (re assurance and observation)).*
- Flexible flat foot is diagnosed by the fact that the arch is restored by dorsiflexion of the big toe or tip toeing and that the subtalar joint motion is not restricted.
- The condition in most cases is asymptomatic (rarely associated with pain over the talar head), but usually the family is concerned about the deformity.
- Treatment:
  - ○ No need for treatment if the child is not symptomatic.
  - ○ Soft inserts (medial arches) can be tried with children who have pain.
  - ○ Those who fail non operative treatment with pain over the talar head (not generalized foot pain), can be treated calcaneal lengthening osteotomy with trapezoidal graft procedure.

Dorsal Bunion:
- Dorsal translation of the first ray.
- Can occur due to release of peroneus longus or tightness of tibialis anterior.
- Treatment: release of the tibialis anterior muscle and/or transfer of the flexor hallucis longus to the metatarsal neck.

Congenital Vertical Talus (CVT):
- The talus is dislocated plantarly from the navicular bone. This will result in rocker-bottom deformity of the foot.
- About half of the cases are associated with syndromes while the other half is isolated pathology.
  - Genetic/ neurologic evaluations is indicated. *(Scenario: newborn with vertical talus, next step?).*
- Diagnosis: by **lateral radiograph of the foot in maximum plantar flexion**.
  - The talus does not lie in line with the metatarsus even with maximum plantar flexion of the metatarsal bones (the navicular is not ossified at birth and cannot be appreciated in the radiographs at birth).
  - This will differentiate a congenital vertical talus from the oblique talus with talonavicular subluxation (oblique talus will line up with the metatarsals when the forefoot is plantar flexed)
- Treatment was classically by extensive soft tissue release. More recently, serial casting followed by limited surgery (Achilles tenotomy and peroneal lengthening, open reduction of the talo-navicular and pinning) became more popular.

Calcaneovalgus deformity:
- Foot deformity in the newborn in which the foot is severely dorsiflexed and everted.
- Differential diagnosis: CVT and posteromedical bowing
- Treatment by observation and possible stretching.

Cavus Foot (See Also Cavus Foot in Foot And Ankle):
- Pathology:
  - High arched foot (plantar flexion of the first ray).
    - The foot will be resting on two pillars only (the heel and first ray). In order to keep the 5th toe on ground, the heel will turn into varus (cavo-varus foot) (tri-pod theory).
    - In the early stages of the disease, the varus will be reversible (with correction of the first ray plantar flexion), later on, it becomes fixed.

- Coleman block test is used to assess the flexibility of the hindfoot varus in cavus foot (**assess flexibility of the hindfoot**).
  - Most cavus feet are due to neurological condition.
    - Most common cause in US is Charcot Marie Tooth (CMT). Other causes: Polio, spina bifida, intra-thecal anomalies.
    - Patient will require neurological consult if the cause is unknown.
  - Tibialis anterior muscle becomes weaker than peroneus longus muscle, this will cause **plantar flexion of the first ray**. Also the peroneus brevis will become weaker than tibial posterior muscle this will cause inversion.
  - Cavus foot can be associated with lateral ankle instability:
    - Patients presenting with ankle instability have to be assessed for presence of cavus foot. If this is the case, the surgeon has to address the cavus component (first ray dorsi-flexion osteotomy and/or calcaneal osteotomy) in addition to reconstruction of the ligament.
- **Treatment:**
  - Initial treatment for flexible deformity is non operative:
    - Brace: lateral heel wedge with well for first metatarsal head or with lateral forefoot post to elevate the lateral side of the forefoot) and therapy for strengthening of the weakening muscular units. _(Scenario: 14 years old, cavovarus foot, family history of CMT, minimal symptoms, treatment? (Brace and therapy)) (Same scenario: what type of brace?)_
  - Surgical treatment:
    - **Soft tissue procedures**: plantar fascia release (partial), transfer of the EHL to the 1MT neck with fusion of the hullux IP (Jone's procedure, will help to dorsiflex the 1st Metatarsus), peroneus longus to brevis transfer (will weaken the strong longus which will decrease the plantar flexion the 1st ray and strengthen the weak brevis which will enhance the subtalar eversion).
    - Bony procedures:
      - For reversible heel varus (assessed with Coleman block test): dorsiflexion osteotomy of the first metatarsal or the medial cuneiform (in pediatric patient, the growth plate of the 1st metatarsus is proximal unlike all other metatarsal bones, so medial cuneiform osteotomy is easier). _(Scenario: 13 years old boy, CMT, reversible heel varus, did not tolerate the brace, treatment? (first ray osteotomy, plus soft tissue (some or all of the following: plantar release, EHL transfer to the 1st MT neck, longus to brevis transfer))). (CP with cavus, plantar flexed first ray, clawing of the hallux, pain under the first metatarsal head and a rigid first tarsometatarsal joint, failure of non operative,_

management? (1st MT base (or medial cuneiform) osteotomy with Jone's procedure)).

- ▪ Irreversible heel varus (or partially reversible): add calcaneal osteotomy (a lateralizing calcaneal osteotomy with proximal translation to correct heel varus). Proximal translation of the posterior tuberosity will help to improve the increased calcaneal dorsiflexion and pitch, improving the lever arm for the gastrocnemius soleus). *(Scenario: 17 years' female with family history of high arch, presenting with cavus, not corrected with Coleman block test, failed non operative, treatment? (Peroneus longus to brevis transfer, medial cuneiform dorsal closing wedge (or plantar opening wedge) osteotomy, and lateralizing calcaneal osteotomy), EHL transfer to the 1st MT neck with 1st IP fusion)).*
- ▪ Planter fascia release as a solo procedure cannot fully correct cavus foot deformity.

Sever's Disease (Calcaneal Apophysitis):

- Clinical presentation: activity-related heel pain, tenderness over the posterior heel (calcaneal apophysis), positive lateral calcaneus squeeze test and a tight Achilles tendon. Radiographs are non specific.
- Treatment is by reduced activity, if no improvement, casts for few weeks.

Kohler's Disease:

- Osteochnondritis of the navicular bone, in children between 3-6 years old.
- The child will complain of foot pain.
- Treatment: If the symptoms are minimal, the child can be observed. If symptoms are more severe: **short leg weight bearing cast immobilization**.

Accessory navicular:

- Present in about in 10% of normal feet, and in most cases it is asymptomatic.
- Clinical presentation: focal foot pain (over the bony prominence) and tenderness over the medial aspect of the navicular bone.
- XR (external oblique view): 3 types:
  - o Type I: separate small ossicle (about 2-3 mm) not connected to the main navicular (usually asymptomatic).
  - o Type II: larger ossicle (about 1 cm) with a cartilaginous synchondrosis to the navicular bone.
  - o Type III: the ossicle is bony fused to the navicular tuberosity.
- Treated initially non operative (show modification, arch support, short term lower leg weight bearing cast), if fails, simple surgical excision. NO need for advancing the

posterior tibia tendon (Kidner's procedure). *(Scenario: 10 years old girl, flexible pes planus, pain over a prominent navicular bone, XR shows accessory navicular, treatment? (cast for 6 weeks)).*

Adolescent Hallux Valgus (Adolescent Bunion)

- Pathology:
    - Metatarsus primus varus (varus deformity of the 1st metatarsal-medial cuneiform joint) is the main pathology.
    - Increased flexibility of the first tarso-metatarsal joint
- Treatment:
    - Initial treatment is non operative
    - Recurrence is high with operative treatment. Delaying the operative treatment as much as possible is preferred.
    - If the patient fails non operative treatment, surgery is usually by double osteotomy (proximal osteotomy to correct the increased inter-metatarsal angle (due to metatarsus primus varus) and distal osteotomy to correct the increased DMAA) (Fig 16).
    - Fusion of the 1st tarso-metatarsal joint (Lapidus procedure) can be done if the main pathology is hyper mobility of the 1st TMT joint.

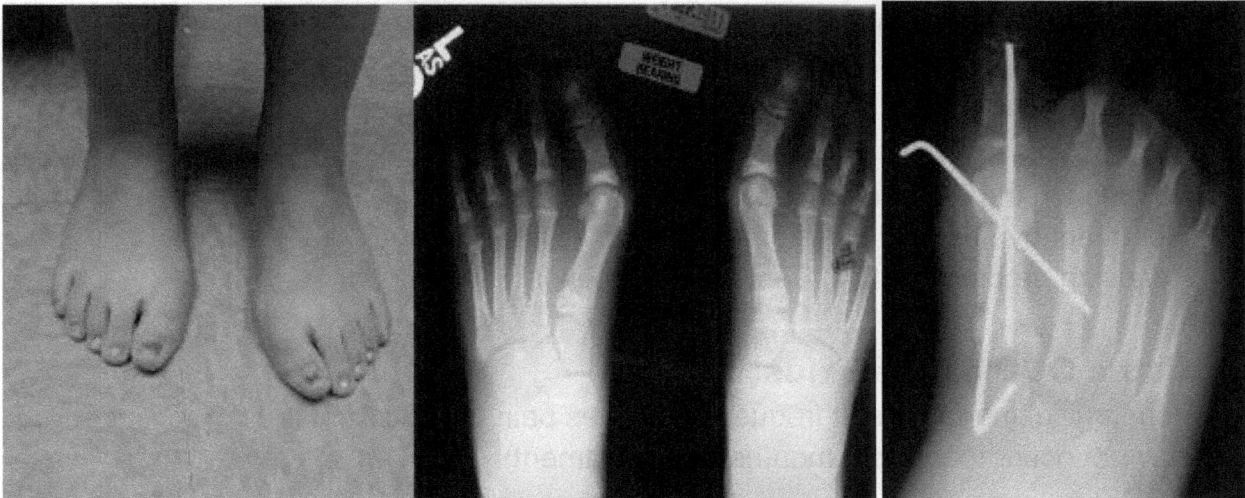

Fig 16: 10 years old girl with bilateral adolescent hallux valgus (more on the left). XR shows increased both inter-metatarsal angle and DMAA. Double osteotomy was done to correct the deformity.

Congenital longitudinal epiphyseal bracket (Delta physis):

- Pathology: C shaped epiphysis on one side of the phalanx/metatarsus (instead of the end of the bone). The phalanx/metatarsus will grow sideway rather than longitudinal causing obvious progressive deformity.
- Can occur in the hand or the foot.

- Treatment:
  - Surgery is indicated because non operative treatment will result in progressive deformity.
    - Excision of the bracket to correct deformity and possible restoration of longitudinal growth.
    - Osteotomy and/or lengthening may be needed if resection alone does not lead to sufficient growth or deformity correction.

Polydactyly:
- Post axial polydactyly (on the lateral aspect of the foot)
  - Autosomal dominant inheritance, more in African Americans.
  - Usually not associated with other congenital anomalies (similar to post axial hand polydactyly).
  - No need for further tests or assessments (other than excision).

Overlapping fifth toe:
- Can be managed conservative by changing foot ware.
- If this fail, surgical treatment:
  - Dorsal and plantar racquet-shaped incision around the fifth toe, EDL tenotomy and dorsal capsule of MTP joint release (Butler procedure).

Curly Toe:
- Common in the 3rd and 4th toes.
- Treatment by observation (most cases are asymptomatic).
- If causing problems with shoe wear: long flexor tenotomy.

Pediatric OCD of The Talus:
- Nonsurgical management frequently relieves pain (despite that radiographic healing may not occur for up to 6 months after treatment)

Shoulder:
Sprengel's Deformity:
- Due to failure of caudal migration of the scapula. There may be cartilagenous, fibrous or bony (the omovertebral bone) connection between the scapula to the cervical and thoracic spine.
- Clinical presentation:
  - One scapula is higher than the other side (unilateral cases) or the neck is broad (bilateral cases).

- o About one third of cases are associated with Klippel-Feil syndrome.
- o Limited shoulder range of motions (especially abduction). The omovertebral bone can limit shoulder abduction to about 90°.
- Treatment:
  - o Observation: if the deformity is not severe and there is minimal functional loss.
  - o Distal advancement of the scapula with excision of the omovertebral bone (Woodward procedure): if there are significant functional limitations.

Little Leaguer's Shoulder (Epiphysiolysis of The Proximal Humerus):

- Due to overuse (excess throwing). The pathology will occur in the hypertrophic zone of the growth plate.
- Clinical presentation: the child will complain of shoulder pain in his/her dominant shoulder with decrease velocity of throwing. On examination, tender ROM of the shoulder, especially internal rotation.
  - o Pain will be during late cooking or deceleration phase of throwing.
- XR: Physeal widening (occasionally, there will periosteal bone formation around the proximal physis), metaphyseal sclerosis.
- Treatment: rest from the throwing activity until the patient is pain free. Then the child should not throw more than the recommended pitch counts for age and should not be playing in two teams. *(Scenario: 11 years old boy, in two teams, complaining of shoulder pain, XR presented, what is treatment?)*

Elbow (See Upper Extremity Sport Injury Chapter):

Radio-Ulnar Synostosis:

- Abnormal bony fusion between proximal ulna and radius, this will lead to severe limitation of pronation-supination.
- XR (Fig 17) will shows bony fusion between the radius and ulan with possible radial head dislocation.
- Treatment for unilateral cases is observation. For bilateral cases, if the condition is asymptomatic or minimal complaints, observation. If deformity is severe and limiting the use of the upper extremity, osteotomy to put the hand in more functional position (pronation for dominant hand and supination for non dominant hand).

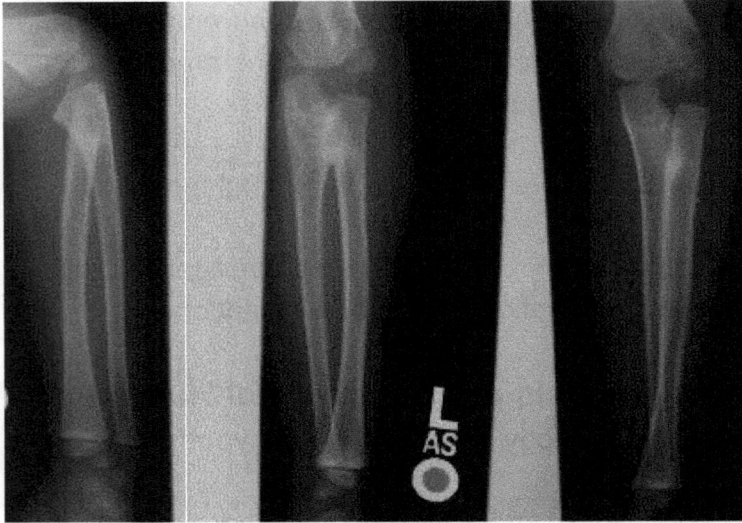

Fig 17: 7 years old boy, brought by parents due to inability to perform certain movement after being enrolled in karate. XRs of the forearm (AP, lateral and oblique) show proximal radio-ulnar synostosis.

Congenital Radial Head Dislocation:

- Cosmetic deformity (painless mass over the posterior aspect of the elbow) is the most common complaint in patients with a developmental radial head dislocation.
- Other complaints include: clicking, limitation of forearm supination/ pronation (rarely there is mild pain associated with condition).
- XR will show dislocated radial head. The radial head is usually convex (dome shaped) (in contrast to missed Monteggia fracture dislocation).
- Treatment:
  - Non operative treatment is the mainstay. Excision of the radial head can be done after skeletal maturity if the patient/ family prefer. Excision of the radial head does not result in increase in the range of motion.

Osteochondritis Dissecans (OCD) of The Elbow:

- Occurs in children older than 10 years old.
- More common in children involved in throwing activity as a result of lateral compression and axial loading of the lateral elbow during throwing activity.
- Mainly affects the capitellum. It may also affect the radial head.
- Clinical presentation:
  - Early stage: intermittent pain and loss of extension.
  - If the condition progress to development of loose fragments, it will cause catching or locking.
  - Examination reveals a small joint effusion, tenderness over the lateral elbow and pain with pronation and supination. Limitation of range of motion can occur with advanced stages.

- Imaging:
  - XR will show the radiolucent lesion of the capitellum.
  - MR arthrogram: if the dye can be seen surrounding the margins of the lesion, this indicates unstable lesion (poor prognostic sign).
- Treatment:
  - Initial treatment for non separated lesions: rest from throwing activity (about 6 weeks). Child can resume play when he/she is asymptomatic and examination shows restoration of painless range of motion.
    - If the child continues to have pain despite adequate rest: arthroscopic drilling for non separated lesion.
  - Separated lesions require either fixation or excision.

Panner's Disease:

- Osteochondritis of the capitullem affecting children younger than 10 years of age.
- Occurs in the dominant elbows.
- More common in boys between 5 and 10 years old.

Hand:

- The signaling centers of the developing upper limb:
  - There are three signaling centers which control the development and guide the growth of the upper extremity.

Signal center	Limb control	Consequence of disruption
Apical Ectodermal Ridge (AER)	Proximal to distal development	Transverse deficiencies with a shortened limb (example: transverse amputation)
Zone of Polarizing Activity (ZPA)	Radial to ulnar direction (pre-and postaxial development).	Duplication or absence of digits (example: mirror hand)
Wingless Signaling Center (Wnt) (arises from the dorsal ectodermal ridge).	Dorsal-palmar limb development.	Example: Nail–patella syndrome

Radial Club Hand:

- Complete or partial absence of the radius with radial deviation of the wrist and hand.
- Can be associated with multiple general congenital anomalies: e.g. VACTRL, TAR (thrombocytopenia Absent Radius), Fanconi Anaemia. Holt-Oram syndrome.
  - Order CBC (to detect Fanconi anemia, which usually occurs at the age of 6 years). *(Scenario: 3 months with radial club hand, next step? (Order CBC)) (Question: most common associated anomaly? (hemopoietic system))*
- Treatment:

- o Correction of the deformity around the age of 4-8 years old by bringing the wrist on line with the forearm (centralization).
- o The most common complication of the centralization recurrent deformity.
- o In cases with elbow fusion or contracture, it is not recommended to correct the deformity (the child will not be able to bring his hand to his mouth).

Ulnar Club Hand:

- Not associated with general medical problems, but it is usually associated with other skeletal anomalies. _(Scenario: 4 months with ulnar club hand? next step? (skeletal survey XR))_

Hypoplastic Thumb:

- May be associated with abnormalities of the heart, spine, and gastrointestinal tract.
- Stability of thumb CMC is the most important factor in determining reconstruction procedure in cases of thumb hypoplasia:
  - o Stable joint can be reconstructed, while unstable joint is better to be amputated then reconsructing the index finger to be the new thumb (index pollicization)
- **Classification:**
  - o **Type I:** the thumb is small with normal components.
  - o **Type II:** Thenar hypoplasia with metacarpophalangeal joint instability (deficient ulnar collateral ligament).
  - o **Type IIIA:** Type II features, plus extrinsic tendon abnormalities and hypoplastic metacarpal, **stable** carpometacarpal joint.
  - o **Type IIIB:** as type IIIA with **unstable** carpometacarpal joint.
  - o **Type IV:** floating thumb (small numb)
  - o **Type V:** complete absence
- **Treatment:**
  - o **Type I:** no treatment needed.
  - o **Types II, IIIA:** thumb reconstruction.
  - o **Types IIIB, IV, V:** pollicization (with amputation of the thumb if present).

Congenital Trigger Thumb:

- **Pathology:**
  - o Triggering and flexion deformity of the IP of the thumb. A Nodule (Notta nodule) can be felt at the base of the thumb over the MCP joint of the thumb.
  - o The condition can be congenital (present at birth) or can be developmental (developing shortly after birth).

- Initial treatment if the child is less than one year old is observation (spontaneous recovery is possible). Stretching exercises/splinting can be tried (questionable efficacy).
- If no spontaneous correction by the age of one year (or patients presenting older than one year): treatment is by surgical release of **A1 pulley**.
- The neurovascular structure that is most likely to be injured while performing a trigger thumb release is the radial digital nerve.

Trigger Fingers:
- Usually multiple fingers affected.
- Can be associated with trisomy 18 or mucopolysaccharidoses.
- The pathology is usually related to more distal triggering at the flexor digitorum profundus passes through sublimus decussation (at the level of A2 pulley, not A1)
- Treatment: excision of one sublimis head to allow the FDP to glide more smoothly.

Congenital Clasped Thumb:
- Flexion deformity of the thumb at the level of MCP joint (in contrast to trigger thumb which is at the level of IP joint).
- Due to absence or hypoplasia of EPB or EPL or both

Syndactyly:
- Can be simple (no bony connection) or complex (with bony connection).
- Can be partial (not the entire length of the two adjacent finger attached) or complete (fusion between the entire length of the two adjacent fingers).
- Can be associated with congenital syndromes (Poland or Apert syndromes).
- Basics of surgical treatment:
  - One syndactyly at a time (to avoid possible bilateral arterial injury of the finger with resultant gangrene).
  - Start with edge syndactyly (thumb/index and small/ring) (around the age of 9-12 months). Central syndactyly can be delayed to the age of 2-3 years.
  - The limit for proximal dissection is the artery bifurcation (not nerve).
  - Most common complication after surgical correction: web creep.

Clinodactyly:
- Lateral curvature of a digit, most commonly affecting the small finger.
- If the condition is mild, no treatment is needed. If the deformity is severe, osteotomy of the phalanx.

Polydactyly

- **Thumb duplication (Pre-axial polydactyly):**
  - **Wassel Classification:**
    - I: bifid distal phalanx.
    - II: duplicated distal phalanx.
    - III: bifid proximal phalanx.
    - IV: duplication of proximal phalanx (most common type).
    - V: bifid metacarpal.
    - VI: duplicated MC.
    - VII: triphalangism (autosomal dominant inheritance)
  - Common in Caucasians.
  - Type VII can be associated with other congenital anomalies (e.g Fanconi anemia, cleft palate, Holt Oram syndrome.
  - **Surgical treatment:**
    - Treatment is more than just amputation of the extra digit. Surgery should consist of ablation of the more hypoplastic skeletal elements and soft-tissue (collateral ligament, thenar muscles) reconstruction of the more developed one.
    - If there are two equal digits: excision the radial digit and reconstruct the radial collateral ligament of the ulnar thumb.
- **Post axial polydactyly (on the ulnar side):**
  - Common in African American.
  - Usually inherited as autosomal dominant.
  - Usually not associated with other congenital anomalies, no other investigation needed.

Pediatric Flexor Tendon Injuries

- Commonly missed and presenting late (requiring staged reconstruction).
- After repair: immobilized for longer periods than adults (4 weeks) using mitten cast (less concern for stiffness).

Macrodactyly:

- Treatment by Epiphysiodesis when the digit reaches length of the same gender parent.

Madelung Deformity:

- Caused by impaired growth of the volar and ulnar aspect of the distal radial physis.

- Can be associated with Turner syndrome or Leri-Weill dyscondrosteosis.

Pediatric Spine:
Spondylolysis:
- Pathology:
  - Defect of the pars interarticularis. Most common location is L5.
  - Present in about 5% of the general population.
  - The condition is developmental (incidence increases from childhood to adulthood).
- Clinical presentation:
  - Most patients with spondylolysis are asymptomatic.
  - Low back pain:
    - More in adolescent. Common in activities with knee extension (gymanist, football, diving)
    - Pain increases with hyperextension.
    - Associated with hamstring tightness, negative straight leg raising.
    - Not every case of back pain with XR picture of spondylolysis is due to the spondylolysis. It may be muscular back pain.
- Diagnosis: radiographs can show the defect (scotty dog collar sign: osteolysis of the pars inter articularis) (Fig 18), if XRs are normal, then order bone scan with SPECT (most sensitive imaging modality, can differentiate between chronic and acute cases).
- The initial management should include restriction of physical activity. Once the athlete has no pain, he/she can return to the sport. Short term bracing can be used *(scenario: 14 years old gymnast, back pain, with extension, XR normal, most sensitive test for diagnosis?)*

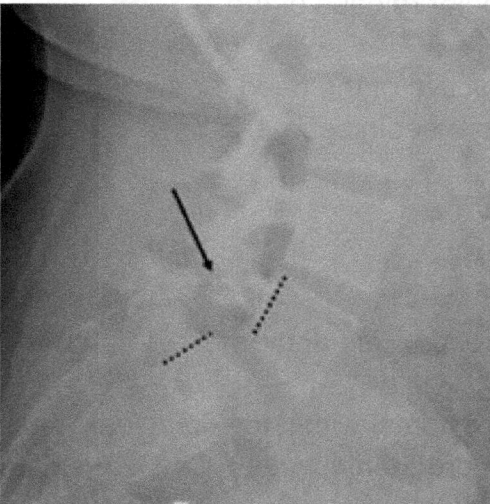

Fig 18: 13 years old boy presenting with back pain with activity, pain increase with back extension. XR of the lumbo-sacral spine lateral view shows spondylolysis (arrow) at the level of L5 and stage I L5-S1 spondylolisthesis (dotted line) with L5 about 20% anteriorly translated in comparison to S1

Spondylolisthesis:

- Pediatric spondylolisthesis is usually "isthmic" type (due to pars defect and associated spondylolysis (see before) (Fig 18).
- Clinical presentation: back pain, hamstring tightness. XR will show the displacement of upper vertebra over the lower one. Commonest level is L5-S1
- It is graded according to the degree of displacement as a percentage of the vertebral width. (I: 25%, II:50%, III:75%, IV:100%).
- Grade I and II: most cases can be treated non operative. The initial management same as spondylolysis. If non operative fails, the treatment is **L5**-S1 fusion. *(Scenario: 16-year-old football lineman low back pain for 3 months, XR shows grade I-II spondylolisthesis L5-S1, management?).*
- High grade spondylolisthesis (Grade III-IV): if non operative treatment fails to control patient's symptoms (high grade slippage is usually progressive), most surgeon will treat by in situ postero lateral fusion of **L4** to S1 with instrumentation. *(Scenario: 16 years old girl, 6 months' history of back pain, hamstring tightness, not able to perform activities, failed non operative treatment. XR grade IV spondylolisthesis. Treatment?)*
- Reduction of a high-grade spondylolisthesis at L5-S1 in a pediatric patient may be complicated by **L5** nerve root injury (reduction of more than 50% of the slippage is not recommended).
- Spondylolisthesis is related to the pelvic incidence (see spine chapter). However, recent studies found that pelvic incidence may not be predictive of spondylolisthesis progression. slip percentage, slip angle, and high-grade spondylolisthesis were predictive of progression of the condition.

Congenital Muscular Torticollis:

- Initial treatment is by stretching exercise. If this fails and the child is older than one year: surgical release is indicated (uni polar or bi polar release of the sternocleidomastoid muscle).
- The extent of muscle fibrosis on ultrasound is predictive of the need for surgery. The more the extent of fibrosis, the higher the chance of needing surgery.

C1-C2 Rotary Subluxation:

- Clinical presentation: patient will present with torticollis.
- XR: asymmetry of the lateral mass of C2 in relation to C1.
- Dynamic CT will show that with head turning, C2 keeps fixed abnormal relation with C1 (C1-C2 does not move with head movement).
- Treatment depend on the time from the start of symptoms: within the first week: anti-inflammatory and soft collar. 1-4 weeks: traction. more than 4 weeks: C1-C2 fusion.

C1-C2 congenital instability:

- Most dysplasias (except achondroplasia) are associated with C1-C2 (atlanto axial instability) instability (especially Morquio dysplasia) *(Scenario: before proceeding with surgery for Morquio patient, what pre-operative evaluation should be done? (Flexion/extension lateral C-spine radiographs))*

Diskitis:

- Common in adolescent.
- Clinical presentation is back pain, tenderness on percussion of the affected area, possible low grade fever, no radicular symptoms. The condition can be missed for few months.
- Blood work: elevated ESR, CRP, WBCs.
- XR: takes 10-14 days to show the characteristic narrowing of the disk space. In early cases, the XR will only shows loss of lumbar lordosis.
- MRI is sensitive and give positive results early in the disease process.
- Treatment: antibiotics according to culture (blood or image guided biopsy) *(Scenario: clinical presentation of diskitis, nest step? (biopsy and culture from the disk space))*

Tuberculosis of The Spine: See Spine Chapter
Infectious sacroiliitis:

- Most common causatives organism is Staphylococcus aureus.
- MRI is the most sensitive imaging modality.
- Treatment is by empirical antibiotic (cultures are difficult to obtain).

Spinal Deformity (Scoliosis and kyphosis):
Congenital Scoliosis

- Pathology: failure of formation or failure of segmentation of the vertebrae.
- Unilateral bar with contralateral fully segmented hemivertebrae has worst prognosis of congenital scoliosis (most progressive curve).
- Assessment of renal, cardiac and spinal cord anomalies should be done (by renal ultrasound, cardiac evaluation/echocardiogram, spinal MRI). Spinal dysraphism is the most common intra thecal associated abnormality with congenital scliosis. *(Scenario: 6 months old with congenital scoliosis and hairy patch in the middle of his lower back, what is the next step? (renal US, cardiac evaluation and entire spine MRI)).*
- Progressive curves will require surgical treatment. For progressive curves related to hemivertebra, the treatment is Hemivertebra excision and limited fusion *(scenario: 6 years old, thoraco-lumbar curve due to upper lumbar hemivertebra, progressive, treatment?)*

Adolescent Idiopathic Scoliosis (AIS):

- More common in female.
- Non painful condition. Normal neurological exam.
- Indication of MRI in idiopathic scoliosis: left thoracic curve, painful curve, curves that are diagnosed before the age of 10 (juvenile and infantile), abnormal neurological exam (abdominal reflex) (all the above have a higher incidence of intra thecal anomalies, eg. Syringomeylia). *(Scenario: 9 years old, XR shows left throracic curve 15 degrees, next step?) (Scenario: 7 years old, 13 degree curve, right thoracic, asymmetric abdominal reflexes, next step?)*
- For AIS, the classical curve is right thoracic scoliosis (convexity to the right).
- Maximal curve progression occurs at peak growth velocity, (about one year before the onset of menarche).
- Treatment:
  - Bracing: proven to be effective in preventing progression in most patients if used regularly (16 hours for Boston Brace). Thoraco-lumbar bracing (without neck extension) is more effective in curves with apex distal to T6. Bracing should be continued until skeletal maturity.
  - Indication of bracing: growing child (more than 2 years of remaining growth (Risser 0-2)) with curve more than 25° or more than 20° with 5° documented progression. *(Scenario: 11 years old girl, referred by school nurse, 26° right thoracic curve, Risser 0, management?) (Scenario: Pre-menarche girls with a curve of 32 degrees, treatment?) (Scenario: 12 years girl with 18° curve, 9 months later 24°, treatment?)*
  - Surgery is indicated for: thoracic curves of more than 50° in skeletally mature children (Risser stage 5) or thoracic Curves of more than 45 in skeletally immature children (Risser stage 1, 2) (lumbar curves > 35° are considered indication for surgery by some surgeons).
  - The standard surgery for scoliosis is posterior spinal fusion of the spine with instrumentation to prevent further progression of the disease.
  - Curves in AIS can be structural or flexible. Curves which can be corrected to less than 25° on lateral bending films are considered flexible and do not have to be fused (will correct with fusion of the structural curve). *(Scenario, 12 years old female, one year post menarchal, 54 ° right main thoracic curve, 35° left upper thoracic and 32° left lumbar curve, on lateral bending radiographs, the curves correct to 15 (upper thoracic), 35 (main thoracic) and 12 (lumbar), treatment? (posterior spinal fusion of the main thoracic curve)).*
  - The most dangerous site for pedicle screw insertion in AIS surgery is concave side at the apex of the deformity (pedicles are smaller and dura is closer)
  - Complication of scoliosis surgery: crankshaft phenomenon in cases of position fixation only (posterior fusion with continued anterior growth) (more common in children under 10 years old with fixation other than pedicle

screws), Superior mesenteric artery syndrome(SMAS), infection: early (most common staph aureus), late (P acne or epidermis).

Neuromuscular Scoliosis:

- Spastic quadriplegic cerebral palsy has around 50% incidence of scoliosis, usually a long C-shaped thoracolumbar curve that may involve the pelvis.
  - o Indication for fusion in these patients is curve progression and loss of function (loss of sitting ability, poor pulmonary function). Treatment is by posterior spinal fusion from T1 or T2 to the sacrum with rigid segmental instrumentation with stabilization to the pelvic. The surgery has the potential to improve the caregiver's perception of the child's comfort.
  - o Progression of scoliosis is common after skeletal maturity in patients with quadriplegic CP.
- Pre-adolescent children with complete spinal cord injury have more than 90% incidence of developing subsequent spinal deformity in the future. Bracing is not effective in treatment of this spinal curve.
- For children with spinal muscular atrophy (SMA): if the spinal deformity is progressing, the treatment is PSF with instrumentation (avoid anterior approach due to effects on the lungs).
- For neuromuscular cases in general fusion should extend to the pelvis (unless the child is ambulatory) to allow adequate control of the pelvis obliquity.

Infantile Idiopathic Scoliosis:

- More common in male
- Risk of progression: Rib overlap of the apical vertebral body or a rib vertebral angle difference (RVAD or Mehta angle) > than 20 degrees (Fig 19).
- The curve is usually left thoracic curve
- If the curve is progressing (> 35°), initial treatment casting (derogation, elongation and flexion), if this fails or if the child cannot tolerate the cast: fusion-less surgery (eg growing rod) to avoid thoracic insuffiency syndrome.
- Fusion-less surgery (e.g. Growing rod): With growth of the child/ repeated lengthening procedures, the distraction force needed increases and length/ correction gained decreases.

Congenital Kyphosis

- The natural history of congenital kyphosis carries the highest risk of paraplegia in spinal deformities in children, especially in progressive deformities that that have an apex at T4-T9 (the watershed area of spinal cord blood flow). Treatment is surgical

- The highest risk of progression is with anterolateral bar with contralateral quadrant vertebrae.
- Treatment: in-situ fusion (posterior).

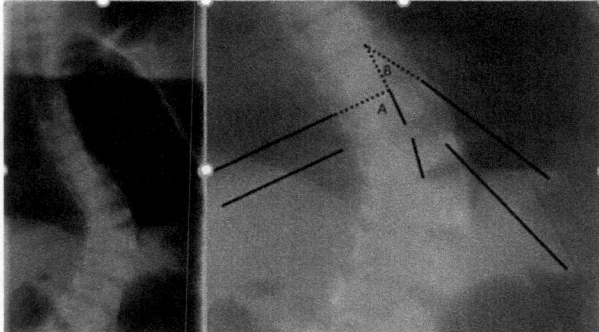

Fig 19: 4 years old boy with infantile idiopathic scoliosis. Right XR is magnification of the middle part of the curve shown on the left. The Rib Vertebra Angle Difference (RVAD) is the difference between the rib vertebra angle (RVA) of the concave (A) and convex sides of the scoliotic curve (B); the RVA is measured on coronal plane radiographs at the

Sacral Agenesis:

- Absence of the sacrum (and possibly lower lumbar vertebrae).
- Without stabilization, progressive kyphosis will develop between the spine and pelvis. The kyphosis progresses to the point that the child will have to use his or her hands to support the trunk during sitting.
- Neurologic deficit is static and present since birth

Scheuermann's Kyphosis (Thoracic Hyperkyphosis)

- More common in boys.
- Rigid kyphsosis, normal neurological exam. The child may complain of mid back pain.
- Diagnosis requires 3 consecutive vertebrae with anterior wedging of more than 5°. XR may also show end plate irregularities.
- Treatment: observation (together with postural exercises) for curves less than 50° (normal thoracic kyphosis is 30-50°). Bracing (extension type spinal orthosis) for curves 50-75° with Risser stage 2 or less. Surgery may be considered for curves when it progresses more than 75°.
    - Correction more than 50% is not recommended (for fear of neurological complications).
    - Surgery usually require posterior spinal osteotomies (see Spine Chapter).

Spinal Trauma
Limbus (Apophyseal) Fracture

- Common in adolescent, equivalent to disc herniation in adult and will cause bilateral radicular symptoms.

- The limbus (apothysis) of the vertebra will have "Salter-Harris" type injury with displacement into the canal.
- XR normal (the apophysis is not calcified yet), CT myelogram or MRI is needed to localize the lesion.
- Limbus fracture usually does not improve with non-surgical treatment (contrary to disc herniation). Management is wide laminectomy with surgical excision of the limbus fragment

Chance Fracture (See Spine Trauma):

- Common in children who suffer motor vehicle accidents while wearing the abdominal seat belt without the shoulder strap.
- Can be bony or ligamentous type: ligamentous one requires surgical fixation.

Odontoid Fracture (See Anatomy Chapter)

- Can be caused by minor trauma, and almost always occurs through the synchondrosis at the base of the dens (fuses at age of 6 years).
- Rarely associated with Neurologic deficits.
- Treatment by closed reduction by neck **extension** and immobilization using a cast, a brace, or halo traction. Nonunion is rare.
- Children younger than 8 years tend to have cervical injuries at C3 and above; children older than 8 years tend to have injuries below C3.

Halo Pin Traction:

- Use more pins (6 pins) a lower insertional torque (2-4 lb/in) is recommended.
- A CT scan of the head should also be considered to assess for the thickest areas of the skull suitable for pin application prior to application

Radiographic Finding in Pediatric Spine:

- The pediatric ADI is normal < 5 mm
- Retropharyngeal space should be less than 6 mm at C2 and less than 22 mm at C6.
- Pseudosubluxation of Upper Cervical Vertebrae:
  - Most commonly seen at C2-3. C3 anterior body will be anterior to the C2 anterior body (the anterior spinal process line will be continuous non disturbed in these cases).
- Atlantoaxial instability: If the ADI > 5 mm (or 10mm in patients with Down's): C1-C2 fusion should be considered
- Down Syndrome:
  - About 15% of children with Down syndrome will have cervical spine instability.

- Lateral flexion-extension views should be obtained before physical clearance for children with Down syndrome.
- ADI > 5mm in children with Down syndrome is contraindication for contact sports and sports with high risk of neck injury (e.g. Diving).
- Cervical fusion is only indicated for children with myelopathic symptoms of if the ADI > 10mm (high complication rate).
-

- Os odontoideum:
  - May be related to unrecognized C2 injury in early childhood.
  - Flexion/ extension lateral neck XRs will show the instability.
  - Treatment :
    - Observation: if asymptomatic and no instability (but it is contra-indicatino for contact sports).
    - C1-C2 fusion: with intractable pain or with radiographic signs of instability (PADI <13 mm or >5 mm of C1-C2 tranlation).

Tips

- Cavus foot and tarsal coalition can both be associated with ankle instability.
- Bilateral hip dysplasia: arthrogryposis (reduce), high lumber spina bifida or spinal muscular atrophy (observation).
- Initial treatment in most cases of pediatric foot is non operative (eg cast immobilization) (do not start with surgery).

Chapter 6:   Pediatric Trauma

Poly trauma:

- Neurological injuries (followed by orthopedic injuries) are responsible for most of the long term morbidities after poly-trauma in children.
  - o For children presenting with poly trauma, orthopedic management should be done with assumption that the child will have full recovery from his/her other injuries.
- If intra venous access cannot be obtained in poly traumatized child: intra osseous infusion can be used.
- Retropharyngeal space should be less than 7-6 mm, and the retrotracheal space less than 14 mm (see spine chapter).
- If there are multiple bone fractures, treatment is usually by internal fixation (rather than the more common treatment by cast immobilization). _(Scenario: 6 years old, MVC, ipsi lasteral femur and tibia fracture, treatment? (internal fixation for both by flexible nails or plates))._

Salter-Harris injury:

- Occurs through the hypertrophic zone of the growth plate (weakest part of the growth plate).
- Salter-Harris I and II injuries should not be manipulated (closed or open) after 5-7 days from the injury (especially in children who have more than two years of growth left) as this may lead to growth plate injury. Remodeling is expected to correct most deformities at this area. _(Scenario: 11-year-old boy, closed reduction of a Salter-Harris type II of the distal radius 8 days ago, XR show approximately 30° of dorsal angulation, treatment? (observation))._
- Treatment of growth arrest (also see LLD and distal radius fracture)
  - o If there are 2 years or more of growth remaining: CT or MRI to map the area of the arrest.
    - If <50%: excision of the fusion bar.
  - o If the fusion is > 50% or if there is less than 2 years of growth remaining: complete the fusion (and then manage the length disturbance if clinically significant).

Open fractures:

- The general rules of open fracture in adults apply to the pediatric patients. _(Scenario: 10 years old, auto versus pedestrian, 13 cm wound, tibia and fibula fracture, management? (antibiotics, irrigation and debridement of the fractures and application of an external fixator))(Question: most important factor in preventing infection after open fracture in children? (prompt administration of antibiotics))._

Compartment syndrome in children:

- The clinical presentation of compartment syndrome in children:
    - Increase in narcotic requirement.
    - Increase in blood pressure and pulse.
- If suspecting compartment syndrome (tense swelling, the above mentioned criteria): measurement of the compartment pressures can be done.

Lower Extremity Fractures:

Pelvic avulsion fracture:

- Muscles avulsions:
    - AIIS: rectus femoris avulsion.
    - ASIS: sartoris avulsion.
    - Ischial spine: hamstrings avulsion.
    - Iliac crest: abdominal oblique muscles avulsions.
- Management: Non operative treatment (rest, no sports participation until pain resolves).

Hip dislocation:

- Posterior dislocation is more common than anterior dislocation.
- Reduction can be associated with separation of the femoral epiphysis from the metaphysis (catastrophic complication).
    - Complete muscle relaxation is needed to achieve reduction with minimal force application (to avoid the physis separation).
    - Closed reduction should be done as an urgent procedure under general anesthesia. Open reduction is needed if there is failure of closed reduction, or if reduction is not concentric

Fracture Proximal Femur:

- Blood supply in children less than 4 years: both lateral femoral circumflex and medial femoral circumflex (see anatomy chapter). With age advancement, the medical femoral circumflex becomes more important.
- Delbet classification
    - Type I: trans-physeal, type II: trans-cervical, type III: basi-cervical, type IV: intertrochanteric
    - Type I: has the highest incidence of AVN.

- For type I, II and III fracture neck femur: Osteonecrosis is the most common complication (near 100% of transepiphyseal fracture, 50% of transcervical fractures, 25% of basicervical fractures, and 10% to 15% of intertrochanteric fractures).
- Other possible complications: nonunion, varus malunion.
- Treatment:
  - Should be treated as emergency: open or closed reduction; capsulotomy or joint aspiration (decreasing the tension inside the capsule may decrease the rate of osteonecrosis).
  - Surgical fixation options:
    - Screws short of the physis.
    - Smooth pins across the physis when little metaphyseal bone is available (with possible added spica cast immobilization).
    - Side plate and screws (pediatric proximal femoral plate): stronger fixation (especially for trochanteric and basicervical type) (See Fig 1).

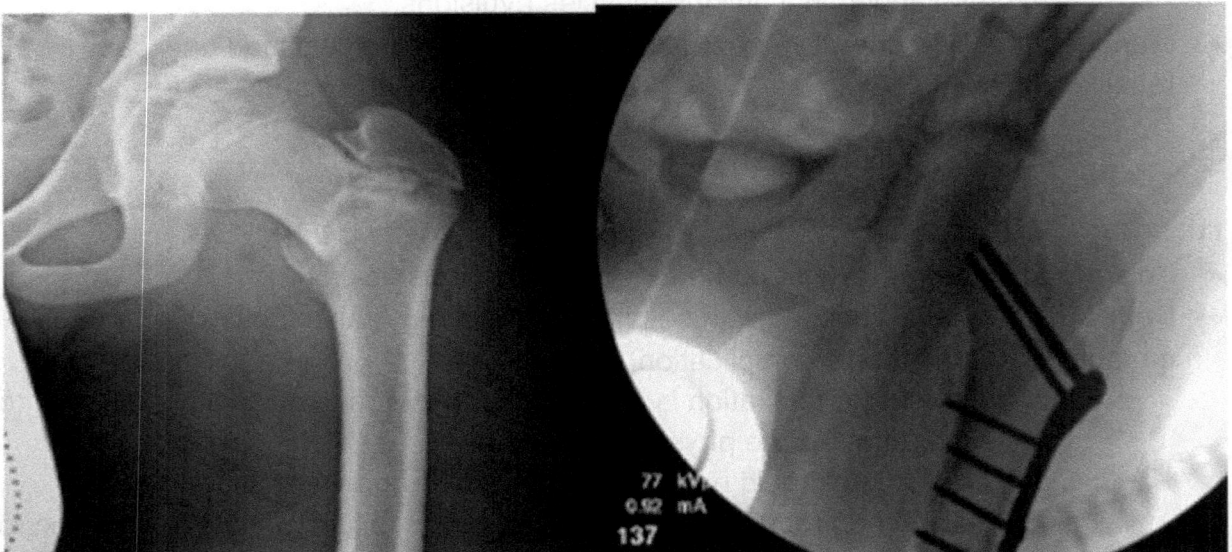

Fig 1: Trochanteric in a 12 years old boy. The fracture was fixed using pediatric proximal femoral plate

Pediatric Femoral Shaft Fracture:

- Femoral overgrowth by about 1 cm is expected in children ages 2- 10 years with femoral shaft fracture.
- Young children (less than 5 years) with minimal shortening can be treated by immediate closed reduction and application of spica cast. **No need for pre casting traction.** *(Scenario: 3 years old, mid shaft left transverse femur fracture, 1.5 cm shortening, treatment?) (Scenario: 4 years old, spiral femur fracture, treatment?).*

- o Avoid 90-90° cast for fear of compartment syndrome.
- o Avoid application of the lower leg part first and use it for traction.
- For very young children (younger than 6 months): Pavlik harness can be used
- Surgical treatment options: elastic nail, rigid nail, submusclar plating, external fixator.
  - o Flexible IM nail (flexible retrograde nail):
    - Best indicated for transverse mid shaft fracture with no comminution (see Fig 2).
    - Has higher complication rate for children heavier than 45 KG (100 pound).
    - To increase the stability of fixation using flexible nail: **increase the diameter of the nail**, use equal sized nails, and contour the nail so the maximum of spread of the two nails is at the site of the fracture.
    - Most common complication is irritation around the knee (related to rod insertion sites) that resolves with rod removal. _(Scenario: 25 Kg boy, transverse non comminuted med shaft femur fracture, flexible nail treatment, most common complication?)_
  - o Rigid IM nail:
    - Piriformis entry nail should be avoided due to possible risk of AVN of proximal femur (injury to lateral ascending cervical artery of the femoral neck (branch from medial femoral circumflex)).
    - The risk is less with "tip of trochanter" entry.
    - Lateral entry nail is the safest entry for rigid nail (See Fig 3). _(Scenario: 13 years old girl, fracture femur, treated with piriformis nail, 6 months after surgery she has hip pain, MRI shows marrow changes, what is the diagnosis? (AVN)) (Scenario: 12 years old, 60 Kg, transverse mid shaft femur fracture, treatment?)_
  - o External fixator:
    - Associated with high incidence of re-fracture after frame removal (especially with transverse fracture types).
    - Used mainly in open fracture or in very unstable poly trauma patient.
  - o Submuscular plating:
    - Best used for comminuted femoral shaft fracture especially in young children (5-12 years old).
- In Summary:
  - o 0-6 months: Palvik Harness.
  - o 6 months- 4 years: immediate casting (no need for pre casting traction).
  - o 5 -12 years:
    - Comminuted: submuscular plating.
    - Non comminuted- transverse- child is less than 45 KGs: flexible nail
  - o Older than 12 years: lateral entry rigid nail (or submuscular plating)

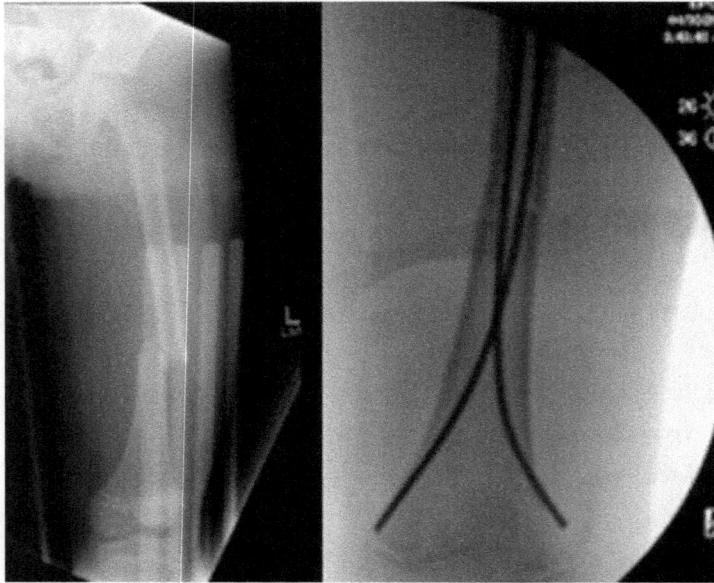

Fig 2: 8 years old girl, weighs 38 Kg, sustained left mid shaft transverse left femur fracture. The fracture was treated by flexible nail with good reduction.

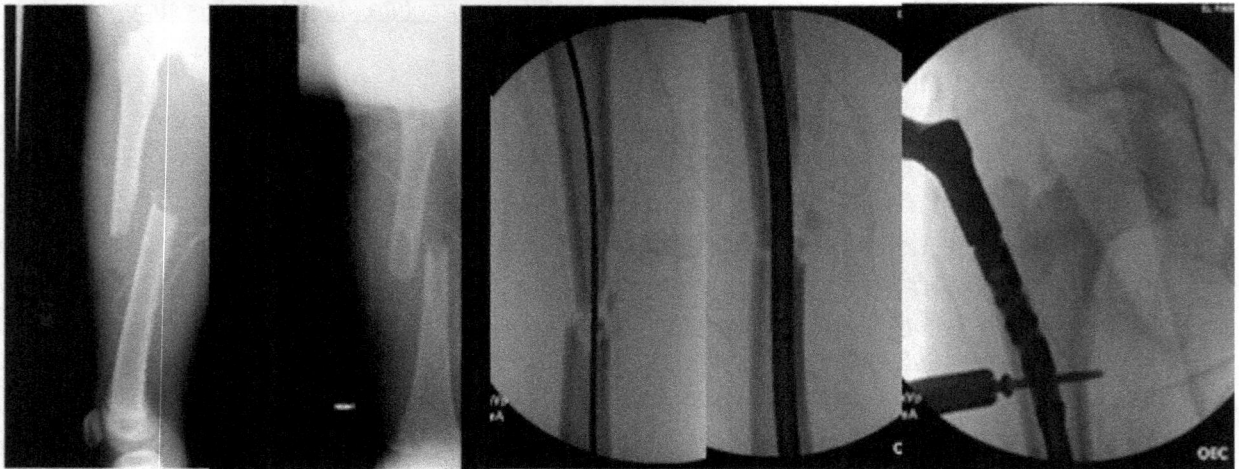

Fig 3: 14 years old boy with right femur fracture, mid shaft with medical comminution; patient was treated by rigid IM nail. Notice the lateral entry of the nail (lateral to the tip of the greater trochanter).

Distal Femur Physeal (Salter-Harris) Injury:

- Displaced SH injury can cause injury to the popliteal blood vessel; urgent reduction is needed.
- The growth plate of the distal femur has prominences called mammillary bodies that interdigitate with distal femur epiphysis. Most distal femoral physeal fracture propagates through multiple layers of the growth plate (as opposed to most Salter-Harris type I and II physeal fractures in other growth plates which occur through the zone of hypertrophy).
  - Distal femur physeal injuries have the highest rate of growth disturbance following physeal injuries (up to 50%)

- **Imaging**:
  - Displaced fracture can be seen in XR.
  - Non displaced fractures: the initial XR can be normal, in these cases (if there is clinical suspicion for the condition), stress views or MRI may be needed.
- **Treatment:**
  - Reduction (closed or open) and fixation with smooth pins across the physis.
    - Cast fixation alone can lead to re-displacement.
  - For S-H II injuries: fixation with metaphseal screws parallel to physis can be done (in cases of big metaphyseal Thurston-Holland fragment) (see Fig 4). *(Scenario: 14 years old, jumping in trampoline, fell and twisted his knee, severe knee pain, pulse is diminished in the foot, XR SH I of distal femur, treatment? (urgent reduction and fixation by K wires, followed by reassessment of the vascularity (do not order further imaging study before reducing the fracture as this may delay treatment))).*
- Growth arrest after distal femur fracture is common (about 50-60%) which frequently causes deformity/ shortening. *(Scenario: 13 years old boy with distal femur fracture, what is the prognosis?)*
  - The older the patient the higher the chance of growth arrest.

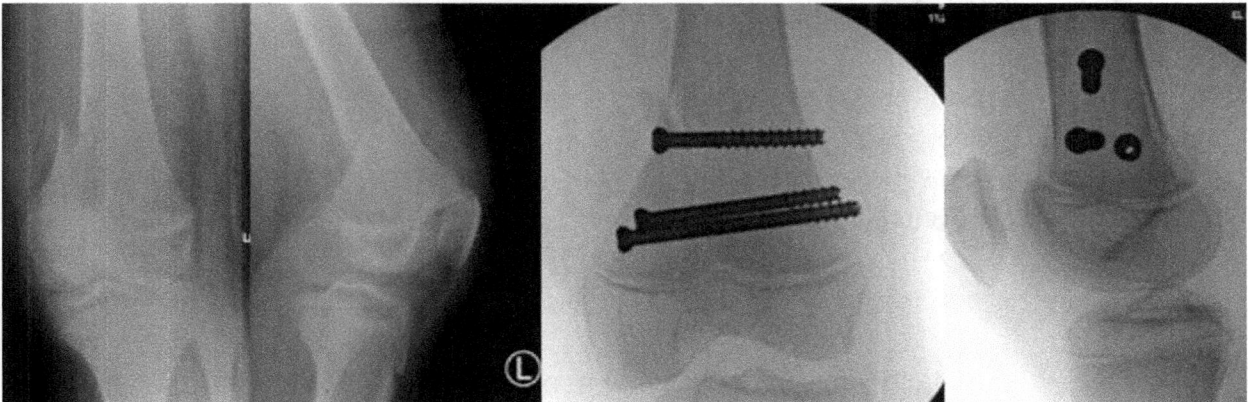

Fig 4: 14 years old boy with all-terrain vehicle (ATV) accident presenting to left knee pain. XR shows S-H type II. Patient was treated with screws in the metaphyseal fragment parallel to the physis.

Sleeve Fracture of The Patella:
- **Pathology:** Avulsion fracture of the lower pole of the patella with periosteum of the anterior patella attached to the avulsed piece (Fig 5).
- **Clinical presentation:** disruption of the extensor mechanism (patient will not be able to do straight leg raising) with hemoarthrosis of the knee joint.
- XR will show superior position of the patella with avulsion fracture, or "sleeve fracture," of the distal pole of the patella (Fig 5).

- o The distal fragment is larger than it appears on the radiograph because it largely consists of cartilage (so it should not be excised).
- Treatment is open reduction and internal fixation (tension band fixation). *(Scenario: 11 years old, fall down while playing football, knee pain and swelling, not able to keep his knee straight when left up by examiner, XR avulsion small lower pole and the rest of the patella is superior, treatment?)*

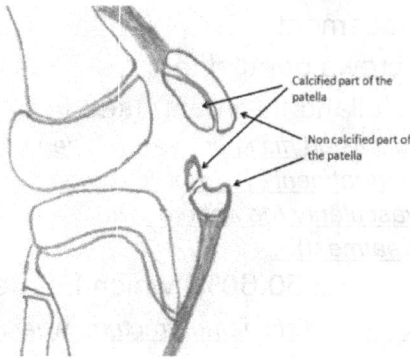

Calcified part of the patella

Non calcified part of the patella

Fig 5: Sleeve fracture of the patella. Noctice that despite the distal segement of the fracture will look small in the XR, it actually has a relatively big segment of non ossified cartilage.

Tibial Spine (Tibial Eminence) Fracture:

- **Classification:**
    - o Type 1: non (or minimally) displaced, type 2: angulated (posterior hinged); type 3: displaced (Fig 6).
- Represent avulsion of the ACL at the tibial insertion.
- Can be associated with entrapment of the anterior horn of the **medial** meniscus underneath type 2 or type 3 spine fractures. *(Scenario: 11 years old, type 3 tibial spine fracture, failure of reduction, what structure may be involved?)*
- Treatment:
    - o Type 2: trial closed reduction and extension casting; if this fails, open or arthroscopic reduction.
    - o Type 3: open or arthroscopic reduction.
    - o The internal fixation is by sutures or intra epiphyseal screws.
- Most common complication after surgical treatment is stiffness and arthrofibrosis.
- Usually associated with asymptomatic laxity of the ACL. This may be related stretching of the ligament at the time of injury.

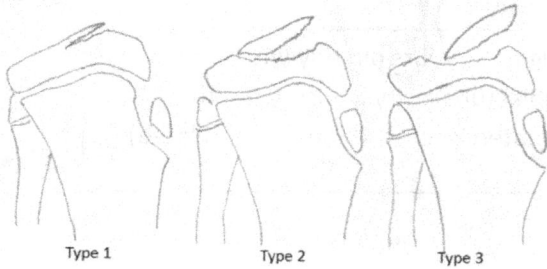

Fig 6:
Classification of
tibial spine
avulsions.

Tibial Tubercle Avulsion:

- **Classification** (Fig 7):
    - Type I: avulsion of the most distal part of the tibial tubercle.
    - Type II: proximal extension without involvement of the articular surface.
    - Type III - Intra-articular fracture in which the fracture line has propagated into the joint.
- Occurs in adolescent near the time of closure of the physis.
- Can be associated with injury to the **anterior tibial recurrent** artery which can cause **compartment syndrome** (of the anterior compartment):
    - Most likely associated complication.
    - Needs urgent fasciotomy of the anterior compartment.
- Treatment by open reduction and internal fixation by screws (Fig 8):
    - Periosteum is usually entrapped in the fracture and will prevent closed reduction.
    - The screws can go across the physis, as there is minimal growth remaining and minimal possibility of having growth disturbance from the screws.
      (Scenario: 14 years old boy, type III tibial tubercle (intra-articular) avulsion, next step? ORIF (not MRI))
    - Type III (extending to the knee joint) can be associated with meniscal injury. Arthroscopy may be needed at the time of open reduction and internal fixation to assess the possible meniscal injury.

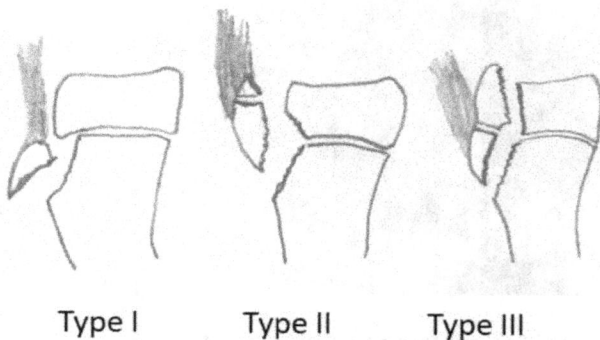

Type I   Type II   Type III

Fig 7:
Classification of
tibial tubercle
avulsions.

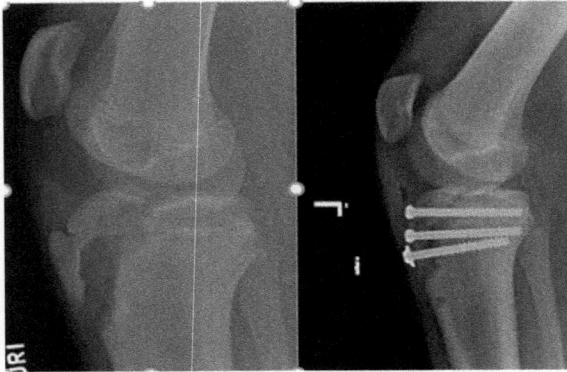

Fig 8: 15 years old boy with type III tibial tuberosity avulsion fracture treated 3 screw (6.5mm cannulated)

Proximal Tibial Physeal Injury:

- Injury to the whole proximal tibial physis (usually SH type I or type II) (in contrast to the tibial tubercle avulsion which is injury to the distal part of the proximal tibial physis).
- Can also be associated with compartment syndrome or vascular injuries.
  - Hyperextension injury has the highest incidence of vascular complication which can cause injury to the popliteal vessels (popliteal vessels are tethered at posterior surface of the proximal tibial epiphysis).
- The initial XR can be normal, in these cases, stress views or MRI may be needed (similar to distal femoral SH injury). *(Scenario: 13 years old boy, playing football, injury to the knee, severe pain, XR normal, management? (admission, neurovascular checks, MRI scan))*
- Treatment is reduction (closed or open) and internal fixation (Fig 9).
  - Smooth pins across the physis (if there is still potential growth from the growth plate) or transphyseal screws (if minimal growth potential is remaining). *(Scenario: 13 years old girl, knee injury will on a trampoline, firm compartments of the leg, difference between compartments pressure and diastolic pressure is less than 30, numbness of the foot, good pulses and good capillary refill, XR: SH type I proximal tibial fracture, treatment?) (N.B.: intact strong pulse is not exclusion for compartment syndrome).*

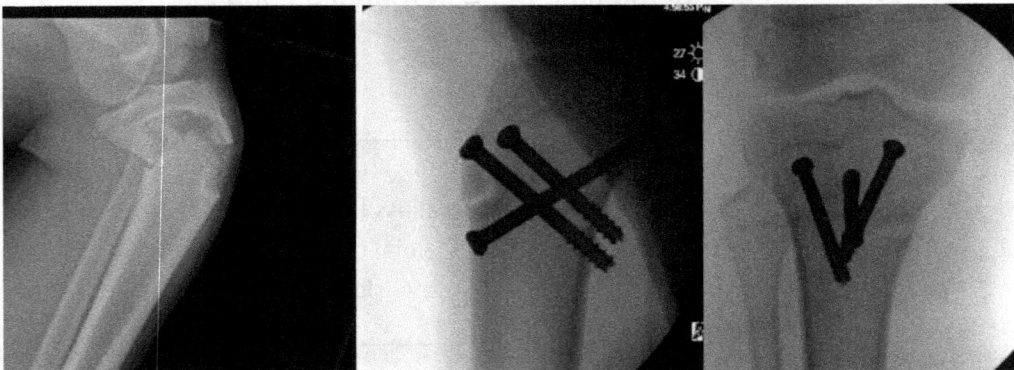

Fig 9: Left XR: 15 years old with proximal tibial physeal Salter-Harris type II injury. Middle and left XR: because patient was approaching his skeletal maturity, crossing screws were used for treatment.

Proximal tibial metaphyseal fracture:

- Gradual valgus deformity can develop after healing (Cozen fracture), this is usually self-limiting and does not need active treatment.
    - Observation of the child is warranted. *(Scenario: 4 years old, fracture proximal metaphyseal tibia, what is the prognosis?)*
    - If the condition does not improve with time, guided growth may be used to correct the deformity (medial proximal tibial physis implant guided growth).

Toddler Fracture:

- Spiral tibial fracture due to twisting injury.
- Usually no history of trauma (the toddler was playing outside when he/she started crying), will be able to walk but with limping, external rotation of the extremity will cause pain.
- XR will show spiral non-displaced fracture on the distal tibia with intact fibula. (Occasionally, XR may be negative) .
- Treated with above knee cast.

Tibial Shaft:

- Tibial shaft fracture can be associated with compartment syndrome.
- Most pediatric tibial shaft fracture can be treated non operatively (closed reduction and log leg cast application).
- If operative treatment is chosen, it can be by plate or flexible nail (rigid nail cannot be used because of the open growth plate proximally).
- For open fracture of the tibia, external fixator is the preferred treatment. *(Scenario: 7 years old, ran over by a car, type IIIB open tibia/fibula fracture, debridement done, fixation by?)*

Ankle Fracture:

- The incidence of growth arrest following physeal ankle injuries is about 50%.
- Type I and II SH injuries of the distal tibia: closed reduction and casting.
    - Operative treatment was not found decrease the incidence of growth arrest.
- Type III and IV SH injuries of the distal tibia: ORIF with an epiphyseal screw parallel to the physis or a meataphyseal screw (if the metaphyseal segment in type IV is large enough) (Fig 10). *(Scenario: 8 years old girl, fall from horse, type IV S-H injury to the distal tibia, treatment? (Open reduction and internal fixation, avoiding the physeal growth plate and joint))*.
    - Medial malleolar SH type IV fractures have the highest rate of growth arrest in pediatric ankle fractures

- ▪ Will result in varus deformity of the ankle.
- **Triplane and Tillaux fracture ankle fracture:**
  - ○ The tibial growth plate fuse over a period of about 18 months: first in the central region, then posteriorly, then medially, then closes laterally.
  - ○ Triplane and Tillaux fractures occur during this period (avoiding growth arrest is **not** the major goal as it is already closing).
    - ▪ The main goal is to restore articular congruity to minimize the development of posttraumatic arthritis.
  - ○ The Tillaux fragment has the attachment of the anterior tibio-fibular ligament.

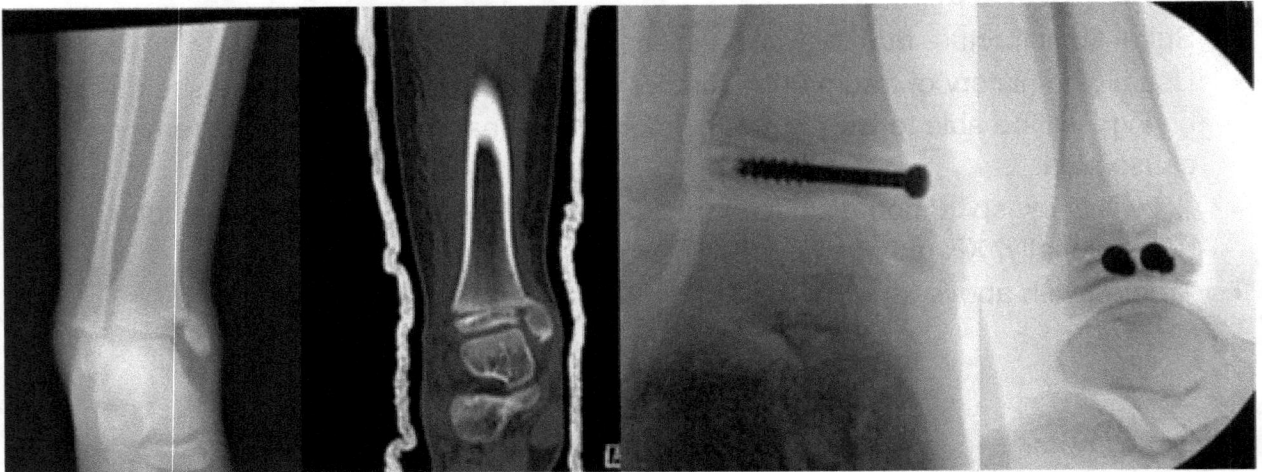

Fig 10: Distal tibia fracture Salter-Harris type II in 11 years old male (XR and coronal CT), treated by two 4.0 cannulated screws in the epiphysis (parallel to the physis).

Foot Fractures:

- In children younger than 5 years of age: proximal first metatarsal (at the site of growth plate) is the most common metatarsal fracture.

Upper Extremity Fractures:
Clavicle Fracture:

- Anatomy: the clavicle is the first bone to ossify, and the medial epiphysis of is the last ossification center to fuse, at age 20 to 25 years (see Sternoclvicular dislocation in upper extremity fracture).
- Displaced clavicle fracture, in children younger than 10-12 years, are treated non operatively (sling immobilization).

- Displaced comminuted clavicle fractures in adolescent (15 and older) are better treated with ORIF by plate and screws.
- Displaced distal (lateral) end clavicle fractures are treated non operative. The coraco-clavicular ligament continues to be attached to the periosteal sleeve and significant remodelling can be expected
  - The injury is usually through the distal physis and AC joint is not dislocated.

Proximal Humerus Fracture:

- 80% of humerus growth comes from the proximal humerus.
- Most of proximal humerus fracture (especially those younger than 10 years old) can be treated by sling for comfort (no need for closed reduction). *(Scenario: 8 years old, fall, proximal humerus fracture, completely displaced, treatment?)*
- Proximal humerus fracture in adolescent (older than 12) with marked displacement/angulation: treatment is closed reduction (due to limited remodeling potential) and percutaneous pin fixation (Fig 11).
- Osteonecrosis of the humeral head can rarely occur in adolescent patients with fracture dislocation of the proximal humerus. Observation is the main line of treatment in these cases.

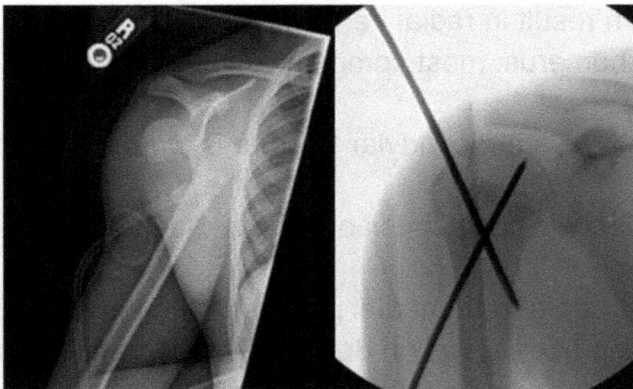

Fig 11: 13 years old boy with right Salter Harris type I proximal humerus fracture displaced 100%. The patient was treated by closed reduction and percutaneous pinning.

Humeral Shaft Fracture

- Humeral shaft fractures in infants and young children heal rapidly with excellent remodeling potential.
- Treatment is immobilization with a coaptation splint and bandaging the arm to the thorax for comfort (a sling and swathe is an alternative).
- If associated with radial nerve palsy: observation for nerve recovery (most radial nerve injuries are due to contusion with high chance of spontaneous recovery).

- o Closed humerus shaft fracture with radial nerve palsy is not an indication for open reduction. *(Scenario: 4 years old, distal humerus fracture, radial nerve palsy, treatment?)*

Supra Condylar Fracture

- Most common pediatric elbow fracture.
- Can be extension type (more common) or flexion type (less common).
- XR of non-displaced fracture: will show posterior fat pad sign
- Modified Gartland classification for extension fractures:
  - o type I: non displaced, type II: angulated (intact posterior cortex), type III: displaced, type IV: completely displaced with a gap (soft tissue interposition) with periosteal disruption.
- Nerve/ vessel injury:
  - o Most common nerve injury with supracondylar in general is anterior interosseous nerve (branch of median nerve); the patient will be unable to flex the DIP of the index and IP of the thumb (unable to do "OK" sign).
  - o Posterior lateral displacement (of the distal fragment) can result in brachial artery and median nerve injuries (by the edge of the proximal fragment), and posterior medial displacement can result in radial nerve injury.
  - o With flexion type supra condylar humerus: most commonly injured nerve is ulnar nerve.
  - o Ulnar nerve injury with extension type supracondylar fracture is almost always secondary to pin placement.
    - ▪ Medial pin inserted with elbow in flexed position is a risk factor for ulnar nerve injury.
    - ▪ To avoid injury of the ulnar nerve from medial pin: insert the pin with relative elbow extension and use oscillation during advancement.
  - o Floating elbow (supracondylar fractures and both bones forearm fracture): have higher complication rate (compartment syndrome and loss of reduction of the both bones treated without internal fixation).
- Malunion:
  - o Displaced supracondylar fracture (especially those treated in a cast) can heal in malunion (**cubitus varus**, elbow hyperextension, and internal rotation) due to collapse of the medial column and rotation of the distal fragment.
    - ▪ The deformity leads to unacceptable cosmetic appearance, no pain and minimal or no functional limitations.
    - ▪ Some long term studies showed that the deformity can result in increased rate of lateral condyle fractures, posterolateral rotatory

          elbow instability and tardy ulnar nerve palsy (due to deformity of the medial distal humerus and possible nerve subluxation).
- Unacceptable appearance is the most common reason to perform corrective osteotomy. *(Scenario: 7 years old, 3 years ago had elbow fracture treated in cast, now has deformity, what is the most common deformity?)*
- Compartment syndrome:
  - Will develop over few hours after injury (not immediately at the time of injury), should not be confused with arterial injury (which happens at the time of injury).
  - Will require forearm fasciotomy.
- Treatment:
  - Type IV, III and some type II are treated by CRPP (closed reduction and percutaneous pinning) (Fig 12, 13)
    - Indication of CRPP in type 2: more than 20° hyperextension or medial impaction. *(Scenario: 4 years old boy, fall from monkey bar, XR: 40° hyperextension with medial impaction, treatment?)*

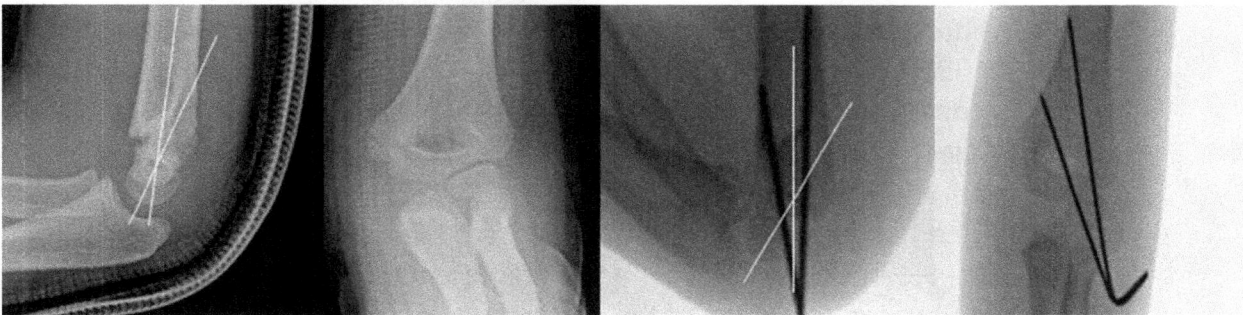

Fig 12: Type II supracondylar fracture with extension of the distal fragement. The shaft condylar angle (normally should be 40°) had decreased to about 15° (indicating 25° extension). Closed reduction and percutaneous pinning was done. The shaft condylar angle regained its normal value.

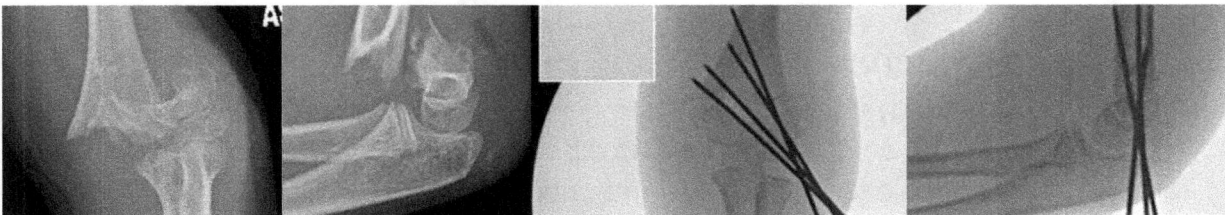

Fig 13: Type III supracondylar fracture (notice the amount of displacement of the fracture). Closed reduction and percutaneous pinning was done with diveregence of the pins.

- o Crossed pins configuration (medial and lateral pins) gives "biomechanically" the maximum rotation stability. Crossing should occur about 2cm proximal to the fracture.
    - Medial pins carry the risk of iatrogenic ulnar nerve injury (see before).
- o Two divergent lateral pins: most common used configuration:
    - Adding third pin will increase the stiffness of the construct (this may play a role in the presence of medial column comminution or slight residual internal rotation of the distal fragment.)
- o Displaced supracondylar fracture with nerve injury: treated as a displaced fracture (CRPP) with observation of nerve function. Recovery usually starts in 6-12 weeks and is completed in 3-6 months in the majority of cases (no indication to explore the nerve in closed injuries). *(Scenario: 5 years old, type III supra condylar fracture, patient unable to do OK sign, treatment?)*
- o Post-operative ulnar nerve palsy after medial pinning (that was not present pre operatively): treatment is removal of the medial pin and observation.
- o Absent pulses with pale and cold hand (unperfused hand): Urgent closed reduction and pinning and reassessment of the vascular condition:
    - If hands become perfused (pink and warm), admit for observation.
    - If after closed reduction, the hand is still unperfused (pale and cold), proceed with exploration of the vessel (anterior ante cubital approach).
- o For pulseless perfused hand (pink and warm): closed reduction and re assessment:
    - If the hand continues to be pulseless but pink and warm: close follow up. No need to explore the vessels (some controversy exists).
- o If after any closed reduction of the supracondylar fracture, the arm becomes pulseless and white, immediate anterior exploration of the arm is indicated (no need for angiogram). If the artery is entrapped in the fracture, release the artery from the fracture area. If the artery is injured, a primary repair or vein graft is needed.

Trans-Physeal Fracture of The Distal Humerus:

- Similar to supra condylar, however, there is no ossific centers of the distal humerus, so the condition can be misdiagnosed as elbow dislocation (which is exceedingly rare in this age population) (See Fig 1 in the pediatric chapter).
- Can be associated with child abuse.
- Management:
    - o Assess for child abuse (involve child protective service).
    - o Closed reduction and percutaneous pinning (no need for MRI or open reduction).

Lateral Condyle:

- Displaced fractures (more than 2 mm in any view) are treated by ORIF (using smooth pins) (Fig 14).
    - Best view to detect displacement is internal oblique view.
- Blood supply to the lateral condyle is from posterior surface, so avoid posterior dissection during internal fixation.
- Non-displaced fractures can be treated nonsurgical with cast immobilization. However, these fractures sometimes displace during cast treatment.
    - Careful follow-up is a must in all fractures treated non-operatively to be able to detect fracture displacement.
    - Arthrography or MRI can be used in non-displaced fractures to assess the articular integrity (fractures with an intact articular cartilage surface are unlikely to displace further).
        - For non-displaced fracture that extend all the way to the articular cartilage (as can be seen by arthrogram or MRI), some surgeons will advocate percutaneous fixation to avoid later displacement (controversy exists).

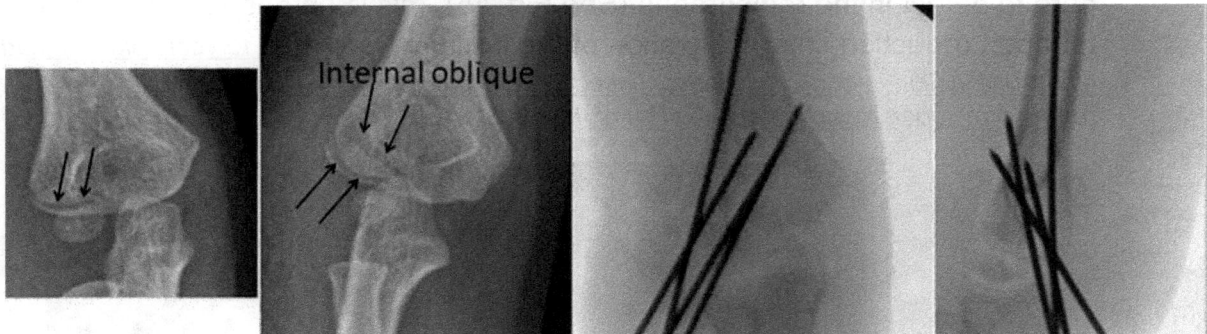

Fig 14: lateral condyle fracture (arrows), intenral oblique shows the displacement of the fracture. Open reduction and internal fixation with K-wires was done.

- Established non united lateral condyle presenting long after the injury (more than few months), treatment by open reduction and internal fixation (with possible bone grafting) (In situ screw fixation and bone graft is a possible alterative) *(Scenario: 7 years old boy, one year ago had elbow lesion that was treated in a cast, presenting now with deformity (cubitus valgus), the treatment now is?).*
- Displaced fractures are prone to develop nonunion.
    - Nonunion can lead to cubitus valgus (continuation of growth from medial side and stoppage of growth from lateral side) which can lead to stretch of ulnar nerve and tardy ulnar nerve palsy (takes few years to develop).

- o Treatment of established nonunion of lateral condyle fracture (debatable)
  - Classic teaching was observation, newer literature suggests internal fixation and bone grafting.
  - The younger the patient and closer the time from the injury (months rather than years), the more the inclination is towards fixation and bone grafting.

Medial Epicondyle Fracture (See Also Shoulder/Elbow Chapter):

- Treatment:
  - o Most medial epicondyle fractures in children can be treated non operatively.
  - o Acute medial epicondyle fractures in **athletes with stresses on elbow** (pitchers) should be treated by ORIF to stabilize the elbow.
  - o If medial epicondyle fracture is widely displaced (>5-10mm) or associated with valgus instability, treatment is ORIF.
  - o Medial epicondyle fracture can be accompanied by elbow dislocation (most common associated fracture with elbow dislocation) that spontaneously reduced. The medial epicondyle can become entrapped in the elbow (can be hard to detect in the radiographs (See Fig. 15), this is an absolute indication for open reduction, internal fixation of the fracture. *(Scenario: 12 years old boy, had elbow dislocation, reduction done, continued to have pain, XR in Fig 15, treatment? (arthrotomy, open reduction and fixation of the fracture)).*

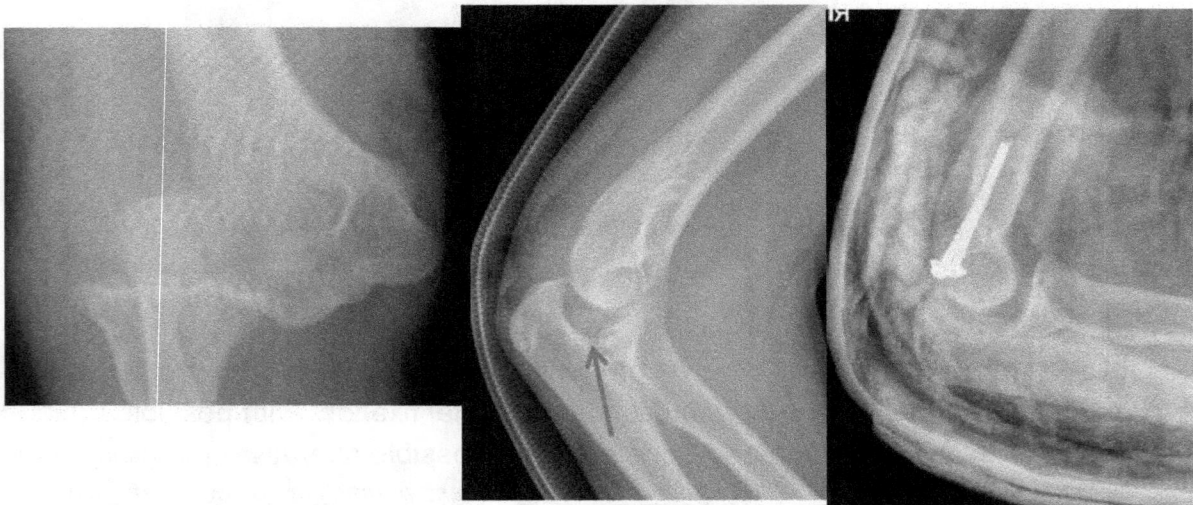

Fig 15: Elbow dislocation (left), after reduction the medial epicondyle can be seen entrapped in the joint (middle). Open reduction and internal fixation was performed with congruent reduction of the joint.

Nurse Maid Elbow (Pulled Elbow):

- Common in young children (2-3 years).
- Clinical presentation: pulling the child arm (e.g. child going to one direction and parent to the other) followed by refusal to move elbow which is kept in flexed pronated position, negative radiographs.
- Treatment by reduction (full supination then flexion).

Radial Neck Fracture:

- Can occur through the metaphyseal bone or through the physis (Salter Harris injury).
- Displaced radial neck fracture (more than 25°): initial treatment by closed reduction.
- If after closed reduction, the fracture is still angulated more than 25°:
  - Operative closed reduction in the operating room using either flexible nail inserted from from the distal radius (Metaizeau technique) or percutaneus K wire hinging the fracture (see Fig 16) then percutaneous internal fixation.
    - Avoid open reduction for complication of stiffness, avascular necrosis and non-union.

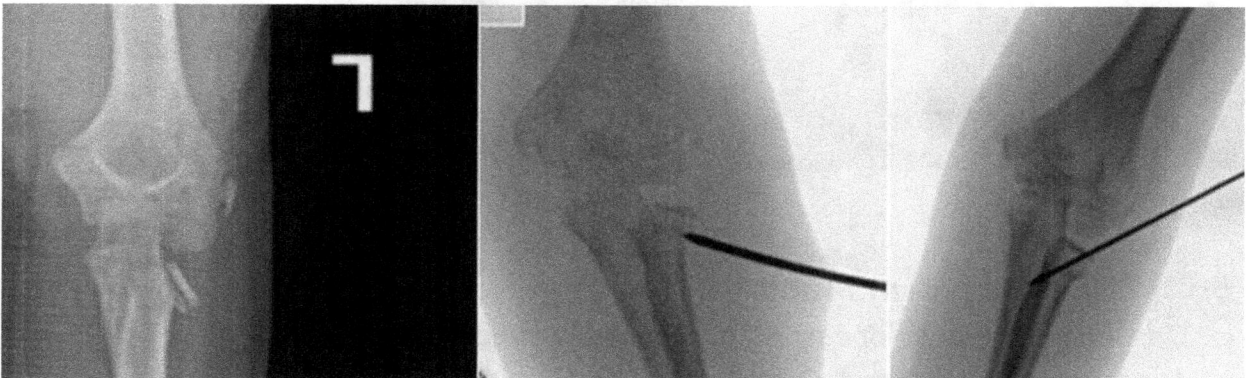

Fig 16: displaced proximal radial fracture. Closed reduction using thick wire to hinge the fracture was done then another wire was passed from the head antegrade to fix the fracture.

Monteggia Fracture Dislocation:

- Fracture ulna with dislocation of the radial head.
- Classified according to the direction of the radial head.
  - Type I (anterior dislocation of the radial head and apex anterior angulation of the ulnar fracture is the most common type of Monteggia in children) (Fig 17).
- **Treatment:**
  - Acute cases are treated by closed reduction of the ulna fracture and radial head dislocation (radial head will usually spontaneously reduce when the ulna is reduced). The position of immobilization in the anterior type (most common

type) is elbow flexion (90 to 100° flexion) and full **supination** (relax the pull of the biceps tendon). Posterior dislocation (less common) is better immobilized with the elbow in extension

- o Ulnar fracture fixation with IM rod or plate may be needed in older patients with unstable fractures/ radial head dislocations (if the radial head cannot be kept reduced in the cast).
- **Missed Monteggia:**
  - o Treatment by ulnar osteotomy (lengthening and angulation); possible open reduction of the radial head.

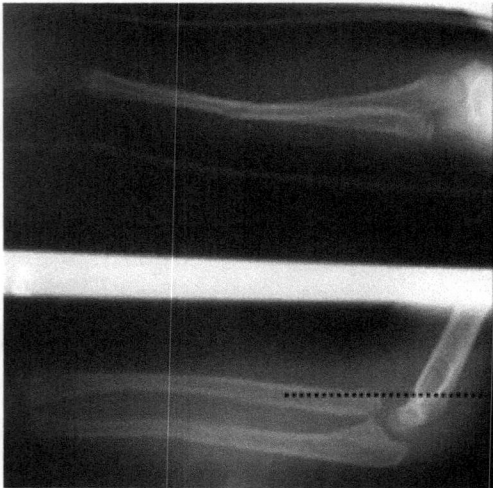

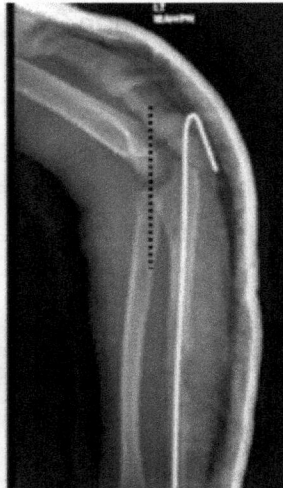

Fig 17: 7 years old boy, wrongly diagnosed with "isolated ulna fracture" 7 days earlier. XR in the clinic showed that the radial head is subluxed (radial head anterior to the capitellum, (dotted line)). Closed reduction and percutaneous pinning was performed, this resulted in the radial head being reduced in relation to capitellum

Both Bones Forearm Fracture:

- Can lead to the development of compartment syndrome.
- Tenodesis of the flexor digitorum to the index, middle, ring or little fingers to the fracture callus can occur causing inability to extend the fingers with the wrist extended, but full extension is possible with wrist flexion (shortened long flexor tendons). *(Scenario: 9 years old, both bones forearm fracture 2 months ago, now unable to extend his ring middle finger with the wrist extended but can extend it with the wrist flexed, explanation?)*
- **Treatment:**
  - o Most cases of both bones forearm fracture can be treated by closed reduction and cast application.
  - o Assessment of rotation: On the AP radiograph, the radial styloid and biceps tuberosity should be oriented 180° to each other; on the lateral view: the ulnar styloid and the coronoid process are 180° to each other.
  - o Acceptable alignment in both bone forearm fractures:

- In children younger than age 9 years: angulations of 15° and malrotation of 45°.
- Children older than age 9 years, acceptable alignment is 10° of angulation and 30° of malrotation.
- Bayonet apposition is acceptable provided that the angular and rotational reductions are within above guidelines.
  - A long arm cast provides better control of deforming forces than a short arm cast.
    - For distal 1/3 forearm fractures: short arm cast can be used.
    - Cast index XR measurement: (forearm width/cast width) should be > 0.8 to ensure good molding and not loose cast.
  - Surgical treatment in adolescent is by IM flexible nail or ORIF (Fig 18). Both have the same rates of union, radial bow reduction and forearm rotation. The flexible nail has shorter surgical time and less blood loss.
    - Loss of forearm rotation is the most common long-term complication for operatively treated forearm fractures.
    - Cast treatment of adolescent patients with forearm fracture is not recommended, operative treatment is preferred.

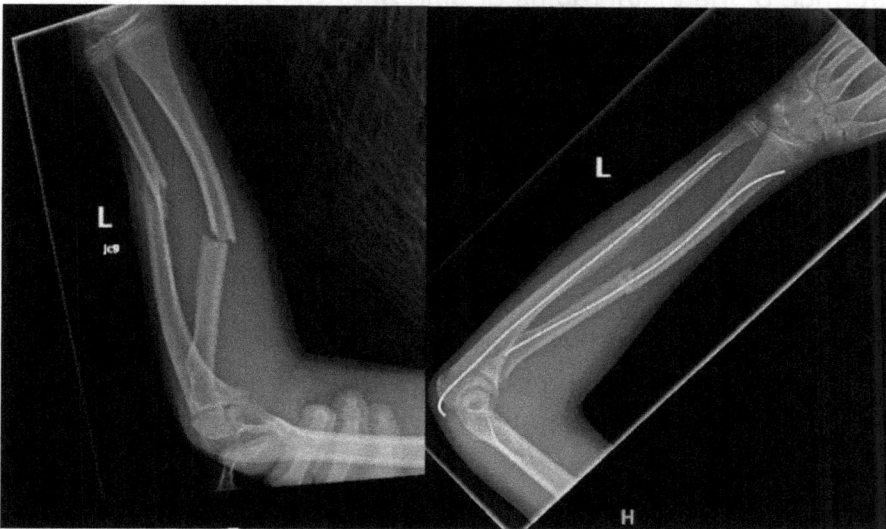

Fig 18: 15 years old boy with radius and ulna fracture. Treatment was done by intra-medullary fixation by flexible nail.

Distal Radius Fracture:

- Accepted alignment: less than 20 dorsal angulations for boys up to 14 and girls up to 12 years' old
  - If the fracture was reduced to acceptable alignment, mold the splint to maintain the reduction. Close follow up to ensure that re-displacement does

not occur. *(Scenario: 7 years, distal radius fracture, reduced, 10° dorsal angulations, next step? (Splint and follow up after one week)).*

- Displaced distal radius injury can cause compression on the median nerve and cause acute carpal tunnel syndrome (See hand chapter).
    - If the condition develops before reduction: treatment is urgent closed reduction and re-assessment.
    - If the condition develops after closed reduction and casting: initial management, is splitting the cast to relieve all external pressure. If this fails, urgent carpal tunnel release will be needed (together with pinning of the fracture to prevent displacement). *(Scenario: 12 years old, displaced type II SH distal radius, reduction under conscious sedation with casting, patient complaining of increase pain and numbness of the hand, splitting the cast fails to control pain, next step?) (N.B. this is acute carpal tunnel and not compartment syndrome, no need for forearm fasciotomy)).*

Distal Radius and Ulna Physeal Fracture:

- Salter-Harris injury of distal **ulnar** physis has high incidence of growth arrest (30-40%) *(scenario: 8 years old boy, fell on outstretched hand, XR SH type II distal radius and ulna, expected complication?)*
- If there is growth disturbance of the distal radius or ulna after SH injury to these growth plate (See pediatric chapter for growth arrest):
    - Treatment is either lengthening of the short bone or growth arrest of the long bone.
    - Growth arrest of the distal radius is hard to obtain (ulnar lengthening may be easier option). Arresting the growth of the distal ulna is easier to achieve. *(Scenario: SH 13 years old girl, SH injury of the distal radius one year ago, follow up XR shows ulna is 2-3 mm longer than the contra lateral side, MRI shows thinning of the distal radius physis, treatment? (epiphysiodesis of the distal ulna)).*
    - CT or MRI mapping of the distal radius growth plate to assess the extent of the growth arrest can be done in young children with potential to correct the deformity by resection of the arrest bar (if the fusion is less than 50% of the growth plate). *(Scenario: 9 years old girl, wrist fracture one year ago, now short radius, management? CT or MRI to assess the extent of growth arrest, if the arrest is not respectable (>50%), lengthening of the radius and epiphysiodesis of the ulna would be the treatment))*

Galeazzi Fracture:

- Fracture of the radial shaft with disruption of the distal radioulnar joint (DRUJ).
- In children is it usually apex dorsal radius angulation (contrary to the usual apex volar angulation of the regular distal radius fracture) with dorsal subluxation of the ulna
- Treatment:

o Most of the cases can be treated by closed reduction and long arm cast in supination (dorsal ulna subluxation is better controlled by supination).

Scaphoid Fractures:

- Scaphoid fractures in children are characterized by:
    - o More common in the distal pole of the scaphoid.
    - o Usually are nondisplaced.
    - o Treatment in cast for 4 to 6 weeks of immobilization. Displaced fracture needs ORIF.

Phalanx Fracture:

- Displaced fracture of the distal part of the proximal or middle phalanx is treated by reduction (open or closed) with internal fixation (Fig 19).
    - o This fracture is furthest away from the physis, so minimal remodeling will occur.
    - o Healed displaced fracture of the distal end of the phalanx will have limitation of the ROM of the IP (by the callus), this should be treated by ostectomy (NOT corrective osteotomy which carries the risk of osteonecrosis) to remove the bony block.

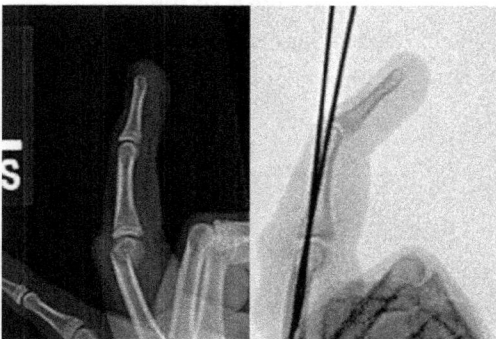

Fig 19: Fracture distal neck of the proximal phalanx of the ring finger in 15 years old boy (notice the flexion deformity of the fracture), treated by closed reduction and K wire fixation.

Seymore's Fracture (Can Occur in Finger or Toes):

- Fracture of the proximal physis of the distal phalanx (Salter Harris injury) with entrapment of the **germinal matrix** in the fracture (open fracture) (Fig 20).
- XR will show apex dorsal angulation of the Salter Harris injury.
- Treatment is irrigation of the wound with open reduction (for removal of the entrapped germinal layer from the fracture) and internal fixation (by pinning) of the fracture and postoperative antibiotics.

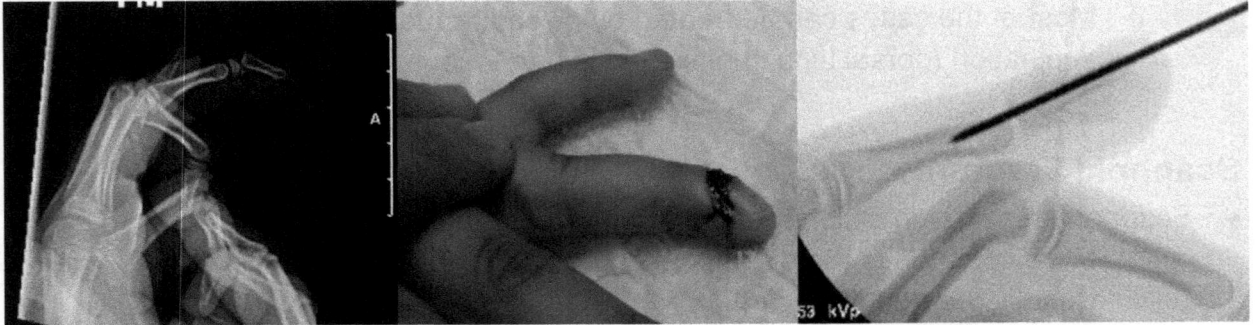

Fig 20: XR and clinical picture of open fracture of the physis of the distal phalanx of the ring finger. Debridement of the wound was done, the germinal matrix was removed from inbetween the fracture ends. Open reduction with pinning was done.

Fracture of The Base of P1 of The Thumb:

- Salter Harris III injury (see Fig 21).
- The fracture fragment has the attachment of the thumb MCP ulnar collateral ligament.
- Treatment of displaced fracture: reduction (open or closed) with internal fixation.

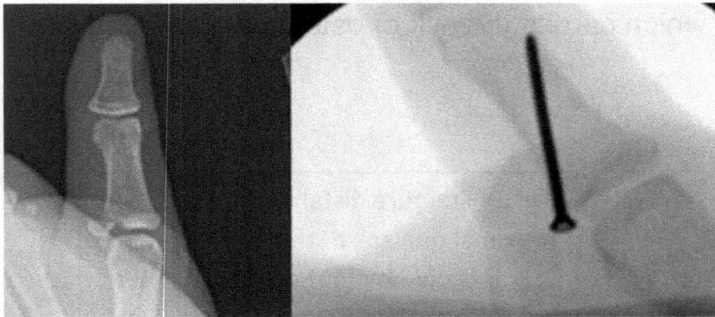

Fig 21: Avulsion fracture of the ulnar part of the proximal physis of the thumb. Open reduction and internal fixation was performed

Extra Octave Fracture

- Salter Harris type II of proximal phalanx of the fifth finger.
- Apex radial deformity.
- Treatment is closed reduction and splinting.

Spine trauma: see pediatric spine

Chapter 7: Musculoskeletal Oncology

General Principles for Musculoskeletal Oncology:

- Conditions causing bone destruction and formation will increase the alkaline phosphatase level in the serum.
- Most common **malignant primary** bone tumor: multiple myeloma, osteosarcoma, then is Ewing's sarcoma (some pathology references consider multiple myeloma not a "primary bone tumor", hence citing osteosarcoma as the most common primary tumor). Most common primary bone sarcoma is osteosarcoma.
- Age at presentation: musculoskeletal oncology
  - **Children:**
    - **Benign:** Osteoid osteoma, Osteochondroma, Chondroblastoma, unicameral bone cyst (UBC).
    - **Malignant:** Osteosarcoma, Ewing's tumor, Leukemia.
    - **Common lytic lesions in children**: osteosarcoma, Ewing's sarcoma, esinophylic granuloma, NOF (non ossifying fibroma), unicameral (simple) bone cyst (UBC), infection.
    - Osteosarcoma is the most common primary malignant bone tumor in children followed by Ewing's sarcoma.
    - Benign lytic lesions in children: unicameral bone cyst (UBC), ABC (aneurismal bone cyst), NOF, fibrous dysplasia (ground glass), osteofibrous dysplasia.
  - **Adult 20-50 with closed physis:**
    - Common lytic lesion: giant cell tumor.
  - **Above 50**
    - Common lytic lesion: metastasis, myeloma, chondrosarcoma lymphoma.
- Location of the lesion:
  - **Epiphyseal:**
    - Chondroblastoma, giant cell tumor.
- Round cell Blue tumor:
  - Ewing sarcoma, lymphoma, rhabdomyosarcoma, neuroblastoma.
- Most common metastasis site from bone and soft tissue sarcomas are the lungs.

Tumor Genes (See Also Genetic Chapter):

- Translocation

Tumor	Translocation	Fusion protein
Synovial sarcoma	t (X:18)	SYT-SSX
Ewing Sarcoma	t (11:22)	EWS-FLI1
Clear cell sarcoma (clear cell	t (12:22)	EWS-ATF1

chondrosarcoma)		
Myxoid Chondrosarcoma	t (9:22)	EWS-CHN
Alveolar Rhabdomyosarcoma	t (2:13)	Pax3-FKHR
Myxoid liposarcoma	t (12:16)	TLS-CHOP

- o t (11 and 22) (fusion protein EWS/FLI 1) is present in about 90% of cases of Ewing. Primitive neuroectodermal tumor has the same chromosomal translocation t(11;22).
- Classic Osteosarcoma:
  - o Possible mutation of RB (Retinoblastoma) gene and p53 tumor suppressor gene (see section of osteosarcoma).
    - The RB gene is a tumor suppressor gene.
- Supernumerary ring chromosomes are seen in parosteal osteosarcoma.
- Giant cell tumor of bone: can have telomere translocations.
- Li-Fraumeni syndrome (LFS):
  - o A Genetic condition characterized by an increased risk for developing different types of cancer (including soft-tissue sarcomas, breast cancer, leukemia, lung cancer, and brain tumors).
- Jaffe-Campanacci syndrome:
  - o A condition characterized by multiple non-ossifying fibromas, cafe-au-lait spots.
- McCune-Albright syndrome:
  - o Polyostotic fibrous dysplasia, cafe-au-lait spots with serrated borders (coast of Maine) and endocrine abnormalitie.

Stains/ Immunostains:

- Cartilage stains blue in H&E histology.
- Nuclear beta-catenin staining is the most specific immunohistochemistry staining pattern that confirms the diagnosis of desmoid tumor.
- Vimentin positivity indicates that a lesion is a mesenchymal neoplasm (e.g. soft tissue sarcomas), but it is not specific.
- Histochemical staining with S-100: positive in cases of malignant melanoma and Schwannoma stains.
- CD-99: positive for Ewings and other PNET.
- Both epithelioid sarcoma and synovial sarcoma have epithelial elements. Both stain positive for Keratin and EMA (epithelial membrane antigen).

Chemo-Therapeutic Agents:

- See basic science.
- Their main action is to induce "apoptosis" (induced cell death).

Radiotherapy:

- Help with pain control in metastatic lesions.
- Mechanism of action: induces DNA damage by the creation of free radicals.
- Used mainly for soft tissue sacromas, metastasis and heterotrophic ossification:
  - o Metastasis: dose 25 rad
  - o Soft tissue sarcoma: 50 rad for pre-surgical radiotherapy or 60 for post-surgical radiotherapy.
  - o HO: 5 rad within 72 hours of surgery.
- Post-radiation sarcomas:
  - o Occurs in about 1% in patients receiving high-dose radiation.
  - o Diagnostic criteria:
    - Different pathologies of original and secondary lesions, location within the field of radiation therapy, latent period of more than 4 years between treatment and new lesion.

Surgery (Margins)

- Margins:
  - o Intra-lesional: excision of the tumor within its capsule (e.g. curettage of the tumor).
  - o Capsular: Removal of the tumor using its capsule as the margin.
  - o Wide excision: cuff of normal tissue around the lesion.
  - o Radical: excision of the whole compartment.
- Most primary malignant tumors can be treated by limb salvage:
  - o However, tumors associated with pathologic fracture, infection, tumors encasing the neurovascular bundle, and tumors that enlarged during preoperative therapy usually require amputation. _(Scenario:18 years old, osteolytic lesion, biopsy shows osteosarcoma, MRI shows the tumor encapsulating, neoadjuvant chemotherapy is given however follow up MRI shows the lesion enlargement of the lesion despite chemotherapy, next step?)_
  - o With pathological fracture, tumor contamination of surrounding tissues occurs. Amputation with wide margin will provide lowest risk of recurrence.
- The use of osteoarticular allografts after tumor resections around the hip joint is not preferred because of inability to perfectly match femoral head size.
- Avoid any invasive procedures in patients with possible sarcomas (traction pins, Ex Fix).

- Indications of amputation (most of these are relative indications): locally recurrent tumors, expected function after limb preservation surgery is minimal, tumor growth the after preoperative chemotherapy or irradiation, invasion vessels/nerve by tumor, distal extremity lesions (e.g. foot/ankle), inability to obtain adequate margin (e.g. incorrectly done biopsy with contamination of too many tissues), limited reconstruction option (e.g. very young skeletally immature patients).

Staging:

- Enneking staging system:
  - Using this system, malignant tumors are staged using Roman numerals, and benign tumors are staged using Arabic numerals.
  - Benign lesions:
    - Stage 1 tumors are "latent", stage 2 tumors are "active" and stage 3 tumors are "aggressive".
  - Classification of malignant bone conditions (MSTS):
    - IA: low grade malignant intra compartmental (within the cortex)
    - IB: low grade malignant extra compartmental (extends outside the cortex).
    - IIA: High grade malignant intra compartmental (within the cortex)
    - IIB: high grade malignant extra compartmental (extends outside the cortex).
    - III: metastatic lesion (irrespective of the grade)
      - Classic osteosarcoma is high grade sarcoma; most common presentation is IIB (with soft tissue extension)
- The AJCC staging system for bone sarcomas:
  - Based on tumor grade, size, and the presence and location of metastases.
  - Stage I: low grade; Stage II: high grade; Stage III: "skip metastases" (discontinuous lesions within the same bone); Stage IV-A pulmonary metastases; stage IV-B non-pulmonary metastases.
    - Stages I and II are subdivided based on size:
      - A: less than or equal to 8 cm in their greatest linear measurement.
      - B: greater than 8 cm in size.
- The AJCC staging system for soft-tissue sarcomas:
  - Stage I: low grade. Stage II: high grade.
    - T1 for tumor size of less than or equal to 5.0 cm; T2 for a size of greater than 5.0 cm in maximal dimension.
    - (a): superficial tumor; (b): deep tumors (deep to fascia).
  - Stage III tumor: high grade, deep, and large (stage II T2b).

o Stage IV tumor: presence of metastasis (N: nodal; M: distant)
- Most important prognostic factor for bone sarcomas is the presence of metastasis at the time of diagnosis.

Biopsy:

- Patients with suspected malignant tumors are best managed by surgeons with specialized training and expertise in orthopedic oncology.
    - o The biopsy of a possible malignant lesion should be deferred to the surgeon who is capable of definitive management of the patient. *(Scenario: 18 years old, presenting with pain and swelling of the proximal tibia, XR shows destructive lesion, next step? (referral to an orthopedic oncologist for staging studies, biopsy, and definitive treatment)).*
- Types: Fine needle; Core and Open.
- Principles of open biopsy surgery:
    - o Longitudinal incision, avoid critical structures (nerves and vessels)
    - o Direct exposure of the area of interest (No inter-plane dissection) (go through single muscle if possible).
    - o Avoid drains.
    - o Good hemostasis.
    - o Frozen section should be obtained to ensure adequate viable tissue has been obtained (not for definitive diagnosis).
    - o Open can be: incisional Vs excisional.
        - Small lesion (<1.5cm in the hand, or <5cm else ware): excisional biopsy
        - Large lesion: incisional biopsy
        - Deep lesion: incisional biopsy.
- Any large (greater than 5 cm), deep, heterogeneous mass in the extremities should be considered a sarcoma until proven otherwise: Biopsy is needed.
    - o Lesion in the hand that is more than 1.5 cm and growing: incisional biopsy or referral to musculoskeletal oncologist specialist
- The most common detrimental impact of an unplanned excision of a soft-tissue sarcoma (that was excised with the assumption it is a benign condition such as hematoma, ganglion or lipoma) is increased wound complications of the definitive surgery (due to of the need for a wider surgical resection and adjuvant radiation).

Work Up For Suspected Malignancy:

- Blood work:
    - o CBC (complete blood count), CMP (complete metabolic profile).

- o Occasionally, other labs may be needed (e.g. Ca level is suspecting hyperparathyroidism).
- Imaging:
  - o CT and MRI of the whole affected segment.
  - o CT chest (to assess presence of lung metastasis from the primary lesion).
  - o CT chest, abdomen and pelvis (if suspecting metastasis to look for primary)
    - CT chest, abdomen and pelvis can show the primary in about 90% of cases.
  - o Bone scan. (*Scenario: knee XR shows destructive lesion in the distal femur in 25 years old male, next step?) (CT chest, MRI of the lesion and bone scan)) (Scenario: 55 years old, shoulder pain, XR lytic lesion, next step? (CT chest, abdomen and pelvis and bone scan to look for possible primary, MRI of the lesion)).*
- Solitary lytic lesion in elderly:
  - o If there is no history of metastasizing tumor:
    - CT chest, abdomen, and pelvis, bone scan and lab work.
    - If the above work up does not show the origin: bone biopsy.
    - Do not assume a solitary lesion is a metastasis and perform prophylactic fixation by IM nail, this will spread the lesion if it is not metastasis. (*Scenario: 60 years old, osteolytic lesion of the proximal femur with pending pathological fracture, next step?)*
  - o If the patient has obvious multiple bone metastatic lesions (there is wide spread metastasis detected by imaging studies) and the primary cannot be detected by CT of the chest, abdomen and pelvis, no need for **pre** fixation biopsy, and tissue should be obtained at the time of surgery. (*Scenario: 75 years old, bone ache, bone scan shows wide spread metastasis, CT chest abdomen and lung did not define the primary, patient has impending fracture of femur, next step? (femur IM nail and biopsy at the time of fixation (no need for pre-operative biopsy))).*

Individual Bone Tumors
A) Malignant Bone Conditions:
Osteosarcoma

- Osteosarcoma is the most common primary bone malignant tumor (excluding multiple myeloma).
- Types:
  - o Classic, paraosteal, periosteal, telengectatic, secondary (e.g. after Paget's disease).
- Age:
  - o Young age in the 2nd and 3rd decades of life (common in patient younger than 20 years). Secondary osteosarcoma usually occurs in elderly.

- Genetics:
  - Common association with mutation of retinoblastoma gene or P53 (tumor suppressor gene) (see before).
- Pathology (see Fig 1):
  - Malignant osteoid tissue (once there is malignant osteoid tissue, the tumor is osteosacroma, even if there is chondroid or fibroid elements).
  - Affect the metaphysis of the long bone, most commonly around the knee.
  - CT chest will show pulmonary metastases at the time of diagnosis in about 10% to 20% of patients with high-grade osteosarcoma.

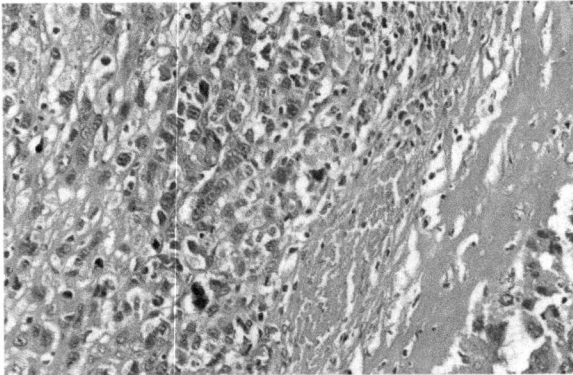

Fig 1: osteoid formation in an osteosarcoma. (From Wikipedia; https://en.wikipedia.org/wiki/Osteosarcoma)

  - In patients with osteosarcoma, stage at presentation (presence of metastasis) has the most important prognostic impact; clinically detectable metastases at presentation have a very poor prognosis.
- Clinical presentation:
  - Classically, osteosarcoma had been described as being presenting by pain (pain preceding the swelling).
- Imaging:
  - XR:
    - Ostelytic-blastic metaphysis lesion (cloud-like matrix, which indicates bone destruction with new bone formation) with soft tissue invasion and cortical destruction (See Fig 2).
    - Mineralization extending into the soft tissue, indistinct margins, and destruction of the normal trabecular pattern. _(Scenario: 25 years old, heal pain and mass of one month, CT shows bone destruction with new bone formation, soft tissue invasion with calcification and periosteal reaction, possible diagnosis?)_
- Treatment:
  - Pre-operative (neo adjuvant) chemotherapy, wide excision surgery, then post-operative chemotherapy.
  - The chemotherapy in osteosarcoma is methotrexate-based chemotherapy.
  - Survival for classic osteosarcoma is about 65%.
- **Parosteal Osteosarcomas:**

- o The most common location of parosteal osteosarcoma is the posterior cortex of the distal femur (very characteristic location in young patients).
- o Heavily mineralized nodular lesion on the surface of the bone.
- o Low grade malignancy with mainly fibrous stroma. Treatment is surgery (wide excision), no need for chemotherapy. *(Scenario: 35 years old, knee pain of 4 months, XR mineralized lobulated lesion that appears to be stuck onto the metaphyseal surface of the distal posterior femur, most likely diagnosis? treatment?)*
- **Periosteal Osteosarcoma:**
  - o Surface lesion, mainly cartilaginous, intermediate to high grade. Chemotherapy is needed (similar to classic osteosarcoma).
- **Telangactitic Osteosarcoma:**
  - o Highly aggressive, XR will show mainly lytic lesion with minimal bone formation (see Fig 3). MRI may show picture similar to multiple fluid levels (Differential diagnosis is ABC, see later).
- **Secondary Osteosarcoma:**
  - o Can occur after Paget's disease, bone infarct, or after irradiation.
  - o Osteosarcoma on top of pagetoid bone has the worst prognosis of all bone sarcoma.

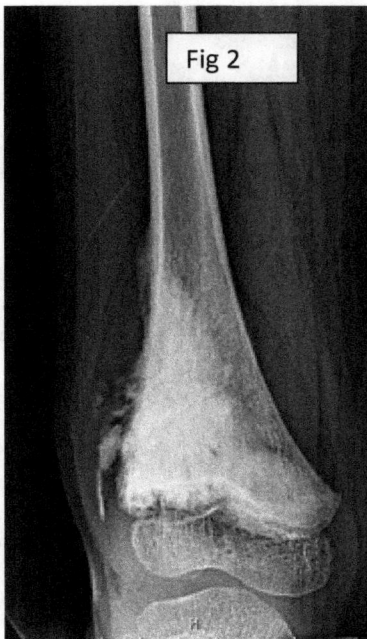

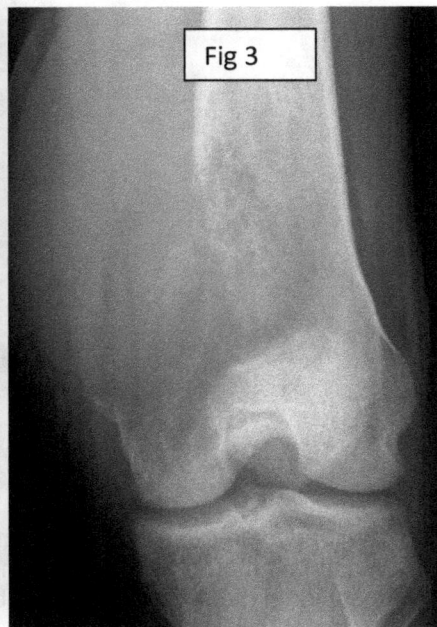

Fig 2 and 3: Two examples of osteosarcoma bone formation. Both figures show distal metaphyseal destructive lesion with soft tissue invasion. Fig 2 shows a lesion that is mainly blastic while Fig 3 shows a lesion which is mainly osteolytic (telangactitic osteosarcoma)

Chondrosarcoma:

- Pathology:
  - o Classic chondrosarcoma: low grade malignancy (rarely metastasize).

- Histology: malignant cellular chondral tissue (bi nuclear cells) (Fig 4).
        - Telomerase activity in chondrosarcoma is related to its grade and recurrence.
    o Location: Pelvis is the most common location. It is common in proximal humerus and proximal femur, and flat bones.
- Imaging:
    o Erosion of the cortex, with calcification (punctuate, arcs and rings). *(Clinical hint: if you see lobulated calcified lesion in elderly that eroded more than 50% of the cortex, think "chodrosacroma", enchondromas do not erode cortex more than 50%).*
- Treatment:
    o Wide excision alone (**the tumor is not chemo or radio sensitive**) (Classic chondrosarcoma has an excellent survival of more than 90%). *(Scenario: Elderly 73 year old patient with shoulder pain for long duration (months), constant, progressive, more at night. Radiographs show osteolytic lesion with calcification, diagnosis?) (Scenario: 60 years old, 9 months of hip pain, XR lytic lesion with calcification, pathology: malignant chondroid tissue, treatment?)*
- **Dedifferentiated chondrosarcoma:** has areas of classic chondrosarcomas and areas of high grade sarcoma. Has very poor prognosis.
- Difference between chondrosarcoma and enchondroma: See enchondroma section.

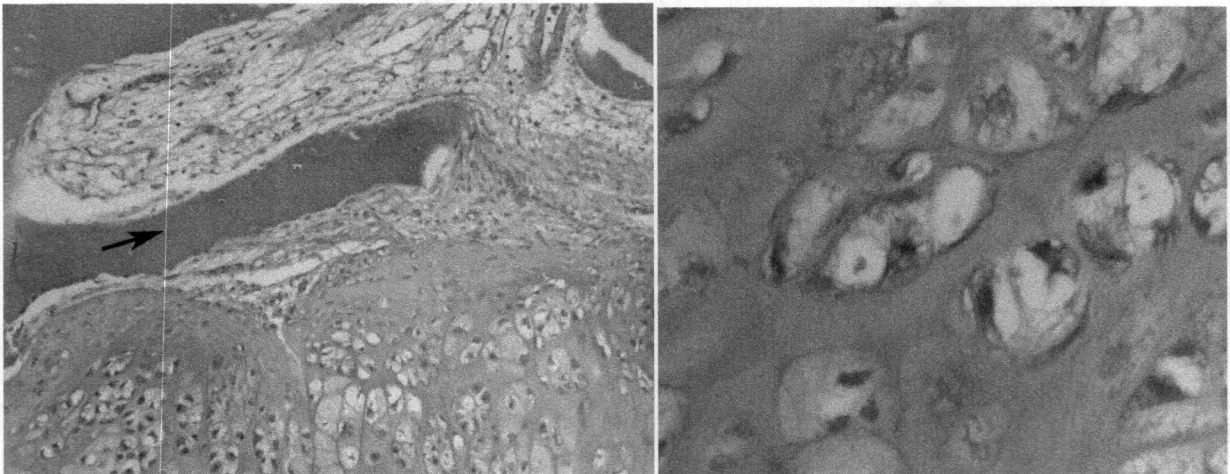

Fig 4 a) Chondrosarcoma. The tumor is present in the lower half of the image and consists of proliferating malignant chondrocytes infiltrating into the bone. The benign bone trabeculae are marked by black arrows (Hematoxylin and Eosin stain; original magnification X100). b) The tumor cells show large nuclei with cytologic atypia. Most lacunae are occupied by two and three nuclei. (Hematoxylin and Eosin stain; original magnification X400) (Courtesy of Dr Nawar Hakim).

Ewing tumor:
- Pathology:

- A neuroectodermal tumor.
- One of the round cell tumor (see before). The cells form pseudorosettes (see Fig 5).
- Immunostains:
    - MIC-2 positive (sensitive and specific marker for neuroectodermal tumor).
    - PAS positive (in contrast to lymphoma) and Reticulin negative (in contrast to lymphoma) (which is another round cell tumor)
    - Vimentin positive (mysechemal marker) and Cytokeratin negative (epithelial marker).
    - **CD99 positive.**
- Diaphyseal lesion (in contrast to osteosarcoma which is more metaphyseal).
- In about 90-95% of patients with Ewing's sarcoma, there is a translocation, t(11:22) resulting in EWS/FLI -1 transcription factor that results in tumor cell proliferation (see tumor genes section above).

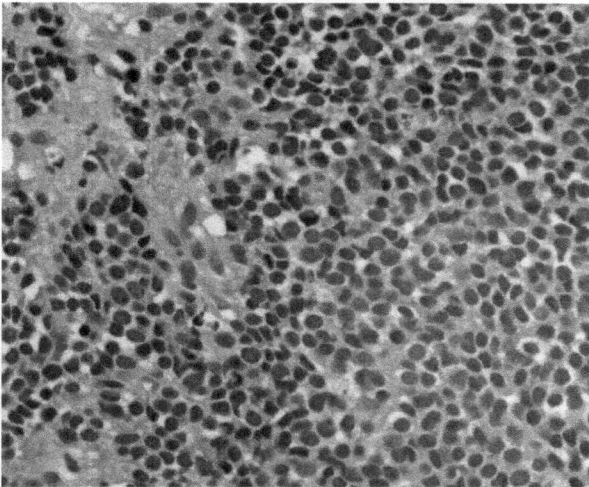

Fig 5 Ewing sarcom of the iliac bone in 16 years old male. The tumor consists of sheets of densely packed tumor cells with small and uniform nuclei, small amount of cytomplasm and indistinct cell membrane (Hematoxylin and Eosin stain, 400 magnifications, Courtesy of Dr Nawar Hakim)

- Clinical presentation:
    - Occur mostly in the first 2 decades of life.
    - Can occur in flat bone (scapula, pelvis), fibula, ulna.
    - Clinical presentation can be similar to infection (fever with increase marker of inflammation).
- Work up/ Investigation:
    - XR: osteolytic lesion (in contrast to osteosarcoma which has new bone formation element), diaphyseal, layers of periosteal reaction (onion skin) (See Fig 6); it can be associated with a large soft tissue component.
    - MRI: to better delineate the lesion.

- o Bone marrow biopsies can be performed as a part of staging (controversial) (to assess the presence of micrometastatic disease in the bone marrow which has a greater risk for recurrence after treatment) *(scenario: 5 years, thigh pain for two months, mild fever, XR: osteolytic lesion of the femur, next step? (MRI))*
- o Biopsy from the lesion: will show the Ewing (round cell) tumor with the characteristic immunostains (see before).
- Treatment:
  - o Chemotherapy followed by surgery (wide resection) or radiation therapy.
    - ▪ Ewing sarcoma is radiosensitive; however, radiation is mainly utilized for nonsurgical anatomic locations. The tumor occurs mainly in young patients and surgery (when possible to obtain wide margin) will cause less morbidity than radian therapy.
    - ▪ Chemotherapy in Ewing tumor is Vincristine, doxorubicin, cyclophosphamide, and dactinomycin-based chemotherapy

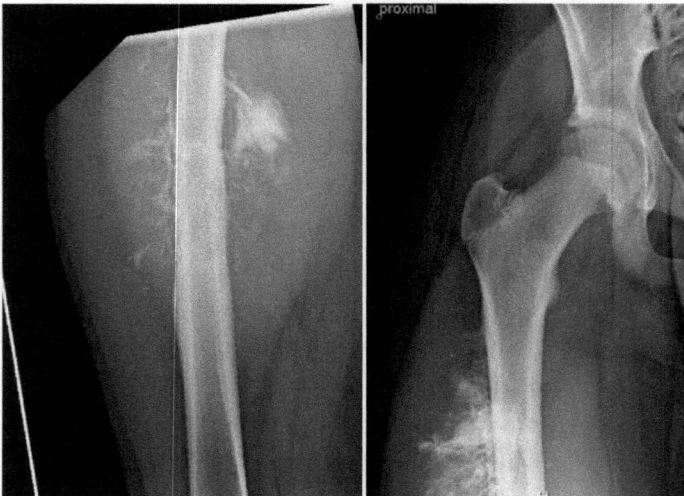

Fig 6: 11 years old with diaphyseal lesion of the proximal femur. Notice the extensive periosteum reaction and the large soft tissue component.

Undifferentiated pleomorphic sarcoma of bone:
- Used to be called "malignant fibrous histiocytoma" (MFH), seen in elderly patients.
- Histologically: Malignant fibrous tissue.
- Treatment: chemotherapy and wide surgical resection.

Neuroblastoma:
- One of the round cell tumors.
- The most common metastatic solid tumor in childhood; can metastasize to bone in children.
- Neuroblastoma arises from neural crest derived cells (nerve tissue in the adrenals, chest, neck, or spine).

Multiple Myeloma:

- Pathology:
    - o **Plasma cells** are the predominant cell type seen on a biopsy specimen.
- Clinical presentation:
    - o Bone pains, possible fatigue (from anemia).
- Lab:
    - o Serum protein electrophoresis and urine protein electrophoresis is used to obtain diagnosis.
        - ▪ Detects kappa and lambda Monoclonal light chains of myeloma.
        (Scenario: elderly patient with XR showing widespread osteolytic lesion, what blood work may give correct diagnosis?)
    - o Normochromic, normocytic anemia, thrombocytopenia.
- Imaging:
    - o XR: multiple lytic punched out lesions.
    - o Bone scan: can be cold in bone scan (15% of cases) due to bone destruction with no bone formation.
- Treatment:
    - o Chemotherapy.
    - o Bisphosphonates (to decrease bone resorption).
    - o Some cases can be treated by bone marrow transplant.
    - o Pathological fracture or impending pathological fracture: see later (same rules as metastatic lesions).

Lymphoma:

- Pathology:
    - o One of the osteolytic lesion in elderly patient
    - o Pathology: blue round cell tumor.
    - o Usually non-Hodgkin B cell subtype. CD **20/45** positive.
    - o Intra-medullary bone lesion with large soft tissue extension and little bone erosion.
- Treatment:
    - o Chemotherapy and/or radiation.
    - o Surgery for pathological fracture. *(Scenario: 60 years old, osteolytic lesion, pathology lymphoma, treatment? (referral to medical oncologist)) (Scenario: 65 years old, osteolytic lesion, CT chest abdomen pelvis lung free, pathology round cell, diagnosis? treatment?)*

Adamantinoma:

- Pathology:
    - o Tumor of epithelial origin.

- Microscopically: areas of epithelial cells (in a glandular pattern) in nests within a fibrous stroma (biphasic pattern of glandular epithelial cells surrounded by spindle cells).
  - Positive stain for keratin (epithelial origin).
  - Low grade malignancy
  - Usually affecting the anterior cortex of the tibia.
- XR will show multiple lucent spots of the anterior tibia (soap bubble appearance) (see Fig 7).
- DD:
  - Osteofibrous dysplasia: occur at younger age, cortical lesion, can be accompanied by tibial deformity.
    -
    - Adamantinoma is believed to be closely related to osteofibrous dysplasia, which may represent a precursor condition.
- Treatment: wide resection alone (no chemo or radio therapy, low grade malignancy)

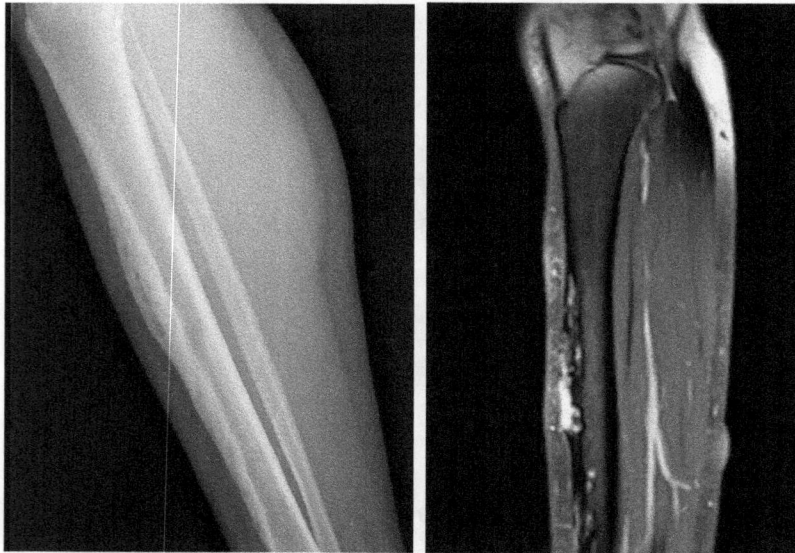

Fig 7: XR and MRI for adamantinoma of the anterior cortex of the tibia. Note the affection of the anterior cortex and the multiple lucent spots of the anterior cortex. T2 scans showing cortical erosion with no soft tissue extenstion.

Chordoma:

- Mid-line tumor that develop in the spinal column, common in the sacrum.
- The cell of origin from notochord remnant.
- Pathology: physaliferous cell (vacuum cell)
  - XR: usually the lesion cannot be seen. CT: shows bone destruction with possible calcification.
- Treatment:
  - Wide local excision. (high recurrence rate)

o The tumor is a radiosensitive tumor; however, surgery with wide local excision is preferred if possible.
- To preserve near normal bowel and bladder function: either preserve S2 on both sides or S2, S3 and S4 on one side.
- Surgery: wide surgical resection, this may require encroachment over nerve roots, bladder or bowl structures.
- Radiation is added if there are positive margins.
- No chemotherapy.

B) Benign Bone Conditions:

Osteoid Osteoma:
- Clinical presentation:
  - o More common in young age (first two decades of life).
  - o Night pain. Etiology of pain: significant inflammatory response to the tumor leading to high levels of prostaglandin production.
  - o In spine: osteoid osteoma will lead to scoliosis with the lesion in the **concavity** of the lesion (see spine chapter).
- Pathology:
  - o Small lytic lesion (the lesion itself is less than 1.5cm) with the reactive sclerosis around the lesion (the sclerosis can be more than 1.5cm).
  - o Histology: immature woven bone, no signs of mitotic figures.
- Imaging:
  - o XR: sclerosis (usually the lesion itself cannot be seen) in plain XR (see Fig 8).
  - o The CT will demonstrate an intra cortical lucent nidus with a small amount of mineralization in the middle surrounded by reactive sclerosis (see Fig 8). *(Scenario: 15 years old, left shin pain, more at night, awakes the patient at night, relieved by ibuprofen, diagnosis?).*
  - o Intensely positive (very hot) in bone scan.
- Treatment:
  - o Options: Surgical excision, radiofrequency ablation (RFA) or medical treatment (the condition is usually self-limiting after about 2 years).
  - o Most effective and least morbidity treatment is by radiofrequency ablation. *(Scenario: 17 years old boy with hip pain, CT showing nidus and surrounding sclerosis, treatment?)*
  - o If the lesion in the hand phalanges, treatment is by curettage as ablation is not preferred for lesions in the digits because of the risk of thermal necrosis of the overlying skin as well as the digital neurovascular structures (relative contra-indication).

- o Lesion close to the cord (lamina of the spine), also treated by curettage to avoid thermal injury to the cord (relative contra-indication).

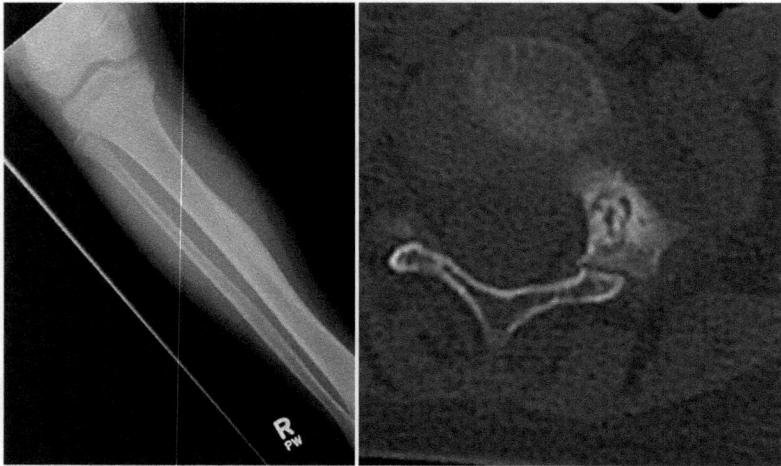

Fig 8: AP pf the left tibia in 11 years old boy with tibial shin pain, notice the sclerosis of the medial side. The lesion itself cannot be seen on the plain XR. CT of the lumbar spine of 7 years old with back pain showing sclerotic nidus surrounded by a small radiolucency. The nidus measures 10 mm.

Osteoblastoma:

- Occurs in young age.
- Similar to osteoid osteoma (however bigger than 1.5 cm) with similar microscopic picture (with osteoblastic rimming of the lesion).
- Common in the posterior element of the spine.
- Treatment: curettage and grafting

Nonossifying Fibroma (NOF, Metaphyseal Cortical Defect):

- Clinical Presentation:
  - o The condition is seen in children. In most cases the condition is accidentally discovered (XR taken for another reason), less often can cause activity related pain.
- Radiograph: osteolytic lesion, metaphyseal, eccentric, with sclerotic margin (see Fig 9).
  - o Jaffe-Campanacci syndrome: Multifocal NOF associated with mental developmental delay and café-au-lait spots.
- Treatment: observation (as the condition should heal spontaneously with gowth). Rarely, if causing symptoms: curettage and bone graft. (_Scenario: 14 year old (boy/girl), sport injury, XR shows the lesion, NO pain prior to injury. Diagnosis? (NOF), treatment? (observation))._

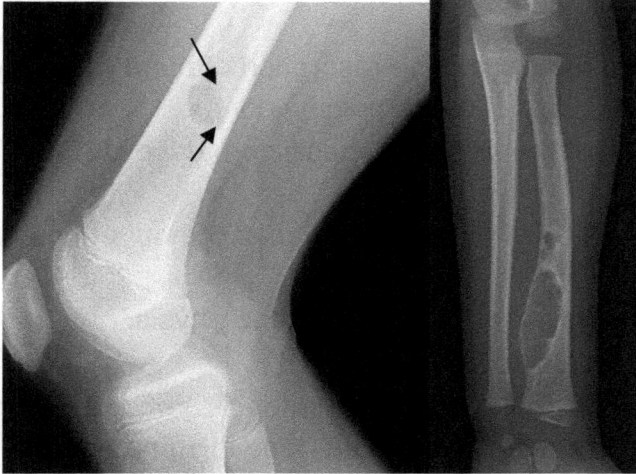

Fig 9: Lateral XR of the knee of 15 years old boy taken after injury during playing (notice the healing NOF which is expected soon to be completely healed. AP of the forearm of 6 years old boy taken after falling. Notice the eccentric lobulated metaphyseal meeting.

UBC (Unicameral Bone Cyst):

- Lytic lesion in the metaphysis, no soft tissue mass; usually present with an associated pathological fracture
- Most common location: proximal humerus.
- XR: metaphyseal, minimal to no expansion of the bone, the lesion is not wider than the width of the growth plate. Falling leaf sign can sometime be seen (see Fig 10). *(clinical hint: UBC is different than NOF in that UBC usually occupies the whole width of the bone (while NOF is eccentric lesion replacing part of the metaphysis) and that UBC is very close (touching) the physis (where NOF is usually separated from the physis by a normal tissue).*
- Treatment:
    - If non symptomatic (accidentally discovered) or with a pathological fracture of the bone: observe (may heal with the fracture). Chances of complete healing with fracture are around 10-25%.
    - If causing symptoms: aspiration and injection (steroid or bone marrow aspirate or bone graft substitutes) or curettage and bone grafting. *(Scenario: 12 years old, fall down on right shoulder, XR shows UBC (osteolytic lesion, no soft tissue invasion, fallen leaf sign, not wider than physis) with pathological fracture, treatment? (sling for comfort))*

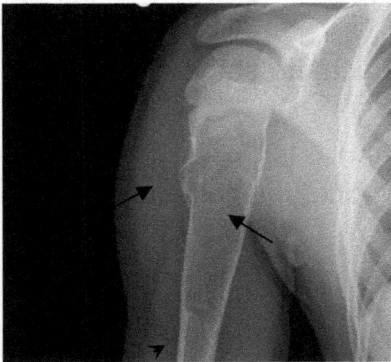

Fig 10: AP of the proximal humerus of 10 years old boy. He had right shoulder pain after falling while playing. The XR shows UBC with pathological fracture (arrows). Fallen leaf sign can be seen (arrow head).

ABC (Aneurismal Bone Cyst)

- Expansile lytic lesion; it usually causes near complete resorption of bone with very thin remaining cortical lining and expansion0 of the remaining cortex.
- Caused by up-regulation/ translocation of the ubiquitin-specific protease USP6 (Tre2) gene.
- Microscopically: spindle cells, giant cells, and blood-filled spaces without endothelial lining.
- XR: expansile lytic lesion in the metaphysis that is wider than the physis.
- MRI: very characteristic multiple fluid levels appearance.
- Treatment is biopsy, followed by intra-lesional excision (extended curettage (use of high speed burr) and bone grafting. Wide resection can be done in some bones like fibula or ilium.
  - Embolization may be done pre operatively to decrease intra-operative blood loss in large lesions.
- Recurrence:
  - High local recurrence rate (up to 50% in some studies).
  - Risk for recurrence: younger age, presence of open physes, type of surgical removal.

Brodie's Abscess:

- Pathology: subacute osteomyelitis, may be associated with a sinus tract.
- Differential diagnosis include osteoid osteoma, intracortical hemangioma, and stress fracture.

Fibrous Dysplasia

- Pathology:
  - Gs alpha gene mutation (GNAS1 gene) affecting the Gsα subunit of the receptor/adenylyl cyclase coupling G proteins (activating mutation) causing deficient inhibition of cAMP and improper formation of calcified osteoid (activating mutation in the gene that encodes the alpha subunit of stimulatory G protein (G(s)alpha)).
    - This will lead to woven bone that does not reach the stage of mature bone.
  - It can be associated to bone deformity (e.g. varus hip).
  - Can be mono-ostotic (one bone affected) or poly-ostotic (multiple bone affected).
  - Micro: low power magnification: Chinese letter appearance (chicken soup appearance).
- Radiographs:

- Ground glass appearance (the lesion appears to fill the bone over the affected length, however it have different density than the surrounding bone) (see Fig 11).
- A metaphyseal/ diaphyseal lesion
- Prominent cortical thinning.
- Possible deformity of the affected bone (e.g. shepherd crook deformity in the proximal femur). *(Scenario: 20 years old, chest XR for pneumonia, proximal humerus lesion affecting the proximal two third of the bone, cortical thinning, ground glass appearance, no prior history of pain, possible diagnosis?)*

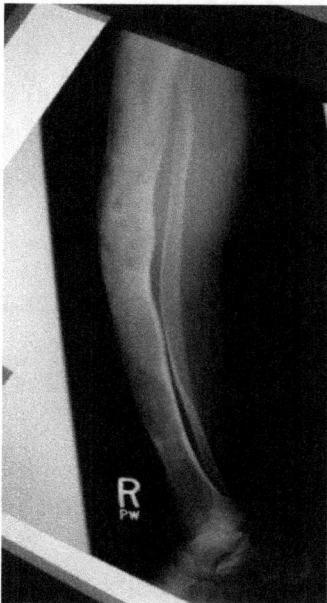

Fig 11: Lateral XR of the right leg in 16 years old boy with poly-ostotic fibrous dysplasia. Notice the deformity of the tibia and ground glass appearance of the affected bone.

- Bisphosphonate therapy can decrease the pain associated with the skeletal lesions of fibrous dysplasia.
- McCune Albright Syndrome:
  - café au lait lesion, irregular border (Cost of Maine), precocious puberty, endocrine abnormalities.
- Less than 1% of fibrous dysplasia can show malignant change to undifferentiated pleomorphic sarcoma or osteosarcoma.

Osteofibrous Dysplasia:

- Pathology:
  - Microscopically is composed of bone trabeculae arranged as "Chinese letters" (similar to fibrous dysplasia) with **prominent osteoblastic rimming.**

- o Osteolytic lesion in the anterior tibia, well circumscribed, minor anterior bowing of the tibia is frequently seen. Can be associated with tibial deformity.
- It occurs at a very young age, usually less than 10 years.
- The lesion is unpredictable in nature, but local recurrence is very high in patients who undergo surgery before 15 years of age. The condition may represent a pre-cancerous condition changing to adamantinoma (see adamantinoma section).

Osteochondroma:

- The cortex of the lesion is continuous with the cortex of the host bone; the medulla of the lesion is continuous with the medulla of the host bone (this can be more obviously seen in the CT)
- The cartilaginous cap can be up to 1cm in children, and about 2-3 mm in adults.
- If osteochondroma changes into malignant, it usually changes to chondrosarcoma (less than 1% (extremely rare) in isolated lesion and about 10% in MHE)
- **Multiple Hereditary Exostosis (MHE):**
  - o Autosomal dominant condition.
  - o Upper extremity can show: ulnar shortening, radial bowing, subluxation of the radiocapitellar joint or the radial head in PRUJ (see Fig 12).
  - o Radiographs: metaphyseal widening and sessile lesions. XR of the forearm can show the above deformities (see Fig 12).
  - o Possibility of change of malignant transformation: about 10%, when this happen, the most common malignant tumor is chondrosarcoma (Secondary chondrosarcoma of low grade).
  - o Most cases are due to mutation of EXT1 or EXT2 (less common EXT3).
    - ▪ Cases that are due to mutation of EXT1 have more affection, more deformity and higher incidence of malignant changes than EXT2.
    - ▪ EXT1/EXT2 are the tumor suppressor genes.

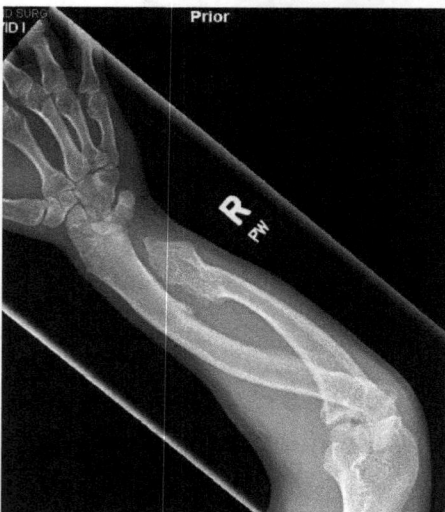

Fig 12: 14 year's old boy with MHE. Notice the multiple sessile osteochondromas, ulnar shortening and radial bowing.

Enchondroma:

- A common bone benign tumor.
- Radiographs will show the characteristic "rings and arch".
- Histology: cartilage tissue, few mature chondrocyte (hand lesions are more cellular than lesions in other areas of the body).
- Treatment: observation if accidently discovered.
  - In the hand: treatment is curettage and bone grafting especially if there pathological fracture.
- Enchondroma Vs chondrosarcoma:
  - Clinical presentation and imaging are more important than the microscopic appearance in differentiating enchondroma from chondrosarcoma.
    - With enchondroma there is no bone destruction, minimal endosteal scalloping (less than 50% of the cortex is eroded)
    - Both can be hot in bone scan.
    - Enchondroma: usually are not painful unless there is pathological fracture (pain can be due to other pathology (eg rotator cuff tear or AC joint injury) *(Scenario: 20 years old, shoulder injury during wrestling, XR shows calcification in the proximal humerus with no scalloping or bony destruction, no history of pain prior to trauma, diagnosis?) (Scenario: 40 years, knee injury, XR circumscribed intramedullary lesion with calcification, MRI no destruction of the cortex, no history of knee pain prior to trauma, treatment? (observation and follow up XR)) (Scenario: 75 years old, shoulder pain with overhead activities, positive Howkin sign, XR shows well circumscribed lesion with calcification, no bone destruction and no cortex erosion, reason of shoulder pain? (RC pathology))*
- **Multiple Enchondromatosis (Ollier's Disease):**
  - Non hereditary.
  - About 10-30% chance of life time malignant change to chondrosarcoma.
  - **Maffucci's syndrome**: is a form of enchondromatosis associated with subcutaneous and deep hemangiomas. The risk of malignancy is about 100% (however, in most cases it is not in the form of sarcomatous transformation of an enchondroma, but it is from internal organ malignancy).

Chondroblastoma:

- Pathology:
  - Epiphyseal (or apophyseal lesion).
  - Microscopically: chondroblasts with grooved nuclei ("coffee-bean nuclei") with surrounding chondroid matrix. There is areas of fine mineralization outlining the stromal cells (chicken-wire or cobblestone appearance)
- Clinical presentation:
  - In young age (usually before closure of the physis).

      o Joint pain, well localized (chondroblastoma usually causes inflammation of the surrounding tissues).
- The MRI scan will show extensive bone edema surrounding the lesion, consistent with chondroblastoma (painful condition).
- Treatment: intra-lesional excision (curettage and bone grafting).

Chondromyxoid Fibroma
- Pathology: 3 components microscopically: spindle cells with a myxoid cartilaginous matrix.
- Lytic eccentric lesion with thin reactive bone surrounding it; which differs from NOF in that:
  - Usually painful.
  - More locally aggressive.
- Common in the upper tibia (anterior cortex) (metaphyseal/diaphyseal area).
- Imaging: Scalloped lytic lesion surrounded by minimal sclerotic rim, locally aggressive, poor border delineation (differential diagnosis NOF).
- Treatment is curettage.

Langerhans Cell Histiocytosis (LCH) (Histiocytosis X):
- Neoplasm of the Langerhans cell.
  - The electron microscope picture will show tennis like-racquet shaped cytoplasmic organelles called Birbeck granules (diagnostic of LCH).
  - **CD1A** immunohistochemistry is very specific for Langerhans' cell in Langerhans cell histiocytosis.
- Langerhans Cell Histiocytosis (LCH) is the new name of group of conditions in the past including:
  - Eosinophilic granulomas: solitary or few, indolent and chronic lesions of bone.
  - Hand-Schuller-Christian disease: multifocal, chronic involvement with classical triad of diabetes insipidus, proptosis, and lytic bone lesions.
  - Letterer-Siwe disease: acute, fulminate, disseminated disease.
  - Hashimoto-Pritzker disease: congenital, self-limiting condition.
- Common in young age (most commonly in children under 10 years). _(Scenario: One-year-old with swelling of the forearm, XR shows osteolytic lesion, diagnosis?)_
- Pathology:

- o Sheets of Langerhan's cells with varying amounts of lymphocytes, PMN cells, **eosinophils** and giant cells (eosinophils are not the neoplasm cell in LCH) (See Fig 13).
  - o Histiocytes have large indented nuclei (coffee bean).
  - o Can occur in the diaphysis or metaphysis of long bone.
  - o Most common bone affected is the skull.
- Imaging:
  - o Osteolytic "punched-out" lesion
    - Can appear well-demarcated or permeative/ aggressive with less defined border.
    - The lesion may cause endosteal scalloping or a periosteal reaction.
    - The lesion arises from the medulla of the bone (central).
    - Can look very similar to other lesions (osteomyelitis, Ewing sarcoma, leukemia).
- In the spine: causes classic vertebral collapse (vertebra plana)
- Treatment:
  - o One lesion: observation, or steroid injection, rarely curettage (**the lesion usually heal spontaneously**). *(Scenario: 5 years old, lytic bone lesion, biopsy shows lesion with esinophilic cells, treatment? (observation))*
  - o Multiple lesion or extra skeletal affection: chemotherapy.
  - o Vertebra plana: treatment observation or brace.

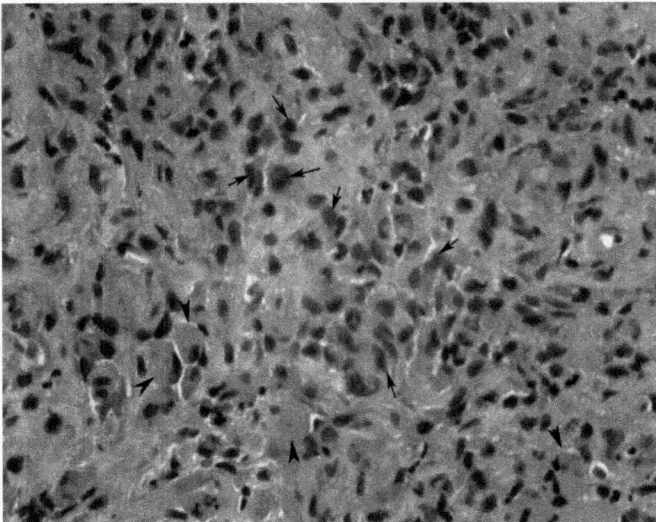

Fig 13: Langerhans cell histiocytosis. The tumor is composed of proliferating Langerhans cells (arrows) in an inflammatory background with predominance of eosinophils (arrowheads). Langerhans cells show elongated or vesicular nuclei and some may show prominent nucleoli. This is an image taken from Hematoxylin and Eosin stained slide (original magnification X400) (Courtesy of Dr Nawar Hakim).

Giant Cell Tumor of The Bone:

- Pathology:

- o Occurs in relatively young age, in the majority of the cases it occurs after closure of the physis.
- o Microscopically: very characteristic appearance of large, multinucleated giant cells in a field of smaller mononuclear stromal cells that look similar to the nuclei of the giant cells (Fig 14).
- o The neoplastic cells in the giant cell tumor are the mononuclear stromal cell (not the giant cell).
  - The osteoclast-like giant cells are directed through the receptor activator of nuclear factor kappa-beta ligand (RANKL) pathway to induce lytic bone destruction seen in this tumor, but the stromal cells are the neoplastic component.
- o Common around the knee and distal radius; can also occur in the sacrum.
- o Despite it is benign; it can metastasize to lung (2% risk of benign pulmonary metastasis in all cases and 6% risk in recurrent cases).
- XR: osteolytic lesion can reach to the subchondral bone.
- Management:
  - o Initial management is biopsy.
  - o Definitive treatment: excision (extended intra-lesional curettage) together with graft or cement application (not mere cement application).
  - o If there is marked collapse of the subchondral bone, curettage and bone grafting may not be possible; in this case, the treatment will be resection with osteochondral allograft. *(Scenario: middle age (30 years old), wrist pain, XR: osteolytic lesion in the radius reaching all the way to the wrist joint, diagnosis? initial treatment? Other study needed? (CT chest)) (Scenario: 25 years old, knee pain of 3 months, XR osteolytic lesion in the distal femur (or proximal tibia) reaching all the way to the subchondral bone), diagnosis?)*
  - o Local recurrence is about 10%

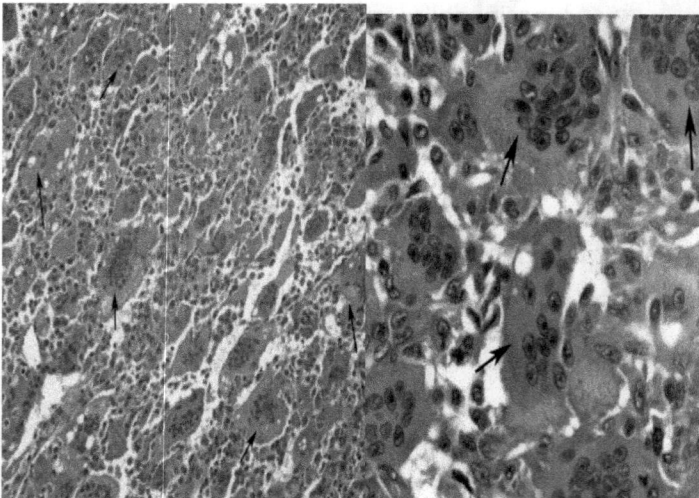

Fig 14: Giant cell tumor of the proximal tibia of a 37 year old male. Left: The tumor shows numerous multinucleated giant cells (black arrows) with mononuclear cells proliferating between the giant cells as part of the tumor (Hematoxylin and Eosin stain; magnification X100). Right: High-power view. Some of the giant cells contain numerous nuclei (black arrows) (magnification X400) (Courtesy of Dr Nawar Hakim)

Synovial lesions:
Pigmented Villo-Nodular Synovitis (PVNS):
- Pathology:
  - Knee is the most commonly affected joint.
  - Microscopically: hemosiderin pigment inside the macrophages.
- Clinical presentation:
  - Middle age.
  - Joint pain and swelling, pain increases with activity and can be alleviated by rest. Classically, the patient will complain of intermittent swelling and pain.
  - Recurrent **hemorrhagic effusion** (aspiration reveals bloody or brownish fluid.). *(Scenario: ankle pain for 6 months, intermittent swelling, XR osteolytic changes on both sides of the joint, biopsy shows hemosiderin, diagnosis?)*
- Radiographs: osteolytic changes on both sides of the joint.
- MRI:
  - Intra-articular nodular masses
  - Low signal intensity in both T1, T2 (characteristic)..
  - Affection of the posterior compartment of the knee.
    - The combination of low-signal intensity areas intra-articular lesions with or without osseous destruction is diagnostic of pigmented villonodular synovitis.
- **Treatment:**
  - Synovectomy
    - Synovectomy (complete) can be arthroscopic or open.
    - Diffuse disease will usually require anterior arthroscopic removal combined with posterior open resection (open resection can give lower recurrence rate that arthroscopic)
    - Recurrent resistant cases may need arthroplasty or radiation
  - Localized PVNS can be treated with localized excision (no need for complete synovectomy or radiation). Most common location for the localized lesion is the anterior knee.

Synovial Chondromatosis:
- Clinical presentation: pain and swelling of the involved joint with possible locking (most common affected joint is the knee).
- Radiographs: multiple calcified masses (loose calcified bodies) in the joint
- MRI: multiple loose bodies.
- Microscopically: benign chondroid tissue (bi-nuclear cells) surrounded by synovial tissue.

- Treatment: complete synovectomy and removal of the loose bodies. *(Scenario: 45 years old, ankle pain and swelling, XR: calcification within the joint, MRI multiple loose bodies, diagnosis?) (Scenario: 25 years old, 18 months' history of hip pain, stiffness and locking, CT shows small ossified masses around the femoral neck, diagnosis?)*

Synovial Sarcoma (see later)

Soft Tissue Sarcoma (STS):
General Rules of STS:

- MRI scan of most STS will show similar picture (low signal intensity on T1 and high signal intensity on T2.)
- Histology is the main method to distinguish between different types.
- Within STS: TIMP (Tissue inhibitor of metalloproteinases) activity is low and MMP (matrix metalloproteinases) and vascular endothelial growth factor are high (this will allow the tumor to invade tissues and metastasize).
- Five soft-tissue sarcomas that can frequently metastasize to the lymph nodes: rhabdomyosarcoma, synovial sarcoma, epithelioid sarcoma, clear cell sarcoma, angiosarcoma.
  - Careful evaluation of lymph node spread and/or sentinel lymph node biopsy plays a role in disease staging and prognosis for these tumors.
  - Lung is the most common site for metastasis for STS (even for the above 5 tumors).
- Synovial sarcoma and rhadomysamrcoma are the most common STS in adolescents and young adults.
- Treatment: **radiation and surgery (wide excision)**.
  - Lesions that are superficial, low-grade lesions, < than 5 cm: can be treated by wide local excision with no need for adjuvant radiotherapy.
  - Lesions that are > 5 cm, high-grade, or deep to fascia: treated by a combination of radiation and surgery.
  - Sarcoma removed without adequate margin (e.g. was thought to be benign lesion (unplanned excision)) is treated with re-resection (if possible). Radiation therapy is generally indicated in these cases. The radiation is used to eliminate microscopic contamination.
    - The most common impact of an unplanned excision is wound complications. This is because of the need for a wider surgical resection and adjuvant radiation.
  - Radiation therapy:

- Pre-operative radiation has the advantage of decreasing the field of radiation and overall radiation dose (5,000 cGy versus 6,600 cGy). The disadvantage is increased wound complication rate (up to 35%).
        - Postoperative radiation has the disadvantage of increased dose applied to a larger treatment field (higher incidence of fibrosis and lymphedema). It has the advantage of lower wound complication rates (about 17% (about half of the pre-operative complication rate)).
        - No significant difference in local recurrence rate between pre and post operative radiation therapy.
    o For STS with resectable pulmonary metastasis or solitary pulmonary metastasis discovered after removal of the tumor, resection of the pulmonary metastasis can be done to improve survival and provide control of the disease.
    o Chemotherapy is not used for treatment of most soft-tissue sarcomas (except rhabdomyosarcoma and soft-tissue Ewing sarcoma).
- Post-radiation fractures: lower extremity STS that were treated with irradiation can develop pathological fracture (average 3-4 years after irradiation).
    o Periosteal excision (during the primary surgery) was found to be a risk factor for fracture after irradiation.

Common Types of Soft Tissues Sarcomas:

- **Malignant Fibrous Histiocytoma (Undifferentiated Pleomorphic Sarcoma) (MFH):**
    o Most common soft tissue sarcoma.
    o Heterogenous picture in MRI.
    o Microscope: multiple atypia.
- **Fibrosacroma:**
    o Microscope: Herringbone pattern (Fig 15).

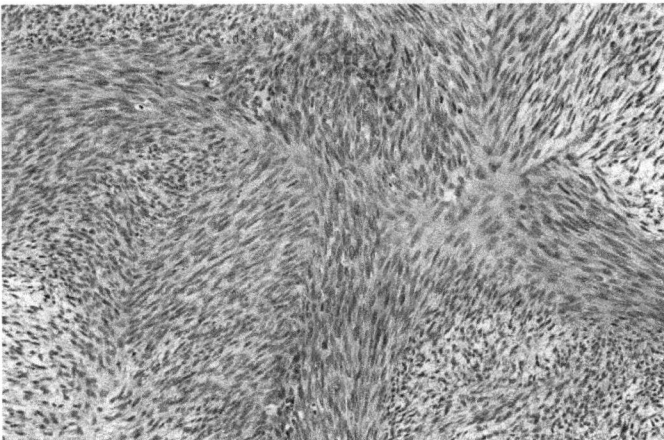

Fig 15: showing high magnification micrograph of the herringbone pattern in a malignant peripheral nerve sheath tumour (from Wikipedia https://en.wikipedia.org/wiki/Fibrosarcoma)

- **Liposarcoma:**
  - Clinical presentation: middle age, slowly growing mass that recently became painful.
  - Microscopically:
    - Lipoblasts (the characteristic cells of liposarcoma): smaller than mature adipocytes, have round, sharply demarcated cytoplasmic lipid (clear) vacuoles (globules) which scallop the nucleus (smaller than vacuoles of mature adipocytes).
    - Myxoid liposarcoma: myxoid background and an interlacing network of fine vessels.
  - MRI: Most of the lesions will have similar appearance of subcutaneous fat with small areas of different signal.
    - T1-weighted: bright signal.
    - Gadolinium with fat suppression: dark signal (from the fat saturation), with some areas of enhancement (other elements of the tumor other than the fat).
    - T2-weighted image: most of tumor will have low signal (as subcutaneous fat) with areas of brightness due edematous tissue within the mass.
    - Difference between lipoma and liposarcoma in the MRI: presence of thick septa and associated nonadipose masses increase the likelihood that the MRI is of liposarcoma and not simple lipoma.
  - **Well-differentiated liposarcoma (WDL)/ atypical lipomatous tumor (ALT):**
    - Lesions with a moderate chance of local recurrence than for ordinary lipoma (up to 50%) with minimal distant metastatic potential.
    - Similar appearance in MRI as regular lipoma (differs than the MRI picture of liposarcoma).
    - Microscopically: mature adipocytes with minimal atypia.
    - Cytogenetic testing (in cases of ALT): supernumerary ring and/or giant rod chromosomes, amplification of the MDM2 oncogene.
    - Lesions in the posterior neck, shoulders and upper back are usually regular lipomas.
- **Leiomyosarcoma:**
  - Pathology: positive immunostaining of smooth muscle actin.
- **Synovial sarcoma:**
  - Can be associated with translocation t(X:18).
  - Epidemiology:
    - Occurs in relatively young patients (3-5 decade).
    - Most common STS to mineralize (calcify).

- Most common STS of the foot and ankle.
- Most common upper extremity soft tissue sarcoma in patients 16-25 years old.
  - XR may show calcification.
  - One of the STS with frequent lymph node metastasis, but lung is still the most common site of metastasis.
  - Histology: Two cell populations: spindle cell and epithelioid (looks glandular).
  - Stains positive for EMA, S-100.
- **Epithelioid sarcoma:**
  - More common in young adults
  - Common in hand (and foot).
    - Most common sarcoma in hand.
  - One of the STS that has frequent metastasis to local lymph node.
  - The tumors can be superficial and may become ulcerated. Deeper lesions are often attached to tendons, tendon sheaths, or fascial structures.
- **Lymphangiosarcomas:**
  - Aggressive angiosarcoma which may arise in a pre-existing lymphedema (Stewart-Treves syndrome: a rare, deadly cutaneous angiosarcoma that develops in long-standing chronic lymphedema)
- **Rhabdomyosarcoma:**
  - More common in pediatric patient.
  - Microscopically: small round blue cell, Desmin positive.
  - Treatment: wide resection of the primary tumor, chemotherapy (responsive to chemotherapy), and radiation therapy.
- **Dermatofibrosarcoma protuberans (DFSP)**
  - Most tumors are superficial and less than 5 cm. Tumor can fungate over a long period of time presenting early as pink plaques surrounded by small capillaries.
  - t(17;22) translocation with the gene PDGFB to the collagen 1 alpha gene.
  - Histologically, the tumor is composed of uniform fibroblasts arranged in a storiform pattern. CD34 positive.
- **Clear cell sarcoma (malignant melanoma of soft tissue)**
  - Compact nests of cells with a clear cytoplasm surrounded by a delicate border of fibrocollagenous tissue with scattered multinucleated giant cells.
  - Positive for S-100 and HMB45 (a melanoma-associated antigen).

Marjolin Ulcer:
- Malignant tumor arising in chronic wounds (usually takes about 20-30 years)

- Pathology: squamous cell carcinoma (not sarcoma). Malignant squamous cells with characteristic keratin pearl (amorphous pink material).

Benign Soft Tissue Tumors:
Desmoids Fibroma (Desmoids Fibromatosis) (Fibromatosis) (Extra Abdominal Desomid):
- Benign lesion with high recurrence rate.
- Pathology:
  - Microscopically: fibroblasts and myofibroblasts (spindle-cell lesion) in a collagenous matrix with low mitotic activity.
  - **Beta Catenin positive**.
  - Very hard lesion with infiltrative nature.
- MRI: Dark in T1 and T2. It has ill-defined invasive-infiltrative nature with marked enhancement with gadolinium administration.
- Treatment:
  - Wide surgical resection. Surgeon has to warn the patient regarding the high recurrence rate.
  - Estrogen receptor inhibitors have been used to treat desmoids tumors.

Nerve Sheath Tumor (Neurofibroma And Schwannoma (Neurilemmoma))
- Exquisite tenderness is a characteristic finding of benign nerve sheath tumors.
- Schwannoma (Neurilemmoma):
  - Benign nerve sheath tumor. Well-encapsulated lesion located on the surface of a peripheral nerve (eccentrically located within the nerve) and encapsulated by the perineurium.
  - Located within the nerve sheath.
  - Usually solitary lesions (in contrast to neurofibromas).
  - Clinical presentation: painful mass (exquisite tenderness); paresthesias or numbness without significant weakness. A positive Tinel's sign in the distribution of the affected nerve.
  - Pathology:
    - Well encapsulated on the surface of a peripheral nerve (nerve sheath tumor).

- Histology shows benign nerve elements including verocay bodies with Antoni A (more cellular) and Antoni B (less cellular, loose myxoid regions) areas.
- Microscopically, Antoni A (a pattern of spindle cells arranged in intersecting bundles) and Antoni B (areas with less cellularity with loosely arranged cells).
- Malignant transformation is exceedingly rare.
  - MRI have characteristic appearance:
    - Target sing: hyperintensity in the periphery while hypointensity in the center on T2-weighted images (due to compactly packed cellular Antoni A regions which is in the central part and loose myxomatous Antoni B regions in the peripheral part).
    - String sign: the eccentric peripheral nerve entering and leaving the lesion resembling a string
  - Treatment: **Marginal excision** with preservation of the associated nerve fibers is the treatment of choice for symptomatic schwannomas (low recurrence rate).
    - Schwannoma are usually easier to remove than neurofibroms.
      (Scenario: swelling in the posteromedial ankle, positive Tinel's sign, treatment?)
- **Neurofibroma:**
  - Neurofibroma is a spindle cell tumor arising within a peripheral nerve (new studies shows it also arise from Schwann cell, but it behave different than Schwannoma)
    - Microscopy: a wavy collagenous matrix ("rope-like") with elongated cells.
    - S100 positive.
  - Can be solitary or multiple (associated with neurofibromatosis type I (NF1) (von Recklinghausen's disease)) (see general condition chapter)
    - In cases of NF1: malignant transformation of a lesion can occur in about 5% of patients (changes to malignant peripheral nerve sheath tumor (MPNST)). While in cases of solitary lesions, malignant transformation is very rare.
  - Treatment: This tumor is more invasive than Schwannoma, so it will require removal of the affected nerve (causing distal nerve affection) (recent studies shows that neurofibromas can also be managed with marginal excision with acceptable recurrence rates).

Lipoma:

- Common types: subcutaneous, subfascial, submuscluar.

- Same signal of the subcutaneous fat in all MRI sequence.
- Angio-lipomal: can be painful (in contrary to other lipomas).
- Management:
    o Large lipoma: excisional biopsy (if you do incision biopsy you may miss small areas of malignant tissue).

Hemangioma:
- Symptoms are intermittent "wax and wane".
- XR may show calcification of the lesion.
- Treatment options: observation, or injection of sclerosis agent (depending on the severity of the condition) (surgical excision has high local recurrence rate). *(Scenario: 30-year-old with a mass on shoulder for the few months which is **intermittently** painful, swelling comes and goes, especially after exercises, icing relieve symptoms, diagnosis?)*

Giant Cell Tumor of Tendon Sheath
- More common in the hands and feet, more common in the palmar/plantar aspect.
    o Associated with decreased ROM for the affected digit. It can become fixed to the underlying bone.
- The tumor has a yellowish-brown color and lobulated areas.
- XR may show bone erosion.
- Microscopically: fibrous stroma with giant cells, histiocytes, and hemosiderin deposition (similar in histology to PVNS).

Elastofibroma:
- Benign lesion, likely inflammatory mass.
- Stains positive for elastin.
- Most common location is deep to the inferior angle of the scapula, sometimes it may occur bilateral.
- Clinical presentation: pain or mechanical symptoms related to its location.
- Treatment: if the lesion is symptomatic, treatment is by excision

Tumor Like Conditions:
Myositis Ossificans

- Lesion in the soft tissue that is more ossified at the periphery than the central part "Zonation Phenomenon" (more mature in the periphery). Separated from the cortex of the bone.
- History of muscle trauma few weeks/ months (e.g. arm wrestling, tackling in football game), followed by appearance of hard mass in the muscle.
- Treatment: most cases can be managed by observation.

Tumoral Calcinosis:
- A hereditary disease of phosphate metabolism (with other renal anomalies).
- Large soft-tissue calcification mass: lobulated, well-demarcated calcification distributed most commonly around the extensor surface of large joints.
- XR: amorphous, cystic, and multilobulated calcification.
- CT can better delineate the mass and will show NO Erosion or osseous destruction

Melorheostosis
- Rare tumor like condition characterized by the classic radiographic appearance of flowing hyperostosis in a long bone "wax falling down the side of a candle".
- This hyperostosis may be on the periosteal or endosteal surface of the bone.

Bone infarcts:
- Opaque patches in the medulla (the diaphysis of long bones) without bony destruction. Most cases are asymptomatic and discovered accidently in the radiographs.
- XR: Central in location (in the medulla of the bones), not expansile, with a characteristic "smoke up the chimney" picture.

Cortical Desmoids (Periosteal Desmoid or Tug Lesion)
- Cortical irregularity reactive-type lesion in the posteromedial aspect of the distal femur, can be bilateral, may be related to microtrauma due to pulling of the adductor magnus or medial gastrocnemius muscle.
- Common in adolescent, usually resolve by the age of 20 years.
- No soft tissue lesion or bone destruction.
- No treatment is required.

Cat Scratch Disease

- Benign and self-limiting illness (lasts about 6 to 12 weeks if no antibiotic therapy was administrated).
- Bartonella Henselae is the proposed etiological agent.
- Clinical presentation:
  - A primary cutaneous lesion about 1-cm papule or pustule at the site of a cat scratch or bite about 3-10 days after the incident.
  - 7-14 days after the onset the skin lesion: development of tender lymphadenopathy (axillary, **epitrochlear**, inguinal). The lymph node can become suppurative.
- **Criteria for diagnosis:**
  - History of cat scratch, positive skin-test to CSD test antigen, characteristic lymph node lesions; and negative laboratory test for other causes of lymphadenopathy.
  - Diagnosis can be made with three of the above four.
- Treatment: medical treatment by antibiotics (eg azithromycin, ciprofloxacin).

Baker's cyst (see Pediatric Chapter)

Ganglion (See Hand Chapter).

Glomus Tumor (see Hand Chapter)

Metastasis:
- **Basic Science:**
  - Metastasis is a complex cascade of events including invasion (of the blood vessels), intravasation, dissemination, extravasation (at the distant site of the metastasis), and tumor-cell proliferation at the secondary site.
    - Metarix Metaproteinase (MMPs) are matrix-degrading enzymes that increase the permeability of the basement membrane, allowing cancer cell invasion and metastasis to occur
    - Integrin is a Cell Adhesion Molecule (CAM) expressed by tumor cells that allows the tumor cell to adhere to the endothelial layer of the host at a distant site (in sending metastasis). Integrin promotes tumor cell from distant areas to attach to bone during metastasis.
- 5 most common primaries which send metastases to bone: lung, breast, prostate, kidney, thyroid.
  - Lung cancer bone metastasis has the shortest mean survival.
- If you detect a lytic lesion in elderly:

- o CT chest, abdomen and pelvis, in addition to bone scan (PET scan can be used as an alternative to bone scan especially if there is history of lung cancer).
- Most common site of metastasis is spine (thoracic spine) (see later).
- Most common primary to metastasis to hand is lung carcinoma.
- Blastic metastasis (radio-opaque in the radiographs): can be of prostate or breast origin. *(Scenario: 80 years old male, pelvic pain, XR and CT scan show multiple blastic lesions in the bone,) what is the source of metastasis? (prostate)).*
- A new lesion in a patient with known remote history of carcinoma but without established bone disease needs to be evaluated before stabilization (CT chest, abdomen and pelvis/ bone scan).
    - o In 15% of cases, the new lesion will not be related to the previous pathology.
    - o Do not assume that the new bone lesion is metastatic disease from the remote history malignancy. *(Scenario: breast cancer 5 years ago, now pain in the hip, XR osteolytic lesion, next step? (CT chest, abdomen and pelvis)).*
    - o If patient presents with multiple bone lesion (multiple bone metastasis), no need for separate biopsy procedure (biopsy can be obtained at the time of stabilization). However, if the patient present with one lytic lesion, and body CT could not detect a lesion, biopsy of the bone lesion is needed before fixation/reconstructive surgery.
    - o History, physical examination, and CT chest, abdomen and pelvis will identify 85% of primary lesions; biopsy is needed when the primary lesion cannot be identified (see above).
- Microscopy of metastatic carcinoma: epithelial cells in a fibrous stroma.
- Bone resorption by metastasis (to create lytic space) is through the common pathway for RANKL activation (see basic science Chapter)
- **Renal cell carcinoma:**
    - o Occasionally renal cell carcinoma can have solitary bone metastasis. In this case the lesion (the bone metastasis) may be amenable to reconstruction (the prognosis is better with solitary lesion but still not as good as a primary bone lesion).
        - Solitary renal cell carcinoma metastasis can be managed by excision and reconstruction.
        - Wide resection of isolated renal cell carcinoma metastasis can improve long-term survival (even if the primary was removed few years before).
    - o Renal cell metastases are very vascular. Pre surgical embolization can help decrease bleeding.
        - Metastatic renal cell carcinoma should have embolization before surgery (excision or fracture fixation).

- Chemotherapy is directed to inhibit the vascular endothelial growth factor (VEGF) pathways (tyrosine kinase inhibitors).
  - Response to radiotherapy is unpredictable (often it is radio-resistant).
  - Patient over age 50 years with hematuria and a large osteolytic bone lesion: this most probably a bony metastasis form renal cell carcinoma.
- **Breast cancer metastasis:**
  - Mixed lytic and blastic lesions.
  - Better prognosis with metastasis which are estrogen and progesterone receptor positive and HER-2 negative (HER-2-positive tumors are less responsive).
- **Prostate cancer metastasis:**
  - Usually (but not always) blastic.
  - Very hot in bone scan.
- **Treatment:**
  - **Radiation therapy (the whole segment):**
    - Help with pain control.
    - Radioactive strontium 89 (89Sr) is used in the treatment of metastatic blastic carcinoma for relief of bone pain. 89Sr is similar to calcium and highly absorbed by osteogenic metastasis.
  - **Bisphosphante:**
    - Significantly reduces metastatic bone pain in about 50% of patients with bony metastasis.
    - Reduces hypercalcemia and bone loss.
    - Reduce the incidence of new bony metastasis.
    - Delays the initial onset of bone complications (time to the first skeletal-related event).
    - Prevent an increase in size of existing bony metastasis lesions.
    - For patient with metastatic diseases on bisphosphante: the incidence of osteonecrosis of the jaw is very small (about 2.5%). Risk factors include longer length of treatment (the most important risk factor), the type of bisphosphonate and previous dental procedures.
  - **Possible prophylactic fixation:**
    - Prophylactic fixation of long bones is recommended for patients with Mirels' score higher than 8 and considered for patient with score of 8.
    - If surgery is done, postoperative irradiation should include that whole operated area to avoid seeding of the hematoma with the metastasis.
    - Preoperative embolization should be used for highly vascular lesions (e.g renal and thyroid metastases) to decrease bleeding.

- Locked nails should be used for long bones (to protect the whole bones).
    - Subtrochanteric pathological fracture (due to metastasis) is treated by statically locked cephalo-medullary long nail.
    - Femoral neck pathological fractures will require prosthetic replacement (not fixation).
    - If patient with metastasis develop hypercalcemia: hydration (with furosemide), bisphosphonates, and evaluation for cardiac arrhythmia. (see general disease chapter/hypercalcemia)

- **Mirels' scoring system:**

	1	2	3
Site	Upper extremity	Lower extremity	peritrochanteric
Pain	Mild	Moderate	Severe
Lesion	Blastic	Mixed	Lytic
Size of the lesion	<1/3 of diameter of bone	1/3-2/3 of diameter of bone	>2/3 of diameter of bone

- **Spine metastasis:**
    - Imaging:
        - 30-50% of cancellous bone must be destroyed before changes can be seen on plain radiographs.
        - "Winking owl" sign: disappearance of one of the two pedicles, indicative of metastasis destruction of the pedicle.
        - After obtaining initial radiographs, the next step is to obtain an MRI with gadolinium (will show possible compression over the cord). (*Scenario: 60 years old, 6 months of mid back pain, increasing, XR diffuse osteopenia and winking eye, next step?*).
    - Management:
        - If no compression over the cord (no neurological manifestations): the treatment is radiation therapy.
        - Patients with metastatic lesion to the vertebral bodies and cord compression (progressive neurological manifestation): the treatment is anterior decompression and instrumented stabilization followed by radiotherapy. Posterior instrumentation can be added to the construct.
            - Radiation therapy alone or radiation followed by surgery lead to inferior outcomes.
            - A patient with a progressive neurologic deficit should have surgery before radiotherapy.
    - Factors associated with instability of the spine due to metastasis: junctional level (C7-T2), osteolytic lesions, and vertebral collapse.

Tips:

- If you see pathology of round cell tumor: think mainly lymphoma (adult) or Ewing (children).
- Osteolytic lesion in the subchondral bone (epiphyseal): chondroblastoma (open physis) or giant cell tumor (closed physis) or clear cell chondrorsarcoma (elderly in the femoral head).
- Lytic lesion in the proximal humerus in elderly, think in chondrosarcoma.
- Lytic lesion mildly expanding the bone in a child in the proximal humerus with a non-displaced pathological fracture, think in UBC, treatment is observation.
- Young patient, ground glass, pathology shows Chinese letter appearance: think in fibrous dysplasia.
- Bone lesion in the posterior spine (lamina), think in osteoblastoma, osteoid osteoma, or ABC.
- Recurrent hemorrhagic effusion: think in PVNS
- Swelling with Tinel's sign, think in Neurolemmoma.
- NOF can be confused by chondromyxoid fibroma (NOF is surrounded by more dense sclerosis).
- Multiple osteolytic lesions in young patient: think in LCH; in adult think in MM.
- Sacral lesion: think in chordoma (midline, most common), GCT (partially to the side) and Mets.
- Lesions which can be treated by injection: UBC, esinophilic granuloma.
- Lesion which can be treated by curettage and bone graft or curettage/cement: giant cell tumor, chondroblastoma, osteoblastoma, chondromyxoid fibroma, aneurysmal bone cyst.
- Malignant bone tumor treated wide surgical resection alone (without chemo): chondrosarcoma, adamantinoma, parosteal osteosarcoma.
- Pelvis diffuse lesion: think in Paget's or blasic metastasis.
- Lesion which can be (sometimes) treated by radiation alone: primary lymphoma of bone, chordoma, solitary plasmacytoma, and Ewing sarcoma.
- **Solitary** lytic bone lesion in elderly with impending fracture: chose CT (chest, abdomen and pelvis) or biopsy if you do not have a diagnosis (do not NAIL it).
- Soft tissue tumors of the wrist: think in ganglion cysts, giant-cell tumors of tendon sheath, and synovial sarcoma.
- Foot/ankle lesion: think in synovial sarcoma, giant cell tumor of tendon sheath.
- Soft tissue mass in children with calcification; think in hemangioma.
- Pelvic or acetabular lesion in elderly patient: think in chondrosarcoma (especially if there is calcification).

- Metaphyseasl lesion in adolescent with bone erosion and new bone formation: think in osteosarcoma
- Lesion behind the scapula in a female patient 50-70 years old: think in elastofibroma (or less commonly lipoma).
- Benign tumors that need wide excision: desmoid tumor.
- Most common soft-tissue sarcoma in the hand/wrist: epithelioid sarcoma.
- S-100 positive: think in nerve tumor (Neurofibroma And Schwannoma), melanoma (clear cell), synovial sarcoma.
- Multiple osteolytic lesion with general disease that decrease calcium (e.g. malabsorption): think in secondary hyperparathyroidism with brown tumor.
- Fluid level in the MRI: think in ABC
- Lesion that is similar to fat is all MRI sequence: lipomatous lesion (lipoma, atypical lipomatous tumor, or low-grade liposarcoma. Treatment is marginal excision (excisional biopsy) (incisional biopsies of these fatty tumors can lead to diagnosic errors, excisional biopsies are the preferred ones).
- Lyic benign asymptotic lesion in a child: think NOF (eccentric, sclerotic margins). UBC is central lesion usually involving the whole width of the bone (without bone expansion) and may cause pathological fracture.
- History of exposure to cat exposure and elbow lymph node enlargement: think in CSD.
- Coffee bean nuclei: LCH and chondroblastoma
- CD: CD99: positive for Ewings; CD34: positive for Dermatofibrosarcoma protuberans; CD 20 positive for lymphoma; CD1A immunohistochemistry positive for Langerhans cell histiocytosis.

Chapter 8: **The Hip**

Imaging:

- The AP pelvic and false-profile views: acetabular pathology (version, coverage assessment, arthritis). False profile view shows the anterior coverage.
- The lateral views (frog-lateral, cross-table): cam lesion of the proximal femur.
- Radiographic findings of hip pathology:
  - Dysplasia:
    - Decreased lateral center-edge angles (normal: 25° to 45°).
    - Decreased anterior center-edge angle on a false-profile radiograph (normal > 20°).
    - Increased Sourcil (Tonnis) angle (normal < 10°).
  - Impingement (see later for more details):
    - Cam: increase alpha angle (See Fig 1).
    - Pincer: acetabular retroversion or protrusion.
- dGEMRIC MRI hip can be used to assess articular cartilage GAG content in acetabular dysplasia:
  - It indicates the health of the articular cartilage.
  - Low GAG content has been associated with PAO failure.

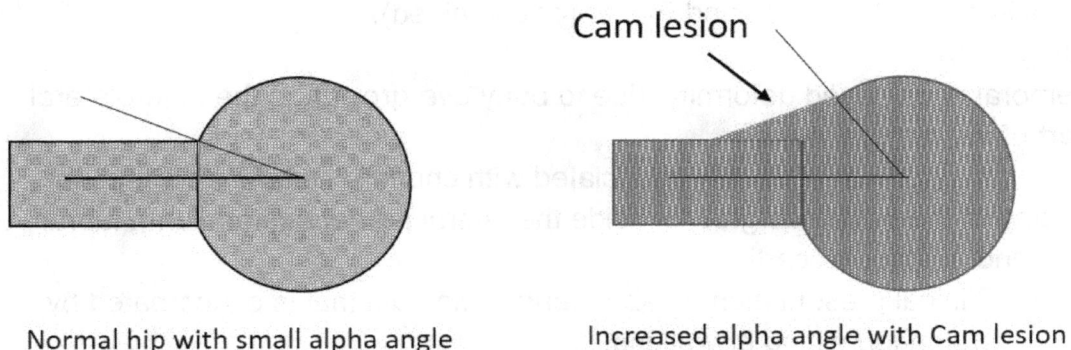

Cam lesion

Normal hip with small alpha angle   Increased alpha angle with Cam lesion

Fig 1: Alpha angle of the hip is the angle between a line from the centre of the femoral head through the middle of the femoral neck and a line through a point where the contour of the femoral head-neck junction exceeds the radius of the femoral head (become non circular). In the cam impingement , the alpha angle is increased (> 55°)

Transient osteoporosis:

- Unknown etiology. Common in **women** in the third trimester of pregnancy and in men in the fifth and sixth decade of life.
- Gradual onset of hip pain with no history of trauma.
- No history of risk factors for AVN (no history of alcoholism or steroid intake).

- o Pain progresses to become severe pain.
- Triad of: sever joint pain, normal XR and CT, and abnormal MRI:
    - o MRI: complete replacement of the marrow signal on T1 weighted images (dark on T1) and increased intensity in T2 of the whole proximal femur (femoral head and neck) (in contrast to AVN which will have focal affection and line of demarcation).
    - o No collapse.
- Self-limiting disease. Treatment is non operative (protected weight bearing and anti-inflammatory drugs).

Femoro-Acetabular Impingement (FAI):

- Abutting the femoral neck against the acetabular edge.
- Clinical presentation:
    - o Patient will complain of pain with activity. The pain is worse with hip flexion, (prolonged sitting, and cycling) and will have positive impingement sign (pain with flexion, **adduction** and internal rotation of the hip).
    - o Decrease range of flexion/ internal rotation of the affected side.
- Two type of impingement: Cam and Pincer (or combined).
- Cam impingement:
    - o Femoral neck based deformity: due to bony overgrowth on the anterolateral part of the femoral neck.
    - o Cam impingement is usually associated with chondro labral lesion (due to forcing of the bone overgrowth inside the lateral part of acetabulum): labral tear and acetabular cartilage delamination.
        - Clinical presentation of labral tear: groin pain that is exacerbated by prolonged sitting or walking.
        - Injury to the acetabular cartilage usually occur in the anterosuperior acetabulum area.
    - o Imaging will show increase alpha angle (Fig 1) (angle at which femoral head leaves the round shape).
        - Normal alpha angle is less than 50°.
        - Other parameters include decreased femoral offset ratio (see fig 1) (normal is > 0.17).
        - XR can show the lesion, but MRI (and MR arthrogram) will better delineate the lesion and show the labral lesion if present.
        - The most sensitive and specific study to detect an acetabular labral tear is an MRI arthrogram of the hip.

- o Initial treatment is non-operative (avoid activities with marked flexion and NSAIDs). If this fails to control the symptoms: treatment is femoral neck osteochondroplasty (and possible labral **repair**) (see sport lower extremity).
    - This can be done either arthroscopically (for small lesions) or by open surgical dislocation for big lesion. The surgical dislocation will require di-gastrics trochanteric flip osteotomy (trochanteric osteotomy with attachment of both the abductors proximally and the vastus lateralis distally to the mobile piece of the trochanter). The capsule will then be open anteriorly in Z pattern to avoid injury to the blood supply of the femoral head.
    - Labrum can be shaved or repaired (repair may lead to better results possibly by improving joint lubrication by creating better sealing effect and preventing egress of synovial fluid from the joint space).
- Pincer impingement:
    - o Acetabular based deformity: either deep acetabulum (eg protusio) or retroverted acetabulum.
        - Retroverted acetabulum will show in pelvis XR as "cross over sign" and prominent ischial spine. (Fig 2). *(Scenario: patient with hip pain and positive impingement sign, what will be XR findings? (either cross over (pincer) or abnormal bony prominence(cam)))*
        - Deep acetabulum: increase lateral center edge angle (normal < 45°).

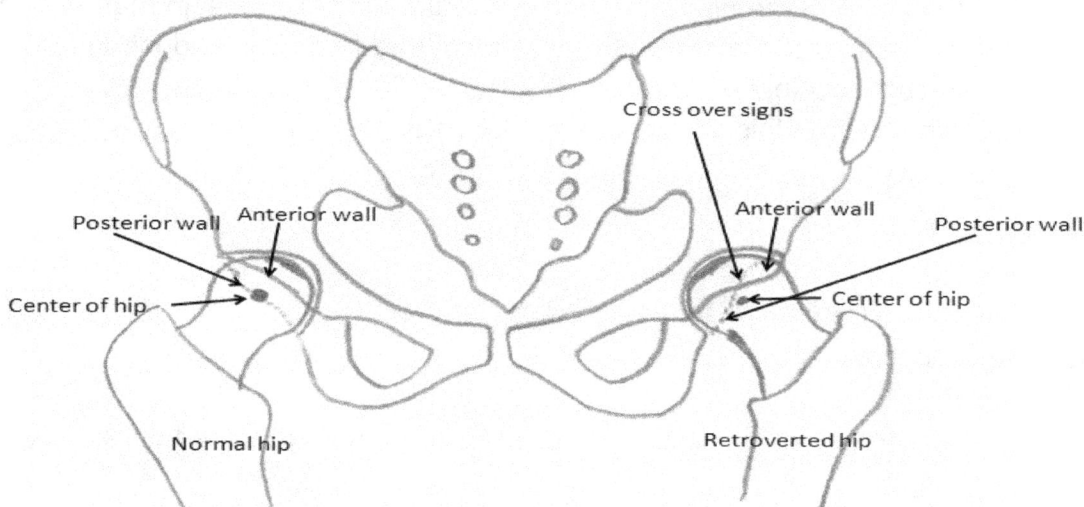

Fig 2: Right hip shows normal version with anterior wall covering about 1/3 of the femoral head and the posterior wall passing close to the center of the head. On the left side, threre is retroversion with corss over sign. The anterior and posterior walls cross each other on the upper part of the femoral head.

- o Treatment:

- Similar to cam impingement. Surgical treatment is by resection of the pincer lesion from the acetabular side to avoid recurrence. If the cause of pincer impingement is retroversion of the acetabulum, osteotomy should be done (reverse Periacetabular osteotomy (reverse PAO)).
- FAI surgery is not indicated if there is established hip joint arthritis.

Hip arthritis:

- Common causes of hip arthritis:
    - Mechanical: hip dysplasia, impingement (common causes of OA).
    - Inflammatory: rheumatoid, Ankylosing Spondylitis.
    - Others: AVN, post LCP, post traumatic.
- Dysplastic hips:
    - Patients with DDH (dysplasia) have the following pathology:
        - Acetabulum: shallow, anteverted, lateralized, and deficient anteriorly, laterally, and superiorly.
        - Femoral head and neck: small head, short anteverted neck, small offset, increased neck-shaft angle, posteriorly placed trochanter, narrow canal.
    - Nerve injury in dysplastic hip undergoing THA: see later (under THA section).
    - In dysplastic hips with high dislocation (Crowe III and IV):
        - Reduction of the hip to the native acetabulum will result in marked lengthening of the extremity. This may lead to difficult reduction of the hip and possible nerve palsy.
        - To overcome this problem: subtrochanteric femoral shortening osteotomy.

Hip osteonecrosis (AVN/ ON)

- The Ficat classification:
    - Stage I:
        - XR: normal, MRI: abnormal signal. Bone scan: increased uptake.
    - Stage II:
        - XR film: mixed osteopenia and/or sclerosis and/or subchondral cysts and lucencies. (No subchondral fracture (crescent sign) or collapse). MRI and bone scan: abnormal.
    - Stage III:
        - XR: crescent sign (Subchondral fracture line) and eventual cortical collapse. MRI: will show the changes seen in XR.

- o Stage IV:
    - XR: Collapse of subchondral bone and severe deformity of the head with secondary degenerative changes **affecting both sides of the joint**.
- MRI:
    - o T1: crescentic, well-defined band of low signal within the superior portion of the femoral head (represent the reactive interface between the necrotic and reparative zones).
    - o T2: the subchondral lesion shows high signal intensity inner border with a low signal intensity peripheral rim (double-line) along with edema extending into the femoral neck.
- The Size of the lesion is the most important factor determining development of symptoms and progression of the disease.
    - o The best prognosis is: small lesions with sclerotic margins.
- Management:
    - o Early diagnosis and intervention improve the chances for the success of head-preservation techniques.
    - o Stage I and II: Hip preservation.
        - Drilling of the lesion, bone graft (autograft, vascularized bone graft or bone substitute) or medical treatment.
        - Bisphosphonates can decrease the risk of collapse and hence decrease pain.
        - Bone grafting can be by vascularized free-fibula bone graft: Donor site morbidities include tibial stress fracture (can be detected by MRI) and ankle instability.
        - If after hip preservation surgery, the femoral head continues to collapse: proceed with arthroplasty.
    - o Stage III and IV: THA.
        - Hemiarthroplasty outcomes are inferior to THA due to acetabular erosion by the femoral head (proximal migration and protrusio).
        - Cementless THA is preferred in cases of AVN of the hip (including cases of sickle cell disease)

AVN of the femoral head in patients with sickle cell disease:

- Untreated AVN of the femoral head in patients with sickle cell disease has more than 75% likelihood of progression to pain and collapse.

- Femoral canal perforation is the most common complication after THA for sickle cell disease (femoral medullary widening from chronic marrow hyperplasia with adjacent patchy areas of dense sclerosis deviating the broaches).
  - Reaming over a guide-wire can be done to avoid perforation.

Resurfacing Hip Arthroplasty:
- Most prostheses are metal on metal implants.
- Indication:
  - Best results in young, male patients with a diagnosis of osteoarthritis.
- Contraindications:
  - Proximal femoral deformity (eg coxa vara) (cannot correct the deformity by resurfacing), femoral bone cyst (poor fixation), osteoporosis of the neck (higher chance of fracture).
- Advantage:
  - Preservation of proximal femoral bone.
  - Lower dislocation rate than conventional arthroplasty and wider ROM (larger head size). *(Question: Advantage of resurfacing?).*
- Disadvantage:
  - Cannot adjust the offset and length compared to conventional THA.
  - Possibility of fracture neck femur (most common cause for early revision).
  - Requires bigger incision and more surgical dissection than conventional THA (due to preserving most of the head).
- Most common cause of re-operation after resurfacing is femoral neck fracture.
- Higher incidence of failure in cases of ON of the femoral head (especially with large necrotic areas).
- For cases of failed resurfacing: treatment is THA.
- Currently is falling out of favor.

Hip Arthrodesis:
- Hip position: 20° to 30° flexion, 0-5° of adduction (avoid abduction), and 5 to 10° of external rotation.
- Hip arthrodesis long term results show pain and degenerative changes of the lumbar spine, ipsilateral knee, and contralateral hip.
- For patients who had hip fusion for long time, and having back pain, ipsi lateral knee pain, contra-lateral hip: the treatment is fusion takedown and conversion to arthroplasty.

- Function of gluteus medius is the most important predictive factor for the ambulatory status after fusion conversion to THA, this can be assessed by EMG.

Hip Dysplasia (see pediatric chapter for hip dysplasia and osteotomies.

Total Hip Arthroplasty (THA):
Nerve Palsy After THA:
- Most commonly affected nerve injury with THA is the peroneal branch of the sciatic nerve (the common peroneal nerve).
    - Sciatic nerve palsy following THA most commonly affects only the common peroneal nerve branch (inability to dorsiflex the ankle causing foot drop), sparing the tibial nerve.
    - Femoral nerve palsy is the second most affected nerve after the sciatic nerve (especially with anterior approaches).
- Risk factors for nerve palsy after THA:
    - evelopmental dysplasia
    - Post-traumatic arthritis
    - leg lengthening by the THA
    - Posterior approach
    - Uncemented arthroplasty
    - Revision surgery
    - Surgeon self-describing the procedure as "difficult"
    - female gender
- Excessive internal rotation of the hip for prolonged periods (during posterior approach) can cause compression of the sciatic nerve by the gluteus maximus tendon.
- Inflammatory arthritis, AVN and obesity are **NOT** risk factors.
- Only about 40% (less than half) of patient with complete peroneal nerve palsy after THA will show complete recovery of the nerve function
- The recovery time is about one year for partial injury and 1.5 years for complete injuries.
- Initial management (for the first year) is ankle foot orthosis (AFO).
    - For patients with peroneal nerve injury: If the patient is not tolerating the AFO, transfer of the posterior tibial tendon (innervated by posterior tibial nerve) through the interosseus membrane to the tibialis anterior muscle or to the mid foot to act as dorsiflexor.

- In DDH, if excessive lengthening of the extremity is expected during THA (in cases of high dislocations): femoral sub trochanteric shortening osteotomy can be done intra-operatively to help protect against post-operative nerve injury.
- Intra operative protection of the nerve: flexing the knee and extending the hip will decrease tension on the nerve.

Dislocation After THA:

- Possible etiologies:
  - Excess anteverted cups:
    - Less anterior coverage, will lead to anterior hip dislocation (with external rotation and extension of the hip).
  - Excess Retroverted cups:
    - Less posterior coverage, will lead to posterior dislocation (with flexion and internal rotation of the hip).
  - Subsidence of the stem:
    - Stem subsidence can lead to hip dislocation (due to loss of abductor muscle tension and strength). *(Scenario: dislocation few months after THA, immediate post-surgery XR and post reduction XR shows the stem had subsided, reason for dislocation?)*
  - In ankylosis spondyolytis
    - Increased incidence of anterior dislocation (due to hyperextension deformity of the pelvis and the hip).
    - Due to pelvis hyper extension (compensating the lumbar and thoracic kyphosis), the cup position can become more anteverted (if following the anatomy of the pelvis). So, the acetabular component should be adjusted to account for pelvic deformity, building less inclination and less anteversion to avoid anterior hip dislocation.
- Risk factors for dislocation:
  - Female gender, inflammatory arthritis (eg rheumatoid), age older than 70, osteonecrosis, arthroplasty after failed internal fixation for proximal femur or acetabulum, prior hip surgery, trochanteric non union, and posterior approach, abductor weakness.
  - Post traumatic arthrtisis without prior fixation for fracture is not considered a risk factor.
    - **Female gender** is the strongest independent risk factor for dislocation after total hip arthroplasty.
  - Larger femoral head (36mm) have less dislocation rate than small femoral head (the head has to rotate larger distance to come out of the socket) (see femoral head/neck ratio section).

- o Direct lateral approach (Hardinge) has lower dislocation rate than posterior approach.
  - ▪ With posterior approach, reconstruction of the external rotators and capsular attachments can reduce dislocation rate.
- o The use of a larger-diameter acetabular (Jumbo cup) component may lead to soft-tissue overgrowth around the liner, causing impingement and increasing the risk for recurrent dislocation.
- o Medialization of the acetabulum will result in less tension in the abductor and increased instability.
- o Late onset dislocation is most commonly due to wear of the bearing surface.
- o Females and diagnoses other than hip OA are risk factors for late onset dislocation.
- Management:
  - o First time dislocation: especially if there is no component mal position:
    - ▪ Treatment is by closed reduction, education about dislocation precautions.
    - ▪ Hip orthoses are of questionable benefit unless the patient is cognitively impaired.
  - o Three or more dislocations: revision (see later).
  - o Dislocation with mal position of the acetabular component (abducted, too much anteversion or retroversion):
    - ▪ Revision of the acetabular component. *(Scenario: multiple dislocations, XRs show mal positioned cup, treatment?) (Scenario: THA 2 months ago, posterior dislocation, reduction done, post reduction cross table lateral XR shows retro version of the cup. Further treatment should include?)*
  - o Maneuvers to increase the stability of the THA:
    - ▪ Increase the soft tissue tension (distal transfer of the trochanter, increase the neck length, increase the offset (extended offset)), constrained liner, larger femoral head).
  - o If no risk factor can be found for patient with repeated dislocation of THA or the risk factor cannot be corrected (eg. Neurologic abductor weakness, dementia): treatment is by the use of constrained liner (especially if trochanter transfer and larger femoral head failed to solve the problem).
  - o Constrained liner should not be used when there is obvious mal aligned acetabular component. *(Scenario: 70 years old, patient has repeated dislocation of THA, during revision abductor were found to be destroyed from local inflammatory reaction, management? (Constrained liner)).*

Offset:

- Defined as the perpendicular lateral distance from the center of the femoral head to the anatomic axis of the femur (Fig 3).
- Restoration of the offset is important to achieve abductor strength.
    - Failure to restore the femoral offset (decrease offset) will result in weak abductors, Trendelenburg gait and bone to bone impingement (trochanter may abide against the iliac crest during abduction) which may lead to dislocation. *(Scenario: dislocation of THA, XR shows trochanter against the iliac crest, what is the cause? (decrease offset)) (Scenario: patient with THA has Trendelenburg positive sign (sound side sag) (due to weak abductor), what can be the reason? (decreased offset)).*

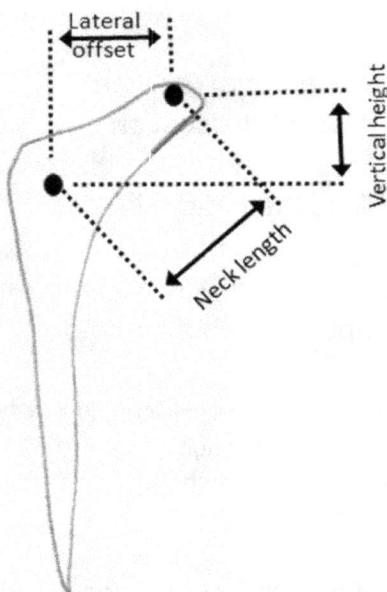

Fig 3: The offset of the prosthesis is the lateral distance of from the center of the femoral head t o the axis of the femur. Increasing the neck length of the prosthesis will result in increase in both offset and vertical height.

- High-offset femoral:
    - Increased soft-tissue tension (improving stability), decrease joint reaction force (Fig 4).
    - Increased femoral offset correlates will decrease in abductor force requirements for a hip balance, consequently decreasing joint reaction forces.
    - Disadvantage is lateral prominence and trochanteric bursitis in thin patients.

- Changing the offset does not affect the leg length.
- Increasing the neck length will increase both the leg length and lateral offset (Fig 3).

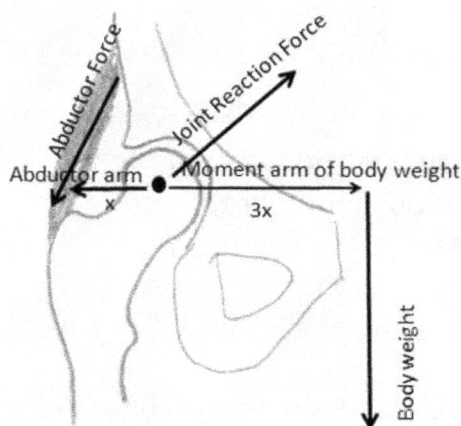

Fig 4: diagram showing forces around the hip joint. The abductor force by its moment arm (x) should equal body weight by it moment arm (3x), so the abductor muscle has to do work which is about 3 times body weight at the single stance. The forces across the hip joint (Joint reaction force) will equal the sum of the abductor

Wear and Osteolysis (in THA):

- Two main types of wear: adhesive and abrasive (abrasive is further sub classified to two body abrasive wear and three body abrasive wear).
- Adhesive wear:
  - Adhesive wear is a phenomenon, which occurs when two materials rub together (frictional contact) with sufficient force to cause the removal of material from the less wear-resistant surface.
  - When the adhesive forces exceed the material strength, material parts are removed from the weaker side.
  - Adhesive wear is the most common mechanism of wear seen in well-functioning hips (*Question: what is the main wear in metal on PE hips?*).
- Abrasive wear:
  - Occurs when a hard rough surface slides across a softer surface.
  - Classified according to the type of contact and the contact environment into two-body and three-body abrasive wear
    - Two-body abrasive wear: projections (asperites) from one surface remove material from the opposed articulating surface.
    - Three-body wear occurs when a third body particle (eg cement piece) is interposed between the bearing surfaces and results in removal of material from one or both of the articular surfaces.
- Osteolysis:
  - Periprosthetic loss of bone secondary to body reaction to particulate debris and it is often clinically silent unless it is accompanied by pathologic fracture or implant loosening.

- o Advanced osteolysis can lead to loosening of the implant. *(Scenario: osteolysis around the femoral stem with loosening, patient complain of pain, cause of pain? (loosening)).*
- o Bisphonsphonate (eg Alendronate) inhibits osteolysis due to wear debris.
- o Wear debris from metal-on-metal will cause **lymphocyte stimulation**; while from metal on polyethylene will cause **histiocytic (macrophage) stimulation**; ceramic on ceramic is the least inflammatory.
- o Stimulated macrophage and/or lymphocyte will result in stimulation of osteoclast (final pathway) by increased IL-1, increased RANK/ RANKL and by increased VEGF gene expression.
    - **Process of PE-induced osteolysis is: macrophage induced osteoclast resorption of bone.** *(Question: **initiator** of the events associated with periprosthetic osteolysis is? (Macrophage))*
- o PE wear findings in the XR: eccentric position of the femoral head within the acetabular cup with decreased thickness of the liner.
- o The biologic response to PE wear debris is dependent on the type and quantity of particles.
    - Particles sized between 0.2 μm and 7-8 μm are the most stimulatory of wear process.
- o Metal on metal articulation leads to smaller wear particles compared to metal-on-PE bearings causing less reactive osteolysis.
- o Linear wear Vs volumetric wear:
    - Large femoral head will have increased volumetric wear and decreased linear wear and vice versa.
    - Radiostereometric analysis (RSA) is considered the most sensitive method for measuring wear in THA: radiopaque tantalum beads are inserted into the bone in certain positions surrounding the implants. These are used to assess the linear wear.
- o Linear wear rate for conventional PE should be less than 0.1mm/year.
    - Wear rates greater than 0.1 mm/year is associated with higher rates of osteolysis. Osteolysis is most closely correlated with wear rate (linear and volumetric)
    - Osteolysis is rarely seen with the wear rate < 0.1 mm per year.
- o Highly cross-linked polyethylene is associated with a reduction in PE wear and osteolysis associated with THA.
- o Retro acetabular osteolysis seen in some cases of THA is commonly due to PE particles tracking through the effective joint space (around the screw holes or screws of the cup)
- o To assess the extent of an osteolysis discovered around the acetabular component in a pelvis AP view, obtain Judet views or get CT scan. *(Scenario:*

hip pain 15 years after THA; Pelvis AP showed supra-acetabular osteolysis, no signs of infection; further assessment is by?)

- Cementless circumferentially coated femoral stems protect against distal femur osteolysis (seal the effective joint space)
    - Proximal noncircumferential porous coating has been associated with a higher incidence of distal osteolysis around the stem.

- Management:
    - For cases of THA with PE wear:
        - Treatment is by liner and femoral head revision. If there is associated retro-acetabular osteolysis: add retro-acetabular grafting. *(Scenario: 60-year-old male, THA 12 years ago, no has pain, radiographs show eccentric position of the head in the cup (due to PE wear), what is the treatment?)*
        - Asymptomatic osteolysis around the well-fixed acetabular component (retro acetabular osteolysis with no radiologic signs of acetabular loosening) is treated by head and liner exchange and retro-acetabular bone grafting.
        - The acetabular cup does not need to be replaced unless found to be loose intra operatively. *(Scenario: routine follow up 12 years post-operative, XR shows retro acetabular osteolysis, patient has no complaints, treatment is?)*
        - Most common complication after isolated liner exchange for PE wear is dislocation of the hip joint. *(Scenario: 80 years old, 10 years THA, no symptoms, routine XR shows marked osteolysis behind acetabular component, CT well fixed parts, treatment? what is the possible complication of this treatment? (Dislocation)).*
        - Asymptomatic osteolysis around a screw in well-fixed acetabular component is treated by revision of the polyethylene liner, removal of the screw, and debridement of the osteolytic lesion with or without bone grafting.
        - If the metal cup is unstable, or if the osteolytic lesion is not amenable to debridement through the screw hole: acetabular component revision may be indicated.

Loosening:

- Femoral loosening:
    - Clinical presentation: Start up thigh pain (pain with first few step), activity related. Subsidence of the stem will decrease the distance between origin and insertion of the abductors causing decrease muscle tension and weakening (limping Trendelenburg gait).
    - XR (Fig 5):
        - Possible osteolysis around the implant.

- For cementless stems: subsidence of the stem, failure of osseous integration with reactive radiolucent line around the implant, hypertrophy of the bone under the collar (in contrast to what happen in cases of adequate bone ingrowth in which there will be stress shielding of bone under the collar), a pedestal formation at the distal tip of the implant.
- Cemented stem: disrupted implant-cement interface, subsidence of the implant, distal cortical reaction around the distal end of the implant.
- Lab: Aseptic loosening: normal WBCs, ESR, C-RP:
  - Aspiration shows WBCs less than 1500/ml.
- Aseptic loosening can be due to osteolysis (period of good fixation then patient started to have pain) or due to failure of initial bony ingrowth (failure of osseointegration) (the prosthesis was always painful) (more common).
- Treatment of aseptic femoral loosening is revision of the femoral component to a **cementless, fully porous-coated (diaphyseal fixation) stem**. *(Scenario: 75 years, 4 years ago had THA, thigh pain for 5 months, activity related, diagnosis?) (Scenario: 65 years old, male, THA 6 months ago, startup pain, XR post op and 5 months later show subsidence of the stem of about 1cm, treatment?)*

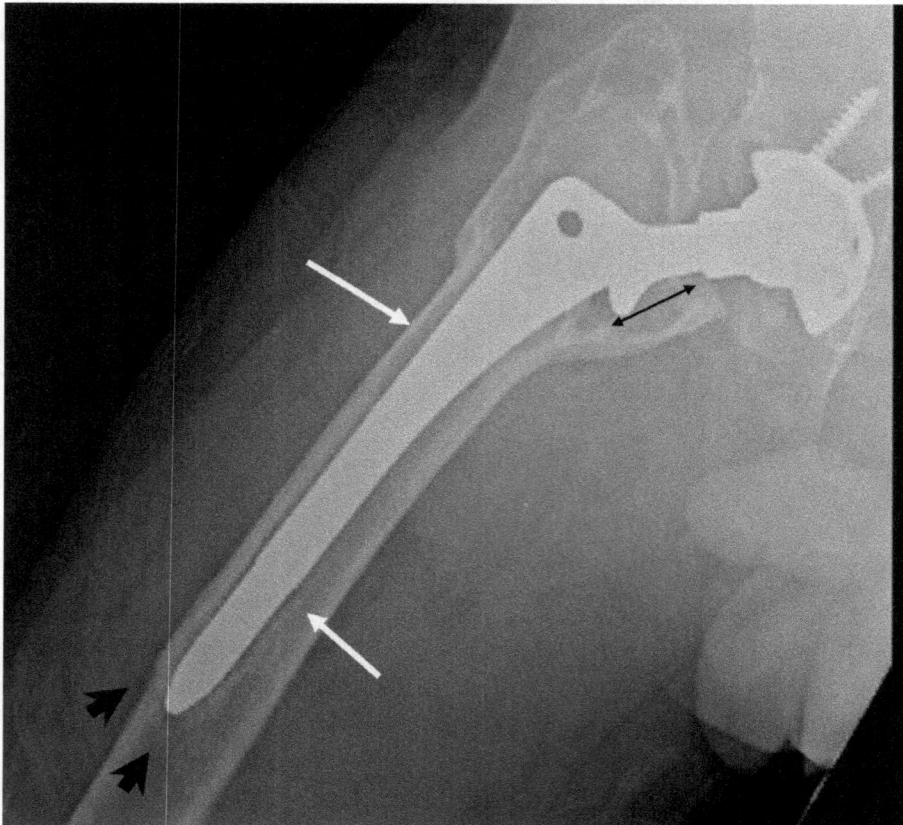

Fig 5: THA done 10 years. Notice the signs of loosening of the cementless stem (severe subsidence of the stem (double sided black arrow), radulcent lines (white arrows), pedestral formation at the distal tip of the implant (arrow heads)).

Arthroplasty After Neck Femur Fracture (See Lower Extremity Trauma Chapter):

- Total hip arthroplasty has higher rate of dislocation (less stability) compared to hemiarthroplasty (bipolar or unipolar).
- Most important risk factor for dislocation of arthroplasty after femoral neck fracture: posterior approach and dementia. (_Scenario: dementic patient had posterior approach for hemiarthroplasty, dislocated few weeks later, what are the important risk factors?_)
- For relatively young and more active (community ambulatory without assistive device) patients: THA (compared to hemiarthroplasty) will provide better long term results, lower pain scores and lower re-operation rate.
- Acetabular erosion and cartilage loss after hemi arthroplasty for neck fracture with hip pain and XR showing loss of joint space, sclerosis and supero-lateral migration of the head of the prosthesis: treatment is by conversion of the hemi (bipolar or unipolar) to THA with insertion of acetabular component. NO need to revise the femoral component if not loose

Basic Science of Arthroplasty:

- **Lubrication:**
    - Three types of lubrication in THA: boundary lubrication, mixed lubrication, fluid film lubrication.
        - Boundary lubrication: the surfaces are largely nondeformable, and the lubricant only partially separates articular surfaces.
        - Mixed lubrication: fliu
        - Fluid film lubrication
- Contact between femoral head and acetabular cup:
    - Slight clearance, not complete congruence, is the most optimal for formation of the fluid film lubrication between the the acetabular cup and the femoral head.
- **Clearance:**
    - Definition: the difference between the diameter of the femoral head and the diameter of the acetabular cup.
    - Clearance of 75 to 150 μm maximizes the fluid film thickness and entrapment between the two bearing surfaces.
    - High clearance will result in increased wear, and low clearance can result in clamping and/or equatorial seizing.
- **Edge wear:**
    - Pore size in the range of 50 to 400 microns is required for optimal bony ingrowth in cemetless prosthesis.

- Stems:
  - o Cemented stems:
    - Stems that are precoated with polymethylmethacrylate have higher rate of loosening and failure.
    - Stiffer stem materials (eg.cobalt chrome) have better performance when used as cemented stems.
    - Smoother corners decrease the rate of failure (decrease stress risers to the cement).
    - The ideal cement mantle is 2-3mm.
    - Antibiotic-impregnated cement causes weakening of the cement (which can increase the risk of aseptic loosening) and the generation of antibiotic-resistant bacteria in the infected implant sites.
    - Osteopenia improves the bone-cement interface in comparison to normal bone (weaker bone will allow more integration and more depth of the cement inside the cortical bone) this will enhance the mechanical integrity.
  - o Cementless stem:
    - There is no clinical advantage to the use of a hydroxyapatite coating on the femoral component for primary total hip arthroplasty over porous coating, however, Hydroxyapatite-coated stems may have a shorter time to biologic fixation.
  - o Stem material: see material chapter
- **Polyethylene (PE):**
  - o Calcium stearate (used to prevent corrosion on PE machine parts) resulted in fusion defects in PE which resulted in lowering the mechanical properties of the PE.
  - o The ideal level of crystallinity is around 50%, a crystallinity over 70% is associated with increased polyethylene failure rates.
- **Methods used to form UHMWPE:**
  - o Ram extrusion (Net shape): the resin of UHMWPE is extruded under heat and pressure to form a cylindrical bar that is then machined into a final shape.
  - o Compression molding: the resin of UHMWPE is shaped into a large sheet that is cut into smaller pieces to use it in machining of the final components.
  - o Direct compression molding: the resin of UHMWPE is directly molded into a finished desired product.
    - Direct compression molding has a lower susceptibility to fatigue crack formation and propagation than other forms of PE manufacturing.
- **Sterilization of PE:**
  - o Methods of sterilization: Irradiation, Ethylene oxide and gas plasma.

- o Ethylene oxide and gas plasma do not create free radicals and there is no effect on polymer cross-linking.
- o Oxidation will occur following polyethylene implantation (in vivo) regardless of sterilization technique.
- o Irradiation in inert gas produce lower oxidation rates and oxidation potential (compared to irradiation in Oxygen); however, some free radicals will still be produced.
- o High dose irradiation (5-15 Mrad) prompts the amorphous regions of the PE to cross-link.
- o With irradiation of PE, free radicals are created leading to cross-linking of the polymer, and a more abrasion resistant and wear resistant PE (but lower mechanical properties). *(Question: how can you increase PE cross links?) (Question: what properties improve with irradiation?)*
  - The amount of irradiation has the greatest effect on the wear properties of PE. The higher the amount of irradiation the greater cross-linking and improved wear characters.
- o Irradiation in oxygen has unacceptably high rates of oxidation and free radical production. Sterilization with gamma radiation in air produces the greatest degree of PE oxidation.
  - PE becomes more brittle with higher rates of early mechanical failure.
  - Increased elastic modulus (stiffer) and decreased strength making the PE vulnerable to delamination (especially with TKA), fracture, and pitting.
- o Oxidation of PE continues during the shelf life if it has been packed in air leading to increase in free radicals
- o To decrease long-term oxidation and residual free radicals: PE can undergo post-irradiation heat treatment (melting or annealing) or addition of antioxidants, such as vitamin E.
  - Remelting and annealing are thermal stabilization methods to reduce free radicals that are formed as a result of the cross-linking process. Both remelting and heat annealing have been shown to reduce wear and osteolysis.
  - Remelting is the heating of the PE above its melting point, changing it from the partial crystalline state to the amorphous state and removing all free radicals, but also worsening it mechnical characteristics.
  - Annealing (heating below the melting temperature) has less effect on the PE mechanical properties than melting (leaves more free radicals). *(Question: what is worst mechanical property (e.g. highest crack propagation under cyclic loading)? Remelted highly cross linked PE)*

- Annealed PE (compared to re melted) has more free radicals, better mechanical characteristics, and equivalent clinical wear.
  - Highly cross-linked ultra-high-molecular-weight polyethylene:
    - Crosslinking dose is increased above the traditional range for gamma radiation sterilization (ie, 2.5 to 4 Mrads)).
    - Has improved resistance to adhesive and abrasive wear but decreased mechanical properties (e.g. decreased toughness, ductility, tensile strength, fatigue strength, and resistance to crack propagation) when compared with conventional UHMWPE. Cross linking improves wear properties but decrease mechanical properties like tensile and fatigue strength.
    - The highly cross-linked UHMWPE generates smaller wear particles than the conventional PE.

Revision THA

- Aseptic loosening of the femoral component: cementless revision of the stem is preferred over cemented revision.
- Polyethylene wear (XR will show superiorly eccentric position of the femoral head) with well-fixed component, see before): treatment is synovectomy and polyethylene liner exchange (no need for more extensive revision work). If there is marked osteolysis behind the acetabulum component: retro-acetabulum bone grafting can be added (See osteolysis section).
  - After PE exchange, there is increased risk of hip dislocation.
- Charnley all-polyethylene acetabular shell has 30% revision for all reasons at 35 years follow up.

Acetabular deficiency:

- AAOS type I defects are segmental, type II are cavitary, type III are combined cavitary and segmental, type IV is discontinuity, and type V is arthrodesis.
- Paprosky classification: Type I: small focal areas of contained bone loss with intact columns and no/minimal distortion of the rim. Type II: distorted/missing rim with adequate remaining bone (column). Type III: Column are not of adequate support.
- Paprosky type I and II acetabular defect (intact columns) are treated with cementless, porous-coated acetabular component with adjunctive screw fixation. No need for Bilobed components or antiprotrusio cage in these cases. *(Scenario: 65 years female, THA 15 years ago, now has pain in her groin that increases with weight bearing, XR shows severe wear and loosening of the cemented, all polyethylene acetabular component with a Paprosky type II acetabular defect. What implant to revise acetabular component?)*
  - If more than 2/3 of the rim is intact, press fit cup can be used with rim fit.

- o Most cases of acetabular revision can be managed by large sized cementless cup (if they have more than 50% of the acetabular bone stock, so long there is no pelvic discontinuity).
- Pelvic discontinuity with minimal bone loss: treated we plate fixation and cementless acetabular cup with screw fixation (anti-prutusio cage can be used for more advanced cases). *(Scenario: acetabular fracture after falling, 5 years post THA, XR shows acetabular fracture and loose cup; treatment is?)*
- Non-contained defects in both the anterior and posterior columns of the acetabulum region affecting greater than 50% of the weight bearing surface or pelvic discontinuity with extensive amount of bone loss and medial wall penetration is best treated by antiprotrusio cage or with structural graft for the defects supported by ilioischial reconstruction acetabular ring component.
- In cases of asymptomatic retro-acetabular osteolysis with well-fixed component: treatment is retro-acetabular bone grafting with change of the head and PE components (see osteolysis).
- Loss of periacetabular (ilium) bone mineral density in the first 2 years following total hip arthroplasty in which a press-fit acetabular component was used is most likely attributable to altered acetabular stress patterns (stress shielding by the implant leading to decrease stress seen by native bone tissue).
- Cancellous bone grafts incorporate more effectively than structural bone grafts (better used in cases of contained cavitary defects).

Femoral deficiency:

- **Paprosky Classificatino**
    - o Type I: intact femoral diaphysis with minimal metaphyseal bone loss.
    - o Type II: intact femoral diaphysis with extensive metaphyseal bone loss.
    - o Type IIIA: > 4 cm of diaphyseal bone preservation for distal fixation.
    - o Type IIIB: < 4 cm of diaphyseal bone preservation for distal fixation.
    - o Type IV: extensive metaphyseal and diaphyseal bone loss.
- **Treatment:**
    - o Paprosky Type I, II, and IIIA defects of the femur (Most cases fall under this category: revision to an cementles, diaphyseal fully coated stem.
        - ▪ If there is more than 4 cm of intact diaphysis available (IIIA), an extensively coated, cementless stem can be used with good results as it will depend on diaphyseal fixation and engrowth (no need to use allograft-prosthetic composites or tumor replacement prostheses for these cases). *(Scenario: 80 years old, THA 10 years ago, having pain for few months, XR shows loose, cemented femoral component with proximal femur deficiency, treatment?)*
    - o Type IIIB should consider a tapered, modular stem and/or bone grafting.

- o Type IV needs tumor prosthesis.
- o If there is extensive osteolysis around the femoral component and the patient is getting thigh pain at rest, revision of the femoral component is needed as early as possible (to avoid peri-prosthetic fracture).

Technical aspects during THA:

- The acetabular quadrants are formed by a line extending from the **ASIS to the center of the acetabulum**, forming anterior and posterior acetabular halves. The second line is drawn perpendicular to the first at the center of acetabulum, forming four quadrants (Fig 6).
    - o The posterior-superior zone is the safe zone for acetabular screw placement during THA. This is followed by posterior-inferior (safe for screws less than 20mm).
    - o Greatest risk of vascular injury with screw placement is in the anterior superior.
        - The most commonly damaged vessels are the common femoral artery and the external iliac artery.
    - o Dangers of long screws:
        - Postero superior: superior gluteal vessels and nerve and sciatic nerve.
        - Anterior-superior: external iliac vessels. *(Scenario: patient after THA have ischemic leg, XR shows long screw, what vessel was injured, what quadrant?)*
        - Anterior inferior: obturator vessels.
        - Posterior inferior: sciatic nerve, inferior gluteal nerve and vessels and the internal pudendal nerve and vessels.
- Minimal-incision technique has the advantage of better cosmetic appearance compared to standard incision. No other advantages could be proven.
    - o If during minimally invasive approach to total hip arthroplasty a femoral periprosthetic fracture occurs, the surgeon should convert it to an extensile approach to adequately visualize the fracture (see complication section).
- The most important predictor of blood transfusion need after THA is the pre-operative Hemoglobin level.
- Combined version: combined ante version of acetabular cup and femur neck should be around 40°.
- Excess abduction or anteversion of the cup can lead to edge loading with accelerated wear.

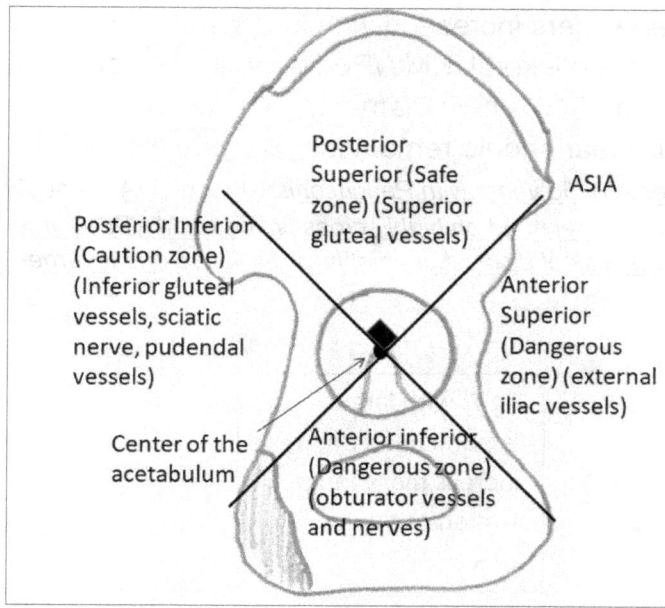

Fig 6: Hip quadrants. A line from the ASIS to the center of the acetabulum will divide the acetabulum to anterior and posterior halves. Then another line perpedicualar to the first line at the center of the acetabulum will divide the anterior and posterior halves to inferior and superior quadrants. Posterior superior quadrant is a safest quadrant followed posterior inferior quadrant.

- For cases with deformity or previous osteotomy of the proximal femur, femoral osteotomy with realignment of the femoral canal and cementless prosthesis that depends on distal fixation is the current preferred technique. *(Scenario: 40 years, had proximal femoral osteotomy for Perthes when he was 9 years old, currently had varus deformity and hip arthritis, what technique for THA?)*
- Primary Cemented cup is used mainly in cases of previous irradiation of the pelvis
- **Head and neck size in THA/ impingement:**
  - A larger femoral head to neck ratio:
    - Can be achieved by bigger size femoral head and not using skirt (Fig 7).
    - With larger ratio, the neck needs to rotate a longer distance before it impinges on the shell wall and levers the head out from the acetabulum. This will result in less dislocation rate and larger ROM *(Question: how to increase ROM or reduce dislocation? (bigger size head, not using skirt))*
    - Skirted neck will decrease the ROM and increase possibility of dislocation (decrease head/neck ratio).
  - The optimal cup position is 45° to 55° abduction.
    - Vertical position of the acetabular component (more abduction) eliminates the benefit of the larger head by allowing dislocation with minimal translation of the head.
  - Minimizing impingement involves avoiding skirted necks, maximizing the head-to-neck ratio and, when possible, using a chamfered acetabular cup and a trapezoidal, rather than circular, neck cross-section (Fig 7).

- ○ Wear rates of regular polyethylene liners increased with increasing femoral head size. Wear rates of highly cross-linked UHMWPE liners are independent of femoral head size between 22 and 46 mm in diameter (i.e. With modern bearings material, the volumetric wear should remain low, despite the increase in head diameter). *(Scenario: 60 years with Parkinsonism, need THA, what bearing to use? (Large diameter metal femoral head on highly cross-linked UHMWPE) (large head due to lower his higher than normal risk of dislocation, highly cross linked due to large head used)).*

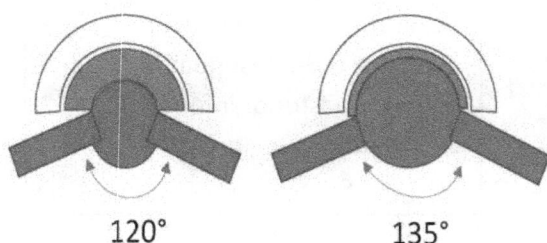

120°   135°

Fig 7: with larger femoral head (right), there is more range of motion of the hip joint.

- **Stress Shielding:**
  - ○ Due to transfer of weight bearing stresses by the prosthesis rather than the bone, the bone is exposed to less stresses leading to decrease bone density of the affected part (indication of good fixation of the component to bone). Absence of stress shielding is an indication of loose stem.
  - ○ Stems with distal coating and distal fixation will result in more stress shielding of the proximal femur leading to more loss of bone content and bone density from proximal femur.
    - Proximal coated stem decreases proximal stress shielding (compared to distal coated).
  - ○ Risk factors for of stress shielding of proximal femur: distally fixed femoral components, cobalt-chrome stems, large diameter femoral components (> than 18 mm in diameter) (factors increasing the stiffness of the prosthesis).
- **Leg Length After THA:**
  - ○ Causes of aberrant LLD (Patient's perceived leg length discrepancy) after THA (the operated side **longer**): Weakness of the hip abductors will lead to ipsilateral trunk lean; this will cause perceived lengthening of the operated side.
    - Radiographs will show equal length of both sides (compare the lesser trochanters on both sides)
- **Renal Failure (End Stage Renal Disease):**
  - ○ High incidence of infection after arthroplasty surgeries.

- o Patient with end stage renal disease and fracture neck femur: treatment with hemiarthropasty will result in less complication than treatment by ORIF.

Metal on Metal (MoM) THA:

- Uses large size head (no PE insert), so risk of dislocation is less (see before).
- Have higher frictional torque than with ceramic on ceramic.
- Will cause increased production of metal ion wear particles and increase level of metals (cobalt and chrome) in the blood and urine.
- There is no correlation between activity level of the patient and serum levels of metal ions.
- **Cup position is important in regard to the amount of wear:**
    - o Contact patch-to-rim (CPR) distance is the distance between the point of application of the joint reaction force and the rim of the acetabular component in the standing position.
    - o Decreased CPR distance (**high abduction angle of the acetabular component**, excessive anteversion of the acetabular component, cup designs with smaller coverage of the femoral head) will result in increased wear.
    - o High wear and elevated serum metal ion levels after metal-on-metal resurfacing hip arthroplasty was shown to be related to acetabular inclination more than 50 degrees (vertical position causes more wear) (see before).
- Clearance plays an important role in wear in MoM bearings. Mixed film lubrication (the lubrication mechanism in MoM) depends on clearances of 100 to 200 μm to maximize the fluid film thickness.
    - o MoM bearings operate in a "mixed lubrication" mode (part of the surface in direct contact and other parts separated by fluid film).
    - o As the diameter of the bearing increases (eg resurfacing), the total sliding distance per step increases in proportion. However, the sliding speed of the bearing surfaces also increases in proportion, which tends to draw in more fluid. This increases the separation of the bearing surfaces and tends to offset the negative effect of the increased sliding distance leading to comparable volumetric wear with other smaller metal on metal implant.
- Compared to metal-on-polyethylene total hip bearing surfaces, the debris particles generated by metal-on-metal articulations are smaller and more numerous.
    - o Metal on metal articulation leads to lower linear and volumetric wear rate and smaller wear particles compared to metal-on-PE bearings, causing less osteolysis than PE wear debris particles (yet, they still can sometimes cause clinical significant osteolysis around the implant).

- o The volumetric wear rate of metal-on-metal articulations is greater than metal-on-ceramic.
  - o The wear rate decrease significantly after the first year "steady state".
- Not recommended for females in childbearing period or for patients with renal insufficiency.
- No proven evidence of increased risk of malignancy.
  - o Patients with metal on metal bearings have increased incidence of certain hemopoietic chromosomal mutations as leukocyte chromosomal aberrations (the clinical significance of that is still not known).
- **Pseudtumour formation:**
  - o Also known as aseptic lymphocyte-dominant vasculitis-associated lesion (ALVAL).
  - o The soft tissue reaction against the metal ion can cause "**pseudo tumor**" which can adversely destroy the soft tissue causing pain of the affected hip and destruction of the hip abductors (limping).
  - o Histological features: predominantly tissue necrosis with infiltration of **lymphocytes** (diffuse and perivascular infiltrates of T and B lymphocytes) and plasma cells.
  - o Clinical presentation: Pain. Obtaining serum trace element levels is recommended. If the levels are high, cross-sectional imaging should be obtained to determine if there is any pseudotumor or tissue necrosis around the hip arthroplasty. *(Scenario: 50 years old, hip resurfacing MOM 7 years ago, 6 months of hip pain, XR normal, markers of inflammation normal, next step? (Serum metal levels and metal-reduction MRI scan))*
  - o Imaging: can be detected by MRI (MARS MRI) *(scenario: THA 5 years ago, Metal on Metal, Pain, next step?) (Question: what condition in MoM can adversely affect revision?)*
  - o Risk factors:
    - ▪ Young, female patients, small components, dysplastic hip, edge loading (malpositioned abducted vertical component) (causing increase amount of particule wear debris, see before).
  - o Lymphocyte reactivity to cobalt, chromium, and nickel did not significantly differ in patients with pseudotumors compared to patients without pseudotumors.
  - o Pseudo tumor formation was found to be a significant poor prognostic factor in revision surgery (marked destruction of soft tissue, abductors and possible nerve invasion)
  - o The pseudo tumor can become infected (increased pain, elevated ESR, and CRP), in this case will need debridement and antibiotics, and eventually two stage revision of the prosthesis.

Ceramic On Ceramic:

- Provides the best wear characteristics.
- Alumina is the most stable ceramic bearing surface in vivo while zirconia has a tendency to change from its stable tetragonal phase to its monoclinic phase in vivo (see materials chapter).
- Disadvantages: squeaking, femoral head failure.
  - The most serious complication of ceramic components is fracture.
    - Revising a ceramic head to a new ceramic head should be avoided because ceramic head fractures can occur if it is placed over a used taper.
  - Squeaking of ceramic bearing:
    - Most common complication related to ceramic.
    - Can be observed in the absence of component malpositioning or hip pain (no need for intervention in these cases). *(Scenario: ceramic THA 18 months ago, no pain, R shows good component position, intermittent squeaking, treatment?)*

Post-Operative Protocols After THA:

- Return to driving: after about 4-6 weeks.
- If the utilized approach is using intra operative anterior dislocation (Smith-Peterson, Watson Jones, lateral Hardinge): post-operative dislocation (if it happens) will be mostly be anterior.
  - Patient should maintain anterior hip precaution (**avoid extension and external rotation and adduction**)
- For posterior approach of hip, the risk of dislocation is mainly posterior dislocation and patient should keep posterior hip precautions (**avoid flexion, internal rotation and adduction**)
- Postoperative ileus following total joint arthroplasty occurs in about 1 % after total joint arthroplasty patients. It is more common after THA than TKA. Risk factors include: older age, male gender, and a history of abdominal surgery (See Ogilivie syndrome in the complication session).
- Anti-coagulation with THA:
  - **The 2007 AAOS guidelines for thrombophlebitis prophylaxis for patients undergoing total hip and knee arthroplasty includes (http://www.aaos.org/research/guidelines/VTE/VTE_full_guideline.pdf):**
    - Use of pharmacologic agents and/or mechanical compressive devices for the prevention of VTE in patients undergoing elective hip or knee arthroplasty

- NO need for routine post-operative duplex ultrasonography screening of patients who undergo elective hip or knee arthroplasty.
- Preoperative risk assessment for DVT, PE and bleeding:
  - For patients who have had a previous VTE, it is better to receive pharmacologic prophylaxis and mechanical compressive devices.
  - Patients with known bleeding disorder and/or active liver disease: it is better to use mechanical compressive devices as a prophylaxis.
- Patients should discontinue anti-platelet agents (e.g., aspirin, clopidogrel) before undergoing elective hip or knee arthroplasty.
- In patients with high risk of bleeding, use inferior vena cava (IVC) filter has conflicting results (cannot recommend for or against).
- Encourage early mobilization.
- Neuraxial (such as intrathecal, epidural, and spinal) anesthesia to help limit blood loss (NO effect on the occurrence of VTE).
- The duration of prophylaxis should be left to discussion between patients and physicians (no definitive period showed advantage over others).

o Use of mechanical prophylaxis (intermittent compression devices) during the hospital stay.
o When warfarin is used as a chemoprophylactic agent, the goal INR is less than or equal to 2 to minimize the risk of bleeding.
o Inferior vena cava filters may be used in selected patients (not routinely).
o If a patient under anticoagulation as a **treatment** for DVT or PE develops hematoma formation, treatment is placement of a vena cava filter, and stopping the anticoagulation, and possible hematoma evacuation. *(Scenario: 50 years old, THA, developed PE, started enoxaparin, few days later, developed hematoma, treatment?)*
o Most DVT occurs in the first week after surgery. Most symptomatic VTE occur between 1-6 weeks post operatively.

Complications of THA
Heterotrophic Ossification (HO):
- Brooker classification (1-4): see Fig 8.
- The process of HO formation begins early post operatively (within days); therefore, prophylactic treatment must be started early
- Risk factors: previous history of HO in the contra lateral hip, ankylosing spondylitis.
- **Prophylaxis:**

- o For patient with high risk of developing HO, recommended prophylaxis is 600 to 800 centigray (rad) of radiation given within 24 hours preoperatively or 72 hours postoperatively.
- o NSAIDs given immediately postoperatively for 7 to 21 days - longer duration has not been shown to be of any additional benefit). Commonly used medication is Indomethacin 75 mg/day for 3 weeks. Selective COX-2 inhibitor were also found to be effective in decreasing the risk of HO.
- **Treatment:**
  - o Nonsurgical management (e.g. extensive physiotherapy) during the maturation phase has limited effectiveness.
  - o There is no role for NSAIDs or radiotherapy as a treatment for already existing HO.
  - o Bisphosphonates only postpone ossification maturation (until treatment is stopped).
  - o Most cases of HO will not clinically affect the ROM and can be managed conservatively. *(Scenario: THA 8 weeks ago, patient is progressing fine with weight bearing and movement, XR Brooker grade 3 HO, what is the treatment at this stage? (Therapy, observation, repeat radiographs, and reexamination in 6-8 weeks, the goal of therapy is to maintain the ROM and not to cure HO).*
  - o **Surgical treatment:** excision of the HO if restricting the ROM of the hip, can improve the functional outcome. Done after maturation of the HO (you do not have to wait until the bone scan turns cold).

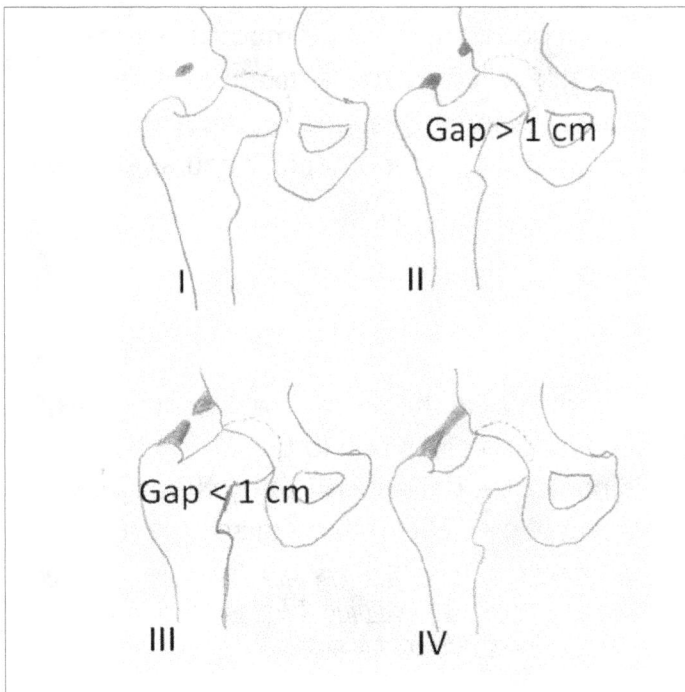

Gap > 1 cm

I   II

Gap < 1 cm

III   IV

Brooker Classifcation for the extent of the HO in cases of hip. Grade I: islands of bone within the soft tissues. Grade II: bone spurs from the pelvis and/or proximal end of the femur, with > 1 cm between opposing surfaces. Grade III: bone spurs from the pelvis and/or proximal end of the femur with bone surfaces < 1 cm. Grade IV shows apparent bone ankylosis of the hip.

Fractures During THA:

- Intra operative fractures of the acetabulum that do not seem to affect stability of the acetabular component can be treated with placement of 2-3 acetabular screws and no changes in post-operative plan.
    - Risk factors for an intraoperative acetabular fracture include underreaming (typically > 2 mm) and placement of a cementless acetabular component.
- Calcar fractures:
    - Risk factor: female gender, cementless stem, minimal invasive approach.
    - Treatment (if discovered intra-operative) by **stem removal**, extension of the incision (if minimal approach was the primary approach), the distal extent of the fracture must be identified, placement of two cables around the calcar and placement of the original stem. *(Scenario: 70 years old female, a cementless THA, the surgeon notices a small crack forming in the anteromedial femoral neck with final implant insertion, management?)*
    - No need to change postoperative weight bearing protocol (patient can be weight bearing as tolerated after surgery). Long-term results are similar to patients without fracture. No increase in subsidence rate.
    - If the condition is discovered in the postoperative XR: If the fracture seems stable and non-displaced: a trial of non-weight bearing and a close follow can be done. Displaced unstable fracture will need revision fixation

Stem Breakage:

- Risk factors: include obesity, lack of proximal bone support and modular stems.
- Mechanism of fatigue stem break is due cantilevel effect (distal fixation).
- Mechanism of failure of modular revision stem is fretting fatigue (contacting components experience cyclic loads while small oscillatory motion occurs between them).

Peri-Prosthetic Fracture:

- **Vancouver classification (Fig 9-10).**
    - Vancouver A: trochanteric fracture proximal to the stem. Treatment by ORIF
    - Vancouver B: fracture around the stem, sub-classified to B1, B2 and B3.
        - Vancouver B1: The stem is not loose, patient **will deny thigh pain** prior to the fracture). Treatment is by ORIF with plate/screws and cerclage cables. *(Scenario: 68 years old, THA 10 years ago, fall down, no prior history of thigh pain, XR does not show obvious loosening, treatment? (ORIF with a plate and screws and augmentation with proximal cables)*

- Vancouver B2 (loose stem): Lucency around the stem or between stem and cement or intraoperative assessment will show it is loose. **Patients will report thigh pain** prior to the fracture that has been increasing in intensity. Treated with revision stem with longer (bypasses the fracture site by at least two cortical diameters) fully coated cementless stem (plus cable fixation of the fracture and possible allograft strut). Most surgeons do not currently use allograft for Vancouver B2.
- Vancouver B3: Stem is loose with very poor remaining bone stock, the patient will report thigh pain prior to the fracture. Treatment is by a long, cementless revision stem **with strut allograft**. An allograft-prosthesis composite (preferred for younger patients) or tumor prosthesis can also be used as alternative techniques. The stem should go distal to all femoral deficiencies by two cortices.

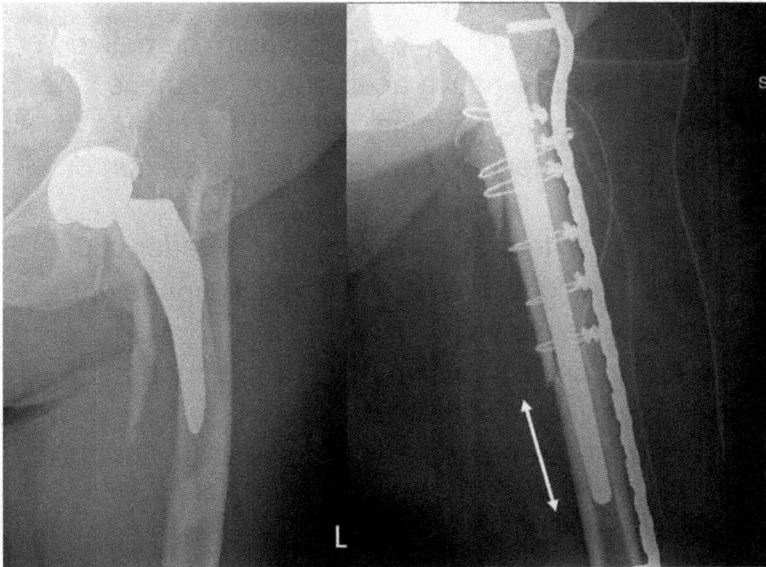

Fig 9: Vancouver B2: Loose stem with lucency around the stem. The fracture was treated with revision with long stem that extends 2 diameters distal to the fracture (double arrow). In this example, plate fixation was added to the construct (Courtesy of Dr Enes Kanlic).

Ogilvie Syndrome:

- Colonic obstruction without an associated mechanical blockage.
- Risk factor: male gender, the use of narcotic pain medications, undergoing hip arthroplasty.
- Radiographs will show dilation of the large intestine.
- Supportive treatment.

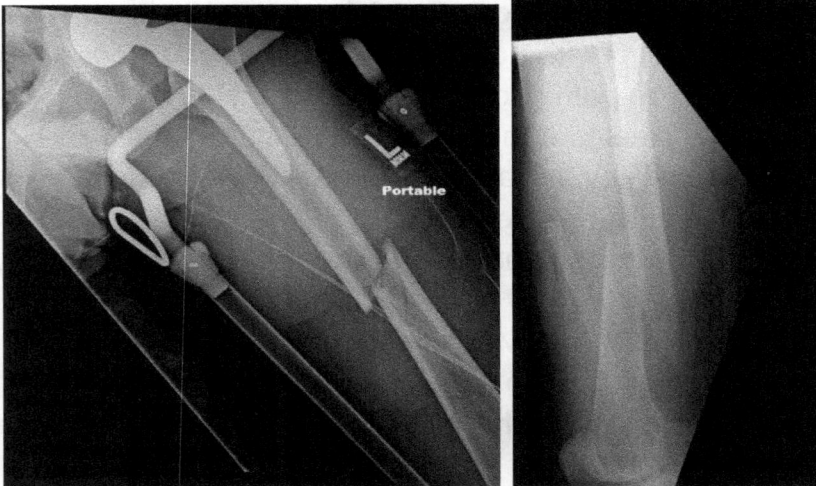

Fig 10: two different examples of Vancouver C THA peri-prosthetic fracture. Both were treated by ORIF of the femur.

Iliopsoas Impingement

- Irritation of the iliopsoas tendon by the acetabular cup.
- Retroverted cup, cups with small amount of antevsion, low cup within the native acetabulum, or large cup relative to the patient's native acetabulum (all these etiologies will cause the anterior edge to be more hanging): will have a large uncovered part that can cause irritation to the tendon during active hip flexion or passive extension.
    - Cross table lateral XR will show the extent of the uncovered anterior cup.
- Confirmation of the diagnosis by injection of local anesthetic in the iliospoas (ultra sound guided) sheath which should alleviate the pain
- Treatment: if the cup is excessively mal position: revision of the cup. If not excessively mal positioned: release of the iliopsoas tendon. *(Scenario: patient with THA, has pain when **climbing stairs or getting up from a seated position** (active flexion), straight leg raising reproduces the symptoms (hip flexion), markers of infection are normal, assessment? diagnosis? Confirmation? Treatment?).*

Post-Operative Infection (Also See TKA Infection)

- Pain is the most common symptoms associated with prosthetic infection.
- Nasal colonization is an independent risk factor for the development of infection with *S aureus* after arthroplasty.
- Most common organism in acute infection is staph aureus, most common organism in chronic infection Staph epidermidis.
    - If the causative organism is MRSA, the patient will have poorer prognosis for eradication of infection and lower functional results compared to infection from MSSA organisms.

- Deep infection is the most common complication after THA done for failed internal fixation after pathologic proximal femoral fracture secondary to malignancy.
- Obese patients have an increased risk for deep infection and wound-healing problems after THA.
- Types of post THA infection (similar to TKA):
  - **Early** postoperative infection (within 2-4 weeks of implantation of the prosthesis:
    - Clinical presentation: continuous discharge from the wound, aspiration will show increase WBC (more than 12,000) (the threshold for early post-operative infection is not well defined, and probably higher for TKA than THA).
    - Treatment is: surgical debridement with isolated femoral head and polyethylene liner exchange.
    - Prolonged post-operative wound discharge is likely a sign of deep infection. It should be **treated aggressive** by return to the operating room for open debridement and irrigation, exchange of modular part (eg PE insert), in addition to appropriate antibiotics based on intraoperative culture results. No need for removal of the femoral or the acetabular component in this stage (or removal of knee implant in cases of TKA). *(Scenario: 75 years old female, THA 11 days ago, serosanguinous wound drainage from the distal part of the wound, treatment?)*
  - **Late** infection (more than 4 weeks):
    - Clinical presentation: pain (in cases of TKA: pain and swelling of the knee).
    - **Markers of infection** (ESR, C-RP, IL-6 and less commonly WBCs) are elevated:
      - CRP and ESR should return to near normal levels at about three weeks and 8 weeks postoperatively respectively (after the index procedure). CRP and ESR are very sensitive for prosthetic infection.
      - IL-6 has been shown to have the highest correlation with infection (its use is now becoming more popular).
    - XR: can be completely normal or it may show signs of deep infection (new periosteal bone formation, osteolysis, and possible scalloping resorption). *(Scenario: 18 months post-operative THA, hip pain, XR shows new bone formation, most probable reason for pain?)*
    - Aspiration of the joint will show increase WBC in the aspirate (**more than 1500/ml with more than 70-75% PMN**), cultures and gram stain can be positive.

- If ESR and CRP are elevated, next step should be joint aspiration *(Scenario: 65 years old male, 6 years ago had THA, recent progressive pain, XR shows lucency around the stem, next step? (markers of infection)) (Scenario: THA 2 years ago, hip pain for the last 4 years, elevated ESR and CRP, next step?)*
- Antibiotics should be stopped for at least two weeks before aspiration. However, pre-operative antibiotic does not affect the result from intraoperative cultures.
- No need for bone scans as a routine exam.
- If ESR, CRP are elevated and first aspiration positive: no need to repeat the aspirate.
- For equivocal laboratory aspiration results (elevated markers of infection with aspirate results less than threshold), a repeat aspiration is indicated. *(Scenario: 60 years old male, one-year post THA, progressive pain, radiographs normal, elevated ESR, CRP, aspirate normal. Next action?). (Scenario: loose THA, increased marker of infection, currently having UTI and receiving antibiotic treatment, next step: aspiration of the hip for cultures three weeks after completion of the course of the antibiotic therapy) (aspiration is better option than Indium labeled WBC)*
- Bone scan can help with late infection. Normally, it stays hot for about one year after surgery. It can also be hot for aspectic loosening.
  - Indium labeled WBC is more sensitive for septic loosening than standard bone scan (Technetium bone scan). However, aspiration is still more specific in diagnosis of septic loosening than the Indium labeled WBC.
- Increased WBCs in the frozen section at the revision surgery for loosening is confirmatory test of infected joint replacement.
- **Treatment is two stage revision (all component).**
  - **First stage is** open debridement with removal of the implants and insertion of an antibiotic spacer, followed by culture specific antibiotic treatment for 6-8 weeks with re assessment of the inflammation markers (after two weeks of antibiotic holiday). *(Scenario: infected THA, first stage done, had antibiotic treatment and infection marker are now normal at the conclusion of the course of antibiotic, next step? (Repeat the test two weeks after stopping the antibiotics))*
  - If markers of inflammation remained elevated despite adequate dosing and time of antibiotic treatment, another session of debridement may be needed before proceeding to revision implant.
  - When the inflammation markers are back to normal (while patient is off antibiotic after finishing his course of treatment), removal of the spacer and implantation of the new prosthesis can be done. *(Scenario: 70 years old male, THA 8 years ago, hip pain for*

3 months, now became persistent, CRP and ESR elevated, hip aspiration is 10,000/ml, 81% PMN, what is the treatment?) (Scenario: 75 years old female, TKA 6 years ago, presenting with increased knee pain and swelling, CRP 12, ESR 75, aspirate shows 3000 WBC/ml, cultures negative, treatment?) (Scenario: loosing of THA, increased marker of infection, negative aspiration, at the of revision surgery there is increased WBC per high power field in the frozen section, but negative gram stain. next step? (removal of the prosthesis, cultures, antibiotic spacer (negative gram stain does not signify absence of infection))).

- Antibiotic cement:
    - Spacers reduce dead space, and deliver high local doses of antibiotics.
    - Increased porosity of the cement will increase elution of antibiotics.
    - The maximal amount of antibiotic to be added to PMMA for optimizing antibiotic elution without deleterious effects on mechanical strength is 5% of the total weight of the PMMA.
    - The antibiotic should be added as a powder, (not a liquid) to avoid affecting the binding and handling properties of the preparation.
    - Most common used antibiotic cement is 3.6 g tobramycin and 3 g vancomycin per 40 g of bone cement.
  - **Late hematogenous infection:**
    - Occurs within **2-4** weeks of systemic infection or source of bacteremia (e.g. dental work).
    - Patient with a well-functioning hip that all of sudden starts to be painful after remote infection or invasive procedure.
    - Treatment as **early postoperative infection** (surgical debridement with isolated exchange of modular component (femoral head and polyethylene liner)).
    - If more than 2-4 weeks since the onset of the hip pain: the hematogenous infection becomes more chronic and treatment better to be two stage revision.
- **Criteria for diagnosis of periprosthetic joint infection (PJI) (Hip and Knee):**
  - One of two major criteria (sinus tract communicating with the prosthesis or pathogen isolated from two separate aspirations) Or
  - Four of six minor criteria (elevated ESR and CRP; elevated joint WBCs; elevated joint neutrophils; purulence of the joint; pathogen isolated in one aspirate; > 5 neutrophil in high power field).

Tips:

- Wear by PE debris: initiator cell (macrophage), final cell (osteoclast)
- Bilateral protusio: think in rheumatoid arthritis or Marfan.
- Early loosening (1-2 years), pain since surgery: think in infection
- Ankylosing spondylitis: think in anterior dislocation and HO.
- End stage renal disease and psoriatic arthritis: think in infection.

Chapter 9:   The Knee

Knee Osteoarthritis (OA) (See Osteoarthritis in General Disease Chapter):

- Imaging: 45° postero-anterior flexion weight-bearing is the most sensitive view to detect early knee OA.
- **AAOS Guidelines (2013) (Some debates exist against these recommendations):**
  - Recommended treatment:
    - Weight loss (for patients with BMI >25), low-impact aerobic exercises, strengthening, self-management programs, neuromuscular education and engage in physical activity consistent with national guidelines.
    - Medication: NSAIDs (oral or topical) and tramadol.
  - Inconclusive treatments (lack of strong supporting evidence):
    - Electrotherapeutic modalities, manual therapy, acupuncture, valgus directing bracing, acetaminophen/opioids, pain patches, steroid injections and PRP.
  - Not recommended:
    - Glucosamine, chondroitin, lateral heel wedges, hyaluronic acid injections, arthroscopic lavage.
- **Hyaluronic acid:**
  - High-molecular-weight polysaccharide.
  - Effective in pain relief in patients with early-to-moderate osteoarthritis.
  - Does not rebuild articular cartilage or alter the natural history of osteoarthritis.
  - Rarely, can result in chemical synovitis (swelling and pain).
- **Surgical treatment of knee OA:**
  - After failure of non-operative treatment of OA (activity modification, injection and NSAIDs).
  - Surgical treatment is usually by total knee arthroplasty (TKA).
  - For medial uni compartment arthritis: unicompartment knee arthroplasty (UKA) or high tibial osteotomy (HTO) can be done (see later).
  - Arthroscopic lavage and debridement for knee osteoarthritis is not effective (especially with absence of mechanical symptoms).
    - Arthroscopic debridement can be considered for arthritic knee with mechanical symptoms (in relatively young people).
    - Arthroscopic debridement should not be done in advanced arthritis or in arthritis with varus or valgus malalignment.

Spontaneous Osteonecrosis of the Knee (SONK):

- **Clinical presentation:** more in females around 60s, with rapid onset of knee pain and no risk factors of osteonecrosis, can occur after knee scope.
- **Imaging:**
  - XR: will show lucency and partial collapse of the femoral condyles.
  - MRI: will show the lesion more obvious.
- **Treatment:**
  - Initial treatment is non operative (self-limiting condition)
  - If non-operative treatment fails: uni-compartment knee arthroplasty (not cartilage repair procedures).

Valgus Producing High Tibial Osteotomy (HTO) (See Also the Lower Extremity Sport Chapter):

- **Indications:** young patients, strenuous jobs, with varus deformity and medial joint pain and medial joint changes in knee radiographs (Ahlback stageI and II changes which is joint space narrowing and obliteration without affection of the subcondral bone), absence of lateral joint pathology.
- **Contraindication:** flexion contracture > 10°, limited flexion (range of motion of less than 90°), inflammatory arthritis, degenerative changes in the lateral and/or patellofemoral compartments, and ligamentous instability.
  - Obesity is relative contra-indication.
  - The ideal candidate for HTO is a thin, active person with a stable knee, unicompartmental knee symptoms, and age younger than 60. *(Scenario: 40 years old, electrician, medial joint pain, XR Ahlback stage II changes, treatment?)*
- **Technique:**
  - Medial opening osteotomy or lateral closing osteotomy.
- **Complications:**
  - Can be complicated by patella baja (especially medial opening wedge osteotomy):
    - Most common complication after HTO.
    - This can cause anterior knee pain
  - Medial opening has more incidence of nonunion (not preferred in smoker).
  - Lateral closing-wedge osteotomy can lead to disruption of proximal tibiofibular (specific complication for lateral closing wedge).
- **TKA after HTO**
  - TKA after HTO can be more difficult to perform than primary TKA due to patella baja, contraction of the patella tendon, shift of the proximal tibial

articular surface in relation to the medullary canal, retained implants, previous skin incisions and scar tissue.

- o Risk factors for early failure of TKA after HTO include obesity, laxity of the knee, mal-alignment, and young age at the time of TKA.
- o Despite TKA after HTO is a more complex procedure than primary TKA, long-term clinical outcomes of both are similar.

Varus Producing Distal Femoral Osteotomy:

- **Indications:** young patients with lateral compartment arthritis (eg after lateral meniscus excision). No patellofemoral or medial compartments symptoms.
- **Contraindications**: patients with prior medial meniscectomy or medial compartment arthritis
- Can be open wedge laterally, closing wedge medially or dome osteotomy. Crescentic dome will produce the least displacement at the osteotomy side. *(Scenario: 40 years old female, long history of knee pain, failed non operative treatment, XR shows 13 femoral-tibial angle in valgus. MRI shows lateral knee compartment cartilage thinning. Treatment?)*

Unicompartment Knee Arthroplasty (UKA):

- **Indications/ prerequisites**: non inflammatory unicompartment arthritis, intact ACL and PCL, no flexion contracture more than 15°, less than 10° varus deformity or 5° valgus deformity, no patellofemoral symptoms (radiographic arthritis findings at the PF joint is not a contraindication), competent medial collateral ligament, more than 90 flexion pre operatively.
- **Absolute contraindication:** deficient ACL, vaurs deformity > 10 degrees, valugs deformity > 5°, joint subluxation of more than 5mm, flexion contracture more than 15°.
- **Relative contraindication:** limited flexion (flexion less than 90°), obesity (currently it is less of a concern)
  - o Osteonecrosis of the femoral condyle is not contra indication.
  - o Asymptomatic patellofemoral XR changes are not contra indication.
- **Surgical considerations:**
  - o A medial UKA should be aligned to allow undercorrection to approximately 0° to 3° of valgus (the normal alignment is 7° valgus) (to protect the lateral compartment from weight bearing stresses).
  - o Can be performed through a smaller incision without dislocation of the patella which will allow faster recovery.

- **Outcome:**
  - UKA (compared to TKA): more closely approximates native knee kinematics, patients have quicker return of function and discontinuation of pain medication, less blood loss, less narcotic use and less length of hospital stay, better postoperative knee scores.
  - UCA leads to better ROM than either TKA or HTO. *(Scenario: elderly, medial joint arthritis, 8 varus deformity, want to be able to kneel (extreme flexion), what type of surgery?)*
  - Higher failure rate in females, osteopenia and high BMI (controversial).
  - Lateral UKA similar results to medial UKA.
  - Low progression of arthritis in the midterm follow up after UKA.
  - **Stress fracture after UCA:** tibial plateau stress fractures after UKA. Patient will present with persistent pain after UKA.
    - More commonly occurs in obese patients (>85 Kg), in association with pin placement during surgery and technical error during the sagittal cut of the tibia.

Patellofemoral Arthroplasty:

- The most common cause of early failure is patellar instability/ mal-tracking.
- The most common cause of late failure is progression of tibio-femoral arthritis.

Total Knee Arthroplasty (TKA):

Approaches for TKA (See Anatomy Chapter):

- If exposure during revision TKA is difficult, and there is a concern that the patellar ligament may avulse from its insertion, the exposure can be extended proximally with a rectus snip or distally with a long tibial tubercle osteotomy.
  - **Quadriceps rectus snip approach**: does not require changes in post-operative plan (weight bearing or ROM) compared to normal medial parapatellar approach. The clinical results are similar to standard approach.
  - **Patellar turndown:** will require change in post-operative rehabilitation protocol by delaying ROM.
  - **Tibial tubercle osteotomy (TTO):** in cases of patella baja, to avoid excess traction on the patella and possible patellar tendon ruptures.

Technique and Applied Anatomy of TKA:

- Mechanical axis of the limb is a vertical line drawn from the femoral head through the center of the knee down to the center of the ankle (used in TKA pre operative planning and template)

- The goal is to have femoral and tibial cut perpendicular to the mechanical axis of femur and tibia respectively.
- The transepicondylar axis of the knee is perpendicular to the AP axis and 3° externally rotated from the posterior condylar line (the posterior condylar axis is 3° internally rotated to the transepicondylar axis) (Fig 1).
  - ○ Valgus knee may have hypoplastic lateral condyle (the trans condylar axis is more externally rotated in relation to the posterior condylar line), failure to recognize that will result in internal rotation of the femoral component (if the component was applied in only 3° of external rotation) (see patellar mal-tracking).

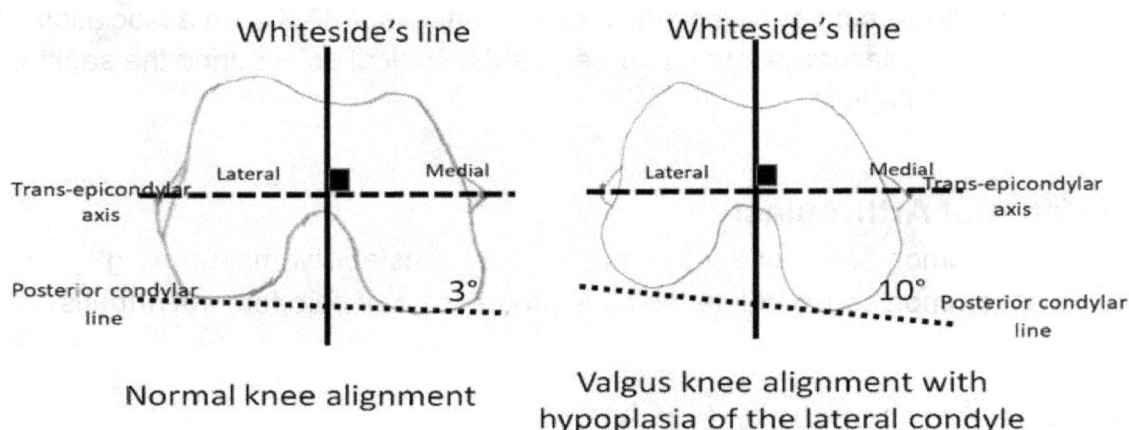

Fig1: The relation between posterior condylar line and transeiphyseal line. The posterior condylar line is 3° internally rotated in relation to the transepiphseal line. In cases of valgus knee with hypoplasia of the posterior lateral condyle, the posterior condylar axis becomes more internally rotated than the normal 3°. Failure to identify this increased internal rotation with valgus knee can result in internally rotated implant.

- The joint line is at the upper level of PE insert.
  - ○ More tibial cutting: lower joint line; while more femoral cutting: elevation of joint line; thicker insert: elevation of the joint line.
  - ○ Elevation of the joint line is associated with disadvantages including anterior knee pain, relative patella baja, restricted knee flexion (especially with CR due to tight PCL), and instability of the prosthesis (see revision).
  - ○ The maximum acceptable joint line elevation is 8 mm (maximum amount you can compensate for by cutting more of the distal femur).
- Appropriate femoral component rotation will create a rectangular flexion gap.

- In normal native knee, the point of contact between femur and tibia moves posteriorly with knee flexion (rollback).
  - In CR knee, due to absence of ACL, the point of contact moves anteriorly with knee flexion (Paradoxical Rollback). This will cause anterior femoral condylar translation in CR knees from full extension to 90° of flexion.
- Closed suction drainage increases the transfusion requirements after TKA (and THA) with no significant effect on wound hematoma, infection, or operations for wound complications.
- If there are multiple scars, use the most lateral scar (blood supply goes from medial to lateral, so the lateral scar will have least effect on the blood supply to the rest of the skin)
- Computer navigation TKA:
  - Can improve the accuracy of placement of TKA components with fewer outliers.
  - Disadvantages: increased surgical time and cost. No studies had shown improved clinical outcomes or implant survivorship.

Knee Prosthesis Design:

- Cruciate retaining (CR), posterior stabilized (PS), constrained condylar, rotating hinge.
- **Cruciate retaining (CR)**
  - XR of CR knee will show NO box on the femoral side (Fig 2).
  - If PCL is tight, this will increase the wear of PE. If release of PCL is excess, it will cause flexion instability.
  - Contra-indication of the CR knee (have to use PS knee instead): absence of PCL, previous history of patellectomy, advanced inflammatory arthritis (rheumatoid, SLE).
  - Relative contra-indication (difficult to balance PCL): flexion contracture, varus or valgus more than 15°. *(Scenario: 48 years old male, previous history of fracture of the knee, now has advanced arthritis, XP presented (no patella seen in the lateral view), what type of prosthesis to use?)*
  - Patients with CR knee and PCL insufficiency or later rupture of the PCL, will have sagittal instability. On examination, there will be a posterior tibial sag, and positive posterior drawer test. Patients will have flexion instability and will have difficulty when going up and down stairs and difficult getting up from chair. *(Scenario: patient had TKA one year ago, having pain and instability, XR shows CR knee prosthesis with posterior knee dislocation (CR does not have femoral box), the reason for symptoms? (PCL insufficiency and knee dislocations)) (Scenario: pain after TKA one year ago, cannot raise from bed or go up and down stairs, reason?) (CR with PCL insufficiency)).*

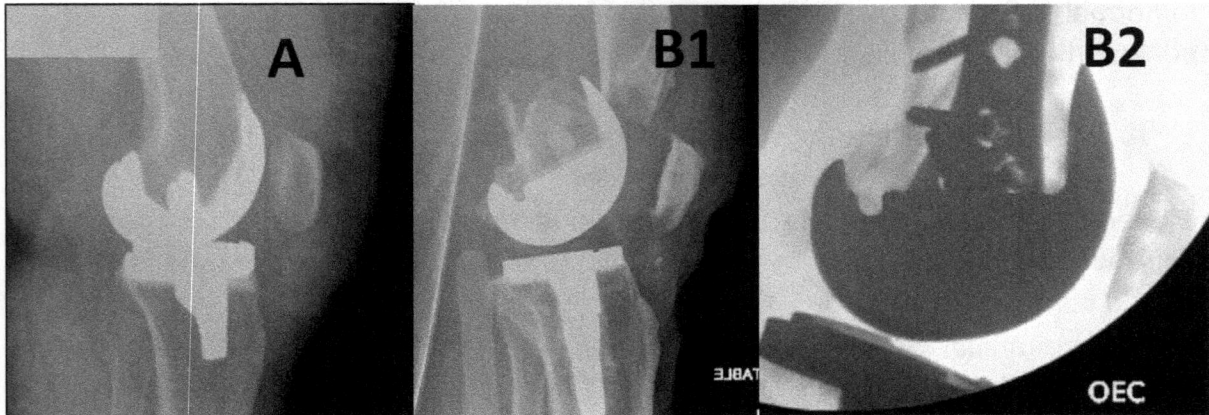

Fig 2: showing the difference between (A) cruciate retaining and (B) posterior stabilized. In PS, periprosthetic femur fractures are usually stabilized with plate fixation (retrograde naili passage can be hindered by the femoral cam).

- **Posterior stabilized (PS):**
    - Posterior-stabilized knees use a tibial post bearing that articulates with femoral box design in flexion to act as a cam mechanism and improve femoral rollback (Fig 2).
    - Flexion instability (the knee is loose in flexion, increased flexion gap) can cause posterior knee dislocation.
        - The femoral component can come out of the post (jump), the femoral cam is translated anterior to the central tibial post causing posterior dislocation.
        - Causes of flexion instability (increase flexion gap) (see also balancing knee cuts section): under sizing the femoral component, anterior translation of the femoral component, increased posterior tibial slope, injury to the popliteus while cutting the posterolateral femoral condyle.
    - PS: the design allows more knee flexion than other designs.
    - The posterior slope in PS should be only around 4° (more slope can cause flexion instability).
    - PCL-retaining and PCL-substituting TKAs both have similar survivorship rates at 10 years' follow-up.
    - Hyperextension of the femoral component in relation to tibial component
        - Can occur with knee hyperextension, insertion of the femoral component in flexion or excess tibial slope.
        - Can lead to impingement between femoral box and anterior part of the tibial post; this will lead to wear of the post and increased backside wear (see below)

- **Constrained knees:**
  - Relies on a large tibial post in a deep femoral box to achieve varus/valgus stability (2°) and rotation stability (2°).
  - Indication: ligamentous instability (varus/valgus) (especially in elderly), moderate bone loss (e.g. neuropathic arthroplasty). *(Scenario: during TKA, the surgeon cut the MCL, in trial there is obvious valgus instability, what type of prosthesis? (constrained condylar)) (Scenario: valgus knee, obvious instability of MCL, what prosthesis? (constrained TKA prosthesis)).*
    - Some controversy exists regarding the use of constrained knees in complete MCL deficiency and Charcot joint, citing the need for hinged prothesis.
- **Rotating-hinge prosthesis:**
  - Constrains anterior-posterior translation in addition to varus-valgus and internal-external rotation.
  - Indication: presence of severe deformity, bone loss, or chronic dislocation, presence of "infinite flexion gap".
  - Hinge total knee prosthesis has a higher rate of aseptic loosening secondary to a high-degree of constraint.
- **Cemented Vs Cementless TKA:**
  - No difference in poly wear between two types.
  - Cementless TKA has increased risk for revision. Loosening of the tibial component was the most common cause of failure.
    - Cemented tibia component (Cementing the metaphyseal and keel portions of the tibial component) results are superior results compared to cementless tibia component.
- **Mobile-bearing TKA (Vs Fixed bearing):**
  - Mobile bearing TKA combines large contact area between tibial and femoral parts (increased conformity) with absence of restrains that may cause stress transfer.
    - This implant design should theoretically reduce polyethylene wear and reduce bone-implant-interface stress (can be used in younger patient and those with higher BMI).
  - Balancing extension and flexion gap in very crucial with mobile bearing TKA as flexion instability can cause posterior knee dislocation.
  - Increasing tibial PE conformity in fixed bearing total knee arthroplasty will increase the contact area, decrease contact stress:
    - Advantage: less risk of polyethylene wear, fracture, and delamination.
    - Disadvantages: limit femoral rollback during flexion and increase shear stress transfer to the implants (in contrast to mobile bearing which has less stress transfer due to movement of the bearing).

Wear (See Also Hip Chapter)

- Wear in TKA prosthesis differs from that in a THA:
  - In TKA: Wear is due to fatigue (pitting and delamination) (THA wear is due to adhesive and abrasive wear). This is due to higher contact stresses in TKA than in THA.
  - The particles isolated from the knee PE are larger and less reactive (in contrast to submicron wear debris particles in THA). This leads to more "osteolysis" in cases of THA than with TKA.
  - UHMWPE sterilized by gamma irradiation in air will cause more wear in TKA (similar to THA) (See hip chapter for more details).
- Risk factors for increase PE wear and PE failure: increasing PE shelf age, younger age of patient, male gender, and a rough tibial baseplate.
- The most common cause for late revision of TKA is PE wear:
  - PE wear can cause osteolysis of the proximal tibia or distal femur (which is a **macrophage** mediated response (similar to THA)).
  - The osteolysis can result in loosening of the components.
  - Polyethylene wear is the most common reason to both focal osteolysis and component loosening at long-term follow up. *(Scenario: 70 years old, TKA 15 years ago, having pain in the last year, labs normal, XR shows loosening, change of position of the TKA, what is the mechanism?)*
  - If this process occurs early (less than 10 years), it is most probably due to technical or implant problem (e.g. mal-tracking, sterilization of PE).
- Backside wear:
  - Backside wear is the PE wear between tibial base plate and PE due to movement between lower surface of PE and tibial base plate causing osteolysis of the upper tibia (by wear debris from the backside of the insert).
    - Wear on the backside of the PE (not on the articular surface side).
    - Modular tibial component (separate base and insert) is easier to apply but leads to this type of tear.
    - Monoblock tibial designs are harder to apply but eliminate backside wear.
- PE wear is commonly related to component rotational impingement (especially with PS designs).
- Early PE wear leading to early catastrophic failure of knee arthroplasty is most commonly related to gamma irradiation sterilization in air and/or shelf storage in air leading to excessive oxidation. *(Scenario: TKA 3 years ago, revision done, picture of retrieved PE showing worn PE on both medial and lateral sides with delamination, what is the cause?)*

- If the PE insert completely wears out, the underlying metal- base plate will be in direct contact with the femoral component, resulting in scratching of the components and release of metal debris; resulting in metallosis of the adjacent soft tissues, reactive synovitis and osteolysis secondary to a host response to both PE debris and metal particles.
  - Patients will complain of knee pain, swelling, squeaking and instability.
- If there is osteolysis without loosening (no pain), it can be either followed up closely (if small) or treated with PE exchange and bone grafting (if large) (so long there is no obvious implant mal position)
  - If there is osteolysis with loosening (pain) the treatment is revision knee arthroplasty (both components and PE). *(Scenario: 65 years, 5 years ago had TKA, No complaint, routine XR shows osteolysis, next step?) (same scenario, has pain for 6 months, next step?)*

Balancing The Knee:

- Commonly used expression:
  - Loose = instability.
  - Lack of extension = flexion contracture = cannot extend= tight extension gap.
  - Lack of flexion = extension contracture = cannot flex = tibia tray lifts-off in flexion = patella impinging on PE= tight flexion gap.
- **General rules:**
  - Proper balancing of a TKA: means achieving symmetrical extension gaps and flexion (usually measured at 90°).
  - Changing the size of the femoral implant, affect the AP diameter mainly (flexion)
  - Distal cutting of femur (joint level): affects extension gap. Posterior cutting of the femoral condyle: affects flexion gap.
  - Posterior tibial slope affects flexion gap (increase slope allow more flexion).
  - Tibial cutting and size of insert: affect both flexion and extension.
    - If more distal tibial cut is used to correct flexion contracture with balanced extension, the TKA will end unstable in extension after the cut. If more distal tibia cut is used to correct extension contracture with balanced flexion, the TKA will end unstable in flexion.
  - Posteriorize or anteriorize the femoral component: affects flexion gap.
  - One strategy to address the selective problem (flexion only or extension only) is to work on the tibial side (which will affect both flexion and extension), then change the other part from balance to opposite (eg flexion instability, can be addressed by thicker insert. This will correct the flexion instability but will cause extension tightness, so add distal femoral cutting elevating the joint line.

- o Little resection of distal femur combined with thin PE can lead to flexion instability (due to thin PE causing wide flexion gap).
    - o Excessive posterior femoral resection will lead to unstable loose flexion gap.
- Flexion contracture: Before proceeding with bony cuts/ implants related solutions, the surgeon has first to (to avoid raising the joint line):
    - o Removal of posterior osteophytes.
    - o Releasing posterior capsule.
- For tight flexion (extension contracture) in CR knee, recessing PCL is an option.

Tabel 1: Balancing flexion and extension gaps (different possibilities):

	Loose flexion	Balanced	Tight flexion
Loose extension	Thicker PE	Distal femur augmentation. (other option is thicker PE with smaller component)	Distal femur augment combined more resection of more posterior femur
Balanced	upsize the femoral component (with use of posterior femoral augments or cement) or move the femoral component posterior. (other option is thinker PE with more distal femoral resection).		Cut more posterior femur, downsize the femoral component, anteriorioze the femoral component or increase the posterior tibial slope. For CR, PCL release or recess.
Tight extension	Upsize the femoral component and resects more distal femur	First: removal of posterior osteophytes and posterior capsule release. If this fails: resect more distal femur	Cut more tibia or use thinner PE

Soft Tissue for Coronal Balance:
- **Tight valgus knee:**
    - o Osteophytes excision (lateral side) then
        - If tight in flexion only: release the popliteus
        - If tight in extension only: release Iliotibial band
        - If tight in both flexion and extension: release lateral collateral ligament.

- The peroneal nerve is at greatest risk for injury during release of the posterolateral capsule with the knee extended (only about 8 mm from the posterolateral capsule with the knee extended).
- In severe valgus with an incompetent or attenuated MCL: consider constrained TKA.

- **Tight varus knee:**
  - The following sequence:
    - Removal of femoral and tibial osteophyte, release of the deep MCL (tibio-meniscal ligament), release of the posteromedial corner, release of the semimembranosus, and partial differential superficial MCL release (anterior part if tight in flexion, posterior part if tight in extension)

Revision TKA:

- The aim is to restore the joint line while maintaining stability.
  - A constraint mechanism that resists varus-valgus loads may be needed (especially if there is ligament insufficiency).
  - Use of stems and augments may be needed (especially If there is massive osteolysis and bone loss) to restore the joint line and maintain stability of the components within the medullary canals.
- If the primary knee fails due to inadequate coronal balance, this will result in PE wear in the narrow side. The treatment is revision of the whole components. Isolated PE exchange will not correct alignment. *(Scenario: TKA, 3 years, in valgus, wear of PE on the lateral side, treatment?)*
- During revision cases, there is tendency to elevate the joint line by applying the femoral component on the remaining bone on the femoral side that is left behind after removal of the prior component (see effects of that in anatomy subheading).
  - The femoral component will be small (causing increased flexion gap) and proximal to where it should be (increased extension gap).
  - Management: the femoral component should be applied more distally (with the use of distal femoral augments) to restore the joint line to more anatomical level and to decrease the size of the extension gap and the femoral component size should be increased (with the use of posterior augments) or posteriorized to decrease the size of the flexion gap.
- For marked bone loss:
  - Either metal augments (preferred for older persons) or Structural allograft (younger patients).
- If the main problem is PE wear and the components are well-fixed without mal-alignment, isolated polyethylene exchange can be considered.

Post-Operative, Rehabilitation and Prognosis

- DVT prophylaxis: see hip chapter.
  - AAOS 2011 guidelines:
    - If a patient has increased risk for bleeding (e.g. liver disease or hemophilia), use mechanical prophylaxis (eg pneumatic calf compressors).
    - If a patient has history of VTE: combined use of mechanical and pharmacological prophylaxis
    - No need for routine screening by duplex.
- For rheumatoid arthritis disease modifying medication: See general disease chapter.
- Both the use of a continuous passive motion (CPM) device and structured physical therapy program following total knee arthroplasty result in equivalent early range of motion.
- Patients with TKA wounds closed in flexion have greater flexion range of motion and required less domiciliary physiotherapy compared to those with wounds closed in full extension. Closing the knee in flexion permits the patients regain knee motion faster with less effort.
- Final ROM outcomes after TKS are not affected by the use of CPM machines postoperatively.
- Females undergoing TKA have longer implant survivorship compared to males, greater improvement in WOMAC scores and equal improvements in SF-12 scores.
- Obese patients (combared to non obeses) have increased risk of complications and after TKA, including infection, loosening, and revision arthroplasty. Survivorship and functional scores in obese patients are lower than non obese

Patellar-Related Aspects of TKA

- To improve patellar tracking:
  - Lateralization of the tibial component.
  - Lateralization o the femoral component.
  - External rotation of the tibial component.
  - External rotation of the femoral component.
  - Medialization of the patellar component.
  - Avoidance of over-stuffing of patellofemoral space (avoidance of small patellar cuts, big patellar components, and anterior translation of the femoral component).
- Risk of patellar mal tracking (lateral patellar tilt and increased lateral subluxation and post operative pain) (opposite of above):
  - Medialization of the tibial component.

- o Medialization o the femoral component.
- o Internal rotation of the tibial component.
  - ▪ Internal rotation of the tibial component results in external rotation of the tibial tubercle and increases the Q angle).
- o Internal rotation of the femoral component (common with genu valgum deformity due to deficiency of the lateral femoral condyle).
- o Lateralization of the patellar component.
- Patellar tracking should be assessed with the tourniquet deflated. *(scenario: after TKA, the patella subluxate laterally despite good component position, next step? (deflate the tourniquet)).*
- Internal rotation of the femoral component during total knee arthroplasty will result in Increased need for lateral release of the patella. External rotation of femoral component decreases the need for lateral retinacular release.
- If mal-tracking of patella is present, CT scan of the knee is best radiographic modality to diagnose the malrotation of total knee components. *(Scenario: 60 years old, TKA few months ago, knee pain, XR show lateral tilt, next step?)*
  - o If the components are determined to be in satisfactory position (CT scan is usually needed to assess this), soft-tissue procedures (eg. lateral retinacular release) can be performed.
  - o If the components (femoral or tibial) were found to be internally rotated, revision of the components should be done. *(Scenario: 67 years old, valgus knee, TKA, persistent knee pain, CT shows the femoral component to internally rotated, treatment?)*
- For patella baja: the surgeon can lower joint line or apply the patella implant in superior patella and trim the inferior patellar bone.
- To surface or not:
  - o Mainly: a surgeon preference.
  - o Absolute indication for resurfacing patella: rheumatoid and other inflammatory arthritis.
  - o Resurface has lower patellar-related pain and higher complication rate and lower patellar related reoperation compared to non-resurface.
- Patellar clunk:
  - o Occurs with certain types of posterior stabilized knee arthroplasties.
  - o Due to the development of a fibrous nodule on the deep aspect of the quadriceps tendon that falls into the intercondylar notch of the femoral component during knee flexion.
  - o Clinical presentation: sharp catching anterior pain aggravated by rising from a chair or climbing stairs.
  - o Treatment: knee arthroscopy to resect the inflammatory nodule.
- After medial parapatellar approach: care should be taken to avoid injury to the superior lateral genicular (by avoiding excess lateral retinacular dissection) as this becomes the main blood supply of patella (see complications section).

Complications:
- **Heterotrophic ossification (HO):**
    - ○ Risk factor for the development of heterotopic ossification (HO)
        - ▪ Obesity, hypertrophic arthrosis (as compared to post traumatic cases), male gender, and ankylosing spondylitis.
- **Stiffness:**
    - ○ If by two months, patient is lacking 90° of flexion or full extension: treatment is manipulation under anesthesia (exclude infection and component malposition first).
    - ○ If there is deteriorating knee ROM, particularly few months after TKA, deep infection should be ruled out.
    - ○ Preoperative ROM is the most consistent predictor of postoperative ROM.
        - ▪ Revision TKA for stiffness and fibrosis only result in small improvement in ROM (pain level may remain the same).
- **Post-operative peroneal nerve palsy**
    - ○ Risk factors: correction of large valgus deformities (>20˚) (most common cause), correction of flexion contracture, aberrant retractor placement intraoperatively (most common cause in absence of valgus deformity), postoperative epidural analgesia, pre-operative diagnosis of neuropathy (centrally or peripherally). *(Scenario: patient with significant flexion and valgus deformity, you should counsel her about which post-operative complication?) (Scenario: TKA for varus deformity, patient had post operative peroneal nerve, most probable cause? (Aberrant retractor placement)).*
    - ○ If discovered in the recovery room: unwrap any compressive dressings and flex the knee, then re-assess.
- **Post-operative patellar tendon rupture:**
    - ○ Mainly due to frying of the tendon. More common after cases of difficult knee exposure (patella baja, revision cases, flexion contracture).
    - ○ Clinical presentation: loss of active knee extension with persistence of passive extension.
    - ○ XR: patella alta.
    - ○ Treatment is by reconstruction with a bone-tendon allograft
        - ▪ The graft should be sutured in maximal tension with the knee in full extension and immobilized in full extension for 6 weeks.
- **Infection after TKA (also see THA/TSA infection)**
    - ○ Classification of TKA infection (similar to THA)
        - ▪ Early post-operative infection (within 4 weeks):
            - • Patient will have increased pain, swelling and discharge.

- Fever or detection of bacteria in the aspirate is not necessary criteria for diagnosis. Lab will not be very helpful as they are normally elevated after surgery (even in absence of infection).
- Treatment is by surgical debridement of the knee with change of the PE insert. No need to wait for the cultures before proceeding to surgery.

- Late infection (see also late infection of THA):
  - Clinical picture, labs and XR: similar to THA.
  - New onset knee pain few months/years after surgery with mild swelling; the wound is usually healed with no discharge. No obvious instability.
  - Next step: blood work (CBC, ESR, C-reactive protein). *(Scenario: 70 year old, TKA 5 years ago, knee pain for 2 years, XR normal, exam shows swelling and good ROM, next step?) (ESR, CRP))*
  - XR: Can be normal. The development of a progressive radiolucency within the first year following TKA is concerning for possible infection. *(Scenario: 65 years old, 9 months follow up, no pain, XR shows progressive radiolucent lines, next step? (Blood work, if elevated, aspiration)).*
  - If the primary surgery (TKA) is less than one year, regular bone scan cannot be used as it will be active from the surgery itself.
  - Treatment standard is by two stage component exchange: resection with implantation of antibiotic impregnated cement spacer followed by re implantation. This treatment has high success rate.
  - If after primary stage, the infection is not cleared (discovered before the second stage by labs or during the second stage by pathology), treatment is by a repeat debridement and placement of another antibiotic spacer.
  - Before proceeding with the second stage (re-plantation), patient has to be off antibiotics for at least two weeks, then either markers of infection (ESR, C-RP) or knee aspiration is done. If there are signs of infection, another debridement is done (rather than proceeding with the second stage) *(Scenario: 70 years old, infected TKA, explanatation done, 6 weeks of antibiotic, next step? (2 weeks' antibiotic holiday followed by either knee aspiration or repeat ESR and CRP)).*
  - Articulating cement spacers are equal to static spacers regarding the rate of infection recurrence, however, they have the advantage of decrease quadriceps shortening, increased ROM for the duration of cement spacer application, better maintenance of joint space and less time for exposure during re-

implantation. Potential disadvantages of mobile spacers include problems with wound healing and an increased risk of cement fracture
- Knee fusion can be considered if there repeated failure of reconstruction especially with failure of extensor mechanism or major soft tissue defect, but it also requires eradication of infection before proceeding.
- Elderly patient with failure of extensor mechanism and MRSA or gram negative infection, may be treated with primary knee fusion
- Amputation is the last resort if infection cannot be eradicated (most surgeon will try twice before considering this).
  - o Risk for periprosthetic infection is higher with TKA (around 1%) than with THA (around 0.7%).
  - o In any case of knee pain, you have to exclude infection.
- **Peri prosthetic fractures:**
  - o Femoral fracture:
    - In most cases the femoral component is well fixed, and the treatment is ORIF (using a fixed angle (locking) plate). If there is relatively large distal fragment (type I), retrograde nail can be used (retrograde nail may not be possible with some closed-box PS femoral component designs (See Fig 2)).
    - Less common, there is loose femoral component or no enough bone stock attached to the femoral component; the treatment will be revision distal femoral replacement (this is best suited for elderly patients due to advantage of early weight bearing). If the femoral epicondyles are going to be replaced with the implant, this will require hinged TKA. Both femoral and tibial components will need to be replaced to convert to the hinged prosthesis.
    - Risk factors: rheumatoid arthritis, neurologic disorders such as Parkinson's disease, chronic steroid therapy, osteopenia, female gender and revision knee arthroplasty. Notching is NOT a risk factor.
  - o **Tibial fracture at the level of the tibial implant with stem loosening:**
    - Revision with a long stem tibial component that bypasses the fracture
  - o **Patellar fracture after resurfaced patella:**
    - Most can be managed non-surgically (if the extensor mechanism is intact).
- **Post-operative skin necrosis with exposed implant or patellar tendon:**

- o Treatment is medial gastrocnemius muscle flap (supplied by medial sural artery) and skin grafting to prevent extensor mechanism disruption and deep infection.
- **Intra operative vascular injury:**
  - o May be related to Homann retractor placement or from the use of the saw.
  - o Post-operatively: the patient will have asymmetrical pulses and poor capillary refill.
  - o Treatment: urgent vascular surgery consultation/ interventional radiologist consultation, and urgent arteriogram.
    - ▪ Vascular perfusion may be obtained at the time of an arteriogram with the use of a stent.
    - ▪ If this fail to re-perfuse the extremity, urgent exploration of the vessel at the level of injury (determined by the arthrogram).
      - If ischemic compartment syndrome develops: four-compartment fasciotomy should be added following revascularization of the extremity (also fasciotomy can be added after revascularization as a prophylactic against re-perfusion compartment syndrome)
- **Extensor mechanism failure:**
  - o Patellar fracture after TKA: if the patient is able to extend the knee, non-operative management (see peri prosthetic fractures).
  - o Chronic rupture of the tendon or avulsion of the tibial tubercle: extensor mechanism allograft.
  - o Intra-operative rupture of the patellar ligament: extensor mechanism allograft.
- **Persistent post-operative wound discharge**
  - o The persistent discharge can lead to infection.
  - o If there is persistent wound discharge after TKA, aggressive treatment is needed (Irrigate and debride the knee (with possible polyethylene exchange) in the operating room).
- **Avascular necrosis of the patella:**
  - o The main blood supply for the patella in the infromedial genicular artery, which is severed in the medial arthrotomy. The superior lateral genicular becomes the main blood supply to the patella.
  - o Adding lateral retinacular release may injure the superior lateral genicular artery causing AVN of the patella.

Tips:
- If after TKA, pain is related to weight bearing, think is mechanical reasons (mal-alignment, loosening, instability). If pain is at rest and activity, think in infection.

Chapter 10:   Foot and Ankle

Examination of the ankle:

- **Silfverskiold test:**
    - Comparing ankle dorsiflexion with the knee extended and flexed.
    - Increase in the dorsiflexion of the ankle by 15° or more with knee flexion is an indication of gastrocnemius muscle contracture (cross both knee and ankle joints, bending the knee will relax the muscle).
        - For muscle lengthening with positive Silfverskiold test (equinus is relieved with knee flexion/ gaining more than 15° dorsiflexion with knee flexion): a gastrocnemius lengthening is sufficient.
        - If ankle dorsiflexion is limited in both knee flexion and extension: the lengthening should be at the level of the Achilles tendon (or both gastrocnemius and soleus muscles need to be lengthened). (*Scenario: 40 years old, ankle arthritis, will have ankle arthroplasty, exam shows -10 dorsiflexion with the knee extended and 10 with the knee flexed, how to approach the equines with the primary surgery? (open gastrocnemius muscle lengthening (not Achilles tendon lengthening))*)
- **Anterior Drawer Test of The Ankle:**
    - If the ankle is in 10-15° of plantar flexion, it will assess the integrity of the anterior talo-fibular ligament. If the ankle is in neutral or slight dorsiflexion, it evaluates calcaneo-fibular ligament.
    - More than 10 mm translation indicates rupture of the corresponding ligament.
- **Lateral Talar Tilt Test (Stress Test Using C Arm):**
    - Measurement greater than 15° indicates rupture of both anterior talo-fibular ligament and calcaneo-fibular ligaments.

Foot and Ankle Arthritis/Fusion/Arthroplasty:

Ankle Arthritis:

- Most common etiology is posttraumatic.
- **Treatment of ankle arthritis:**
    - Initial treatment: non operative (NSAIDS, braces (Arizona brace, or AFO))
    - Operative: fusion, arthroplasty, ankle distraction, debridement of osteophytes, correction of deformity (usually by supra malleolar osteotomy)
        - For end stage disease with failure of non-operative treatment: Arthrodesis or Arthroplasty.
    - **For ankle (tibio-talar) fusion:**
        - The position of fusion is neutral flexion (or 5° plantar flexion in females), 0°- 5° hindfoot valgus, 5°-10° external rotation.
        - Ankle arthritis can lead to subtalar arthritis (long term effect) (notice that subtalar fusion can also lead to ankle arthritis on the long term).

- Heel to toe Rocker sole shoe modification is the most effective modification to accommodate for lost motion after ankle arthrodesis as it helps to create more efficient heel-to-toe gait pattern, increase propulsion at the toe off and normalize gait (see rehabilitation chapter).
  - **Total Ankle Arthroplasty (TAA):**
    - TAA results in better gait mechanics than fusion.
    - The indications of TAA are evolving; however, in general it is more for rheumatoid arthritis and elderly patient with limited activity, less suitable for post-traumatic arthritis (these concepts are currently changing with the development of better new designs).
    - Agility ankle implant has large surface area for bone growth into the tibial component through arthrodesis of the syndesmosis between tibial and fibula. Nonunion of the syndesmosis is associated with failure of the tibial component (not a concern with current TAA designs).
    - Complications: Wound complication, loosening, ectopic bone formation (HO); when ectopic bone formation in the malleolar gutters restricts motion or is a source of pain it may require surgical intervention.
    - Infection after TAA: (see THA, TKA, TSA infections): Flap coverage may be needed if there is wound breakdown.
  - **TTC (tibio-talar-calcaneal) nail:**
    - Will fuse both the ankle and subtalar joints.
    - Because the nail ends in the mid-diaphysis of the tibia, the locking screws or the end of the nail can cause stress riser and fracture; if this happens, the treatment is cast immobilization.
  - **Ankle arthroscopy:**
    - The most common complication of ankle arthroscopy is nerve injury related to portals (See anatomy chapter for specific nerves affection).
    - Synovial fistula after ankle arthroscopy is more common complication with ankle scopes (compared to other joints arthroscopy).

Ankle Osteophytes:

- Repeated dorsiflexion of the ankle (soccer, gymnastics) can cause osteophyte and bony exostosis formation in both the anterior distal tibia and anterior talar neck.
- If this blocks extension, treatment is by debridement of the osteophystes (open or arthroscopic). *(Scenario: 24 years old gymnast, anterior ankle pain, limited dorsiflexion, XR shows anterior osteophytes, treatment?).*

Osteochondral Lesion of The Talus (See Sport Injuries)

- Medial lesion:

- o Atruamtic, posterior, deep.
- o Treatment: for small lesion: drilling. For large lesion or unstable cartilage: medial malleolus osteotomy and osteochondral allograft
- Lateral lesion:
  - o Traumatic, anterior, more superficial.

Hindfoot Arthritis:
- The hindfoot articulations include the subtalar, talonavicular, and calcaneocuboid joints.
- Subtalar joint:
  - o Post calcaneus fracture arthritis of the subtalar joint:
    - Clinical presentation: anterior ankle impingement (pain with dorsiflexion of the ankle, limited ankle dorsiflexion) due to dorsiflexed talus lying horizontally and abutting against the anterior tibia with dorsiflexion.
    - XR: Loss of calcaneal height with horizontal talus.
    - Treated by distraction bone block subtalar fusion. *(Scenario: 40 years old, calcaneus fracture 2 years ago, anterior ankle pain especially during climbing stairs or ascending slopes, XR shows dorsiflexion of the talus, treatment?)*
  - o If there is subtalar arthritis with marked deformity: triple fusion is a better surgical option (compared to isolated subtalar fusion) with possible Achilles tendon lengthening. *(Scenario: 60 years old, valgus deformity, partial correction of the deformity causes pain (arthritis), XR shows arthritis and deformity, treatment?)*
    - Patients with severe rigid hindfoot valgus leading to foot ulceration that is resistant to bracing and custom orthotics and shoes, the treatment is triple arthrodesis (with Achilles tendon lengthening if there contracture of the tendon) *(scenario: 19 years old, spina bifida, valgus feet, stiff, medial ulceration over the talar neck, failed AFO, treatment?).*
  - o Subtalar arthrodesis:
    - Union rate is about 90%. Prior adjacent ankle arthordesis is a risk factor for delayed union and nonunion following a subtalar arthrodesis.
    - The position of fusion is about 7° valgus. The talar- first MT angle should be aligned in AP and LAT views.
    - Fusion will result in about 40% reduction of hindfoot motion.
- Talonavicular arthritis:
  - o Can occur with inflammatory arthropathy.
  - o Arthrodesis of the talonavicular joint eliminates almost all hindfoot motion (80-90% of the hindfoot motion) and it is the most common joint in hindfoot to develop nonunion with attempted fusion. *(Question: what is the joint that has the most impact on hindfoot motion?)*

Midfoot Arthritis (Tarso-Metatarsal Joint):

- Can be due to primary OA (most common), post-traumatic (following Lisfranc injury) or rheumatoid arthritis (symmetrical affection).
- Pain will occur at the terminal stance phase of gait as load is being transferred from the hindfoot to the forefoot.
- Advanced mid foot arthritis: can lead to flat foot deformity. There will be degenerative collapse of the midfoot through the tarsometatarsal joints (loss of the longitudinal arch) with significant forefoot abduction.
    - This is differentiated from PTTD by the ability of the patient to do single stance heel rise.
    - XR will show collapse of the arch at the level of mid foot joints (tarso-metatarsal joints) and not at the level of the subtalar joint (which is the site of collapse in PTTD).
- Initial treatment is non operative.
    - Conservative treatment: shoe modification that includes cushioned heel, longitudinal arch supports and rocker sole to unload the tarsal-metatarsal junction during gait *(scenario: old Lisfranc injury, patient has pain at the terminal phase at push-off and when the patient attempts to climb stairs, XR: mal-united Lisfranc joint, what shoe modification can help?).*
- If non operative treatment fails:
    - Surgical treatment by medial column (navicular-medial cuniform-1st metatarsal) fusion or midfoot fusion (medial cuneiform- 1st MT) with possible Achilles tendon lengthening. Fusion of the midfoot has minimal affection of the foot motion.
    - Fusion of 1st, 2nd and 3rd rays is well tolerated. 4th and 5th rays should be preserved to help the foot to accommodate the floor.

Gouty Arthritis: (See The General Disease Chapter)

- Pain usually at the first MTP
- In chronic cases XR may show osteolytic lesion (gouty lesions).
- Diagnosis: aspiration of the inflamed joint for crystal examination by polarized microscopy (needle-shaped negatively birefringent monosodium urate crystals).
    - The fluid should also be examined for cell count and culture to exclude concomitant infection *(scenario: 50 years old, hypertensive, Hydrochlorothiazide treatment, pain in the first MTP, with redness and swelling, diagnosis?)*

Rheumatoid Arthritis (See The General Disease Chapter):

- Causes synovitis and destruction of the ligament of the MTP joints.

- o This will lead to hallux valgus and dorsal dislocation of the lesser toes MTP joints causing metatarsalgia.
- Treatment:
  - o Hallux valgus: fusion.
  - o Lesser toes dislocations: metatarsal head excision.

Psoriatic Arthritis (See The General Disease Chapter):

- More in females, associated with decreased subtalar motion and second toe dactylitis.
- XR will show a "pencil in cup" DIP deformity.

Big Toe Pathologies:

Hallux Valgus (Bunion):

- Normal anatomy:
  - o Hallux valgus angle (HVA) <15°; 1-2 Inter-metatarsal angle (IMA) <10°; Distal Metatarsal articular angle (DMAA) <15° (Fig 1).
- Pathology:
  - o When the great toe deviates into a valgus position, abductor hallucis muscle becomes flexor and pronator for the toe. This will lead to pronation of the phalanx.
  - o The MTP joint can be congruent or incongruent (this will affect the treatment).
  - o Factors affecting surgical treatment: presence of arthritis, presence of ligamentous laxity, congruence of the first MTP joint, severity of deformity, general condition and co-morbidities of the patients.
- Initial treatment:
  - o Shoe wear modifications should be recommended.
  - o Surgery is not indicated in a patient who has a mild deformity and no pain. *(scenario: 35 years old, bunion, discomfort with tight shoes, management?)*
- Surgical treatment:
  - o For incongruent MPJ: a lateral distal soft tissue release and reconstruction (modified McBride) is indicated (in combination with other procedures).
    - Distal soft-tissue reconstruction (modified McBride) can be rarely performed alone in very mild deformity (less than 30 degrees HVA and 15 IMA) (however, it will be associated with recurrence if done alone in bigger deformities).
  - o For mild cases (IMA is smaller than 14° and the HVA is smaller than 35°) a distal osteotomy is preferred.
    - Distal chevron osteotomy is most often used in a mild hallux valgus with congruent joint and a normal DMAA.

- - A distal soft-tissue procedure may be added if the deformity is incongruent (see before).
  - If mild case associated with increase DMAA, can modify the distal chevron to become bi-planar chevron (to correct both HVA and DMAA). *(Scenario: 60 years old female, hallux valgus, exhausted all non surgical options, XR shows IMA of 11°, HVA 25°, DMMA 20°, congruent MTP angle, what surgery? (bi-planar chevron))*
  - Complication of distal osteotomies (eg. Chevron) is the development of AVN of the first MT (especially if combined with lateral release). Recent data shows that the risk is minimal.
  - The blood supply to the head of the first MT is first dorsal metatarsal artery.
- o Moderate to severe hallux valgus deformities (more than 14° IMA): proximal diaphyseal osteotomy (e.g. scarf osteotomy) is indicated.
  - If associated with non congruent joint: add a distal soft-tissue release to realign the first MTP joint.
  - If associated with increased DMAA (congruent joint): add Aikin osteomty. *(Senario: IM 15°, DMMA 15°, hallux 40°; Scarf osteotomy +/- Aikin can be done)*

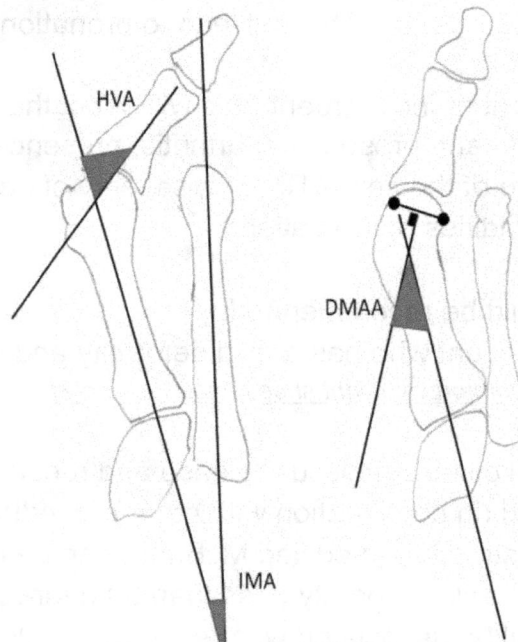

Fig 1: Angles used for assessment of hallux valgus deformity. Inter-metatrsal angle (IMA) is the angle between the axis of the 1st and 2nd metatarsus. Hallux-valgus angle (HVA) is the angle between the axis of the 1st metarsus and proximal phalanx. Distal metaphyseal articular angle (DMAA) is the angle between the axis of the first metarsus and line perpendicular to base of distal articular surface

- o Fusion of the first MTP joint is indicated in cases of advanced osteoarthritis of the 1st MTP joint, rheumatoid arthritis or cases associated with cerebral palsy.

- o Fusion of the 1st tarso-MT joint (Lapidus procedure): in patients with hypermobility of first-ray, metatarsus primus varus or for those who have bunion recurrence after previous surgery.
- o Resection arthroplasty (Keller procedure): rarely done, only with severe deformity in very low-demand patients.
- o Adolescent patients with increased IMA and DMAA: double osteotomy to correct both deformities (after exhaustion of all non operative treatment)
    - ▪ Recurrence is high after surgical treatment for adolescent patients.
    - ▪ If adolescent patient has hypermobility of the 1st ray: Lapidus procedure (1st tarso-MT joint).
- o Severe hallux valgus can be associated with second MTP joint dislocation, clawing and second toe metatarsalgia. Treatment is shortening osteotomy (eg Weil osteotomy) of the second metatarsal with extensor tendon release and dorsal capsular release in addition to treatment of the HV (proximal osteotomy to control the severe deformity (chevron will not provide enough correction)) *(Scenario: severe hallux valgus, dorsal subluxation of the second toe, treatment?)*
    - ▪ Hallux valgus with second toe clawing: have to treat the hallux (even if the hallux non symptomatic) with the treatment of second toe clawing.
- o Complications:
    - ▪ Proximal osteotomy or fusion of the TMT joint can lead to dorsiflexion mal-union with dorsiflexion of the first MT. This will lead to transfer metatarsalgia to the second metatarsal head. *(Scenario: bunion, treatment by Lapidus, now has 2nd MT metatarsalgia, reason?) (Scenario: hallux valgus, treated by proximal MT osteotomy few months ago, now has pain (during push off), XR shows dorsiflexion of the MT, treatment? (plantar flexion osteotomy 1st MT)).*
    - ▪ Resection of both the medial and lateral hallucal sesamoids can lead to great toe "cock-up" deformity. Fibular sesamoid resection (during distal soft-tissue release) can lead to hallux varus.
    - ▪ Recurrence: factors associated with recurrence are: rounded shape of the first metatarsal head, severe lateral displacement of the tibial sesamoid, an increased preoperative IMA, and HVA.
    - ▪ Overcorrection (Hallux varus): if surgery for hallux valgus resulted in late complication of hallux varus deformity, the treatment should be medial capsular release plus split extensor hallucis longus (EHL) tendon transfer to help maintain position and preserve motion at the interphalangeal joint level (transfer part of the EHL tendon into the proximal phalanx, under the intermetatarsal ligament laterally). If the hallux varus is associated with advanced MTP joint arthritis: fusion will provide better results.

- Nerve injury: dorsomedial cutaneous nerve, which is the terminal branch of the superficial peroneal nerve (see approaches section of the anatomy chapter).

Hallux Rigidus:

- Pathology:
    - Decrease ROM of the 1st MTP joint (especially dorsiflexion) resulting in pain during push off.
    - Can result in transfer metatarsalgia, decreased push-off strength and an inverted gait pattern (to avoid weight bearing on the 1st ray).
- Non operative treatment:
    - High toe-box (to accommodate the dorsal ostoephyte).
    - Rigid shank or forefoot rocker bottom sole or **Morton's extension foot insert** (to limit the motion of the first MTP joint during toe-off) *(Question: what is the best biomechanical orthosis for hallux rigidus)*.
- Surgical treatment:
    - If non operative treatment fails to control symptoms: surgery is indicated.
    - If pain at the ends (extreme) of the ROM and not through the mid range and these is negative grind test, treatment is: cheilectomy.
        - If cheilectomy fails to provide 30° of dorsiflexion: dorsal closing wedge osteotomy can be combined with a cheilectomy.
    - If pain is through the whole ROM (including mid range of motion) and there is marked degenerative changes in the joint and grind test is positive: treatment is fusion.
        - For cases of failed cheilectomy: treatment is fusion. *(Question: what is the most important clinical finding predicting the need for fusion vs cheilectomy? (Pain in the mid range of motion of the first MTP)) (Scenario: 55 years old with pain in the big toe with dorsiflexion, negative 'grind' test, and pain at only at the maximum dorsiflexion, initial treatment? (non operative) failed non operative, what surgery?) (Same scenario but pain throughout the whole ROM with positive grind test, treatment?) (scenario: hallux rigidus, had cheilectomy 2 years ago, still having pain, treatment?).*
        - Position of fusion of the 1st MTP joint is 10° of valgus and 15° of dorsiflexion relative to the metatarsal shaft (parallel to the floor so it is barely touching the floor), neutral supination/ pronation.
        - Avoid excessive valgus as it may increase the risk of IP joint degeneration.
        - Other surgical options for advanced cases: prosthetic or interpositional arthroplasty (will preserve motion).

Failed arthroplasty of 1st MTP joint:

- Failed silastic implant in 1st MTP Joint: will cause metatarsalgia and great toe pain.
- It is best treated by implant removal with structural bone grafting (to restore length) and metatarsophalangeal (MTP) fusion. A Keller resection (resection arthroplasty) will exacerbate metatarsalgia.

Intractable Plantar Keratosis (IPK):

- Painful lesion that commonly takes the form of a discrete, focused callus about 1 cm on the plantar aspect of the forefoot. It is usually under the great toe metatarsal head.
- Can occur with neurological lesions that are associated with equines (eg stroke).
- Related to prominent medial sesamoid. XR: will show prominence of the medial sesamoid.
- Initial treatment is non surgical (pad proximal to the IPK to unload the lesion). If this fails to control symptoms: treatment is shaving of the plantar half of the medial sesamoid (to decrease the excessive pressure on the sesamoid while preserving its function)
    - Complete medial sesamoidectomy should be reserved for refractory cases due to potential for complications (hallux valgus).
    - Gastrocnemius release can be added if there is equines contracture.

Sesamoid Stress Fracture:

- Common in runners
- Will complain of foot pain at the 1st MTP joint aggravated with weight bearing. Examination will show tenderness over the sesamoid. Cavus foot (plantar flexion of the first ray) is commonly seen with this condidtion.
- More common with the medial sesamoid.
    - The medial (tibial) sesamoid is larger and more affected by weight bearing.
- Imaging: XR will reveal the fracture of the sesamoid (differential diagnosis is bi-partite sesamoid) and possible fragmentation. Bone scan will show increased uptake over the medial sesamoid (false positive in 25% to 30% of asymptomatic individual). CT can better delineate the fracture. MRI is helpful to differentiate between stress fracture and bipartite sesamoid; also it can differentiate between acute and chronic lesions.
- Treatment:

- o Non operative treatment (similar to treatment of sesamoiditis): stiff sole shoe with rocker bottom contour, pad underneath the metatarsal head, orthotic with a recessed area under the base of the first metatarsal head.
    - Requires longer period, less successful in chronic and displaced cases (not preferred in atrhelets).
- o Medial sesamoidectomy (partial or complete): results in pain relief, and allows return to sports (in about 6-8 weeks). Fracture repair is less predictable.
    - Repair of the capsule in required to avoid deformity (Hallux valgus).
- o Correction of the underlying deformity (cavus) may be needed.

Turf Toe injuries

- Hyperextension of the MTP joint with an axial load applied to a plantarflexed foot.
- Clinical presentation: tenderness at the base of the toe. With severe injury, the hallux will have intrinsic minus position (MTP joint extension and IP joint flexion).
- Can result in hallux rigidus as a late sequelae.
- XR: proximal migration of the sesamoids (indicates a complete rupture of the plantar plate).
- MRI can show the disruption of the sesamoid complex and the proximal retraction. It can also show the disruption of the plantar plate.
- Treatment:
    - o Non-operative: Walker boot or short leg cast.
    - o Indication for operative treatment: retraction of the sesamoids, sesamoid fracture with diastasis, traumatic bunions, or loose fragments in the joint.

Lesser Toes Pathologies:

Claw Toe Vs Hammer Toe Vs Mallet Toe: (See Table 1)

- Claw toe:
    - o Main deformity is hyperextension of the MPJ (usually associated with flexion of both PIP and DIP).
    - o Due to weak intrinsic muscles of the foot and relative strength of the extensor digitorum longus. This will lead to weakness of the plantar plate.
    - o Multiple digits claw toes are usually indicative of neurological etiology, it can also occur after foot compartment syndrome (e.g. following calcaneal fracture).
    - o Treatment of claw toes:
        - Initial treatment: non operative (gel sleeve to relief pressure).

- For flexible claw toe (no fixed contracture at MTP or PIP joints): FDL to EDL transfer (Girdlestone-Taylor operation), the transferred tendon will depress (flex) the MTP. It cannot be performed for fixed contracture.
- For fixed contracture: PIP fusion or PIP resection arthroplasty. EDL lengthening and MTP capsular release can be added.
- If there is long second metatarsal, Weil osteotomy can be added (see below).
- Hammer toe and Mallet toe:
  - Hammer toe:
    - The main deformity is flexion contracture of the PIP (with DIP extension). Most common deformity of the lesser toes.
    - Differentiated from claw toe by the position of the DIP (flexed in claw and extended in hammer).
    - The deformity is more obvious while standing.
    - Initial treatment is non operative, if fails: as claw toe.
  - Mallet toe: the main deformity is flexion contracture of the DIP (with PIP extension) (the reverse of hammer). Treatment is by FDL release (flexible cases) or DIP fusion (rigid cases).

	Claw	Hammer	Mallet
Pathology	Hyperextension of the MTP joint with flexion of PIP and DIP	PIP flexion with extension of MTP and DIP joint	DIP flexion with extension of the PIP and MTP joints
How to differentiate	PIP and DIP flexed	PIP flexed	DIP flexed
Treatment for rigid deformity	PIP resection/ fusion, EDL lengthening and MTP capsular release	As claw toe	DIP fusion/ resection
Treatment of flexible deformity	FDL to EDL transfer (Girdlestone-Taylor operation)	As claw toe	FDL release

Bunionette

- Classification (see Fig 2).
- Treatment:
  - Initial treatment: non operative (wide shoes).
  - Failure of non-operative treatment: surgery according to classification.
    - Increased 4-5 inter-metatarsal (IMT) angle (>12°): diaphyseal osteotomy

- Lateral bowing of the 5th MT: diaphseal osteotomy or distal chevron osteotomy.
- Enlarged lateral condyle of the fifth metatarsal head: lateral condylectomy or chevron osteotomy.
  - Proximal 5th MT osteotomy should be avoided due to healing problems.
  - Lateral condylectomy alone cannot effectively treat increased 4-5 IMT angle or lateral bowing of the distal fifth metatarsal shaft.

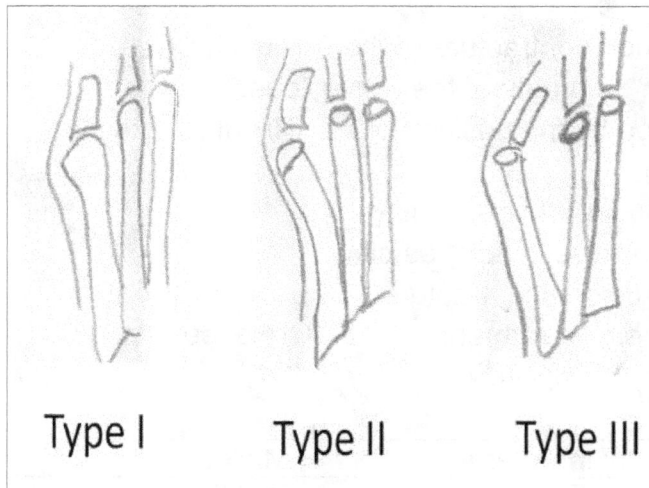

Type I   Type II   Type III

Fig 2: Classification of bunionette. Type I: enlarged 5th MT head; type II: bow of 5th MT in the mid shaft; type III: increased 4-5 inter metatarsal angle (most common type).

MTP Joint Synovitis:

- More common in the second toe.
- Clinical presentation: pain (at the level of MTP joint), swelling and difficulty wearing shoes.
  - Pain with motion of the toe that is less with traction.
- In advanced stages, the supportive ligaments and the plantar plate weaken leading to joint instability.
- Treatment: initial treatment is non operative (ice, rest, NSAIDs, toe splinting).
  - Cases of synovitis associated with long second metatarsal or those with joint instability will require surgical treatment by shortening osteotomy (see below).

MTP Joint Instability:

- Common in the second MTP joint. Can occur with claw tow deformity.
- Treatment: Weil osteotomy (dorsal oblique shortening osteotomy):
  - Will result in decompression of the MTP joint and help relocation of the joint.
  - Has broad surface which decrease the change of nonunion and allow immediate weight bearing.

- o Indications: lesser toes deformity, long or plantar flexed metatarsus, claw toes and recalcitrant metatarsalgia.
- o Done at the distal metatarsal (junction of the metatarsal head and neck). The cut is parallel to the plantar surface of the foot (weight bearing surface), then the metatarsal head is slid proximally (Fig 3).
- o Most common complication is extended or "floating toe" (dorsiflexion contracture at the MTP joint), the toe will not to touch the ground in the standing position.
  - ▪ The intrinsic interossei muscle becoming dorsal to the center of the MPJ causing the development of an extended or "floating" toe.
- o Plantar plate dysfunction can lead to recurrent MTP joint instability after surgical correction.

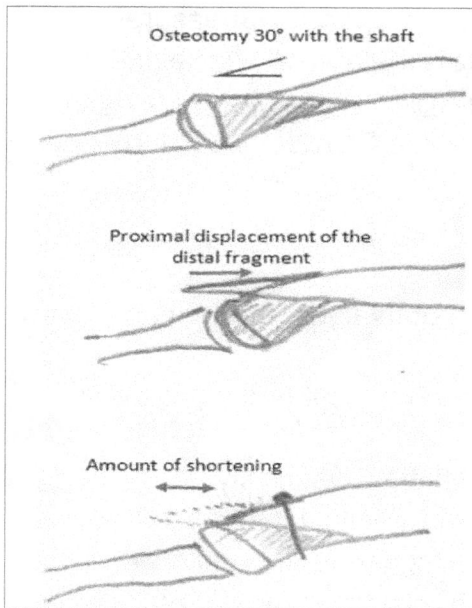

Fig 3: Weil osteotomy for shortening of the metarasal. The osteomy is done parallel to the plantar surface (30° with the shaft of the metatarsus) then the distsal fragment is displaced proximally and internally fixed. The overhanging part of the proximal fragment is excised.

Crossover Second Toes:

- Second toe over the big toe due to attenuation of the plantar plate and lateral collateral ligament leading to instability. This occurs in advanced stages of 2nd MTP joint synovitis.
  - o Should be differentiated from cases of advanced hallux valgus leading to displacement of the second toe (these are treated by addressing the HV).
- Toe drifts toward the big toe and eventually crosses over and lies on top of the big toe.
- Treatment: once drifting of the second toe occurs, surgical treatment is needed (progressive condition).

- Surgery (combination of the following):
  - Capsulotomy of the joint.
  - Flexor-to-extensor transfer (Girdlestone/ Taylor procedure).
  - PIP resection arthroplasty or fusion of the joint.

Freiberg's Infraction:

- Osteochondrosis of the metatarsal head (most commonly in the second), common in adolescent athletes.
- XR will show the flattening of the metatarsal head (early) or fragmentation and osteophytes (late).
- Initial treatment should be non-operative: metatarsal pad, hard sole shoe, CAM boot or short leg walking cast.
  - Surgical treatment only after exhaustion of all non-operative measures.
  - Surgerical options: debridement of osteophytes, metatarsal shortening or dorsiflexion osteotomy. *(Scenario: 16 years old female runner, forefoot pain and swelling aggravated by activities, XR shows fragmentation, treatment? (non-operative first))*

Posterior tibial tendon dysfunction (PTTD)

- **Anatomy and Pathology**
  - PTTD will lead to adult-onset valgus foot (hindfoot valgus, forefoot abduction and collapse of the medial longitudinal arch).
  - Can lead to deficiency of the calcaneonavicular ligament (spring ligament).
  - The spring ligament (calcaneonavicular):
    - Fails in patients with an adult-acquired flatfoot deformity.
    - Extends from the anterior aspect of the sustentaculum tali to the plantar surface of the navicular, supporting the talar head.
  - The posterior tibial tendon has the poorest intrinsic blood supply (watershed area) between its navicular insertion site and the distal medial malleolus.
  - The medial arch depends on dynamic function of PT muscle and static function of calcaneonavicular ligament.
  - Tibialis posterior acts primarily as an invertor of the hindfoot and supinator of the forefoot during the stance phase of gait. Hindfoot inversion will lock the foot and allow it to act as stable platform for foot progression needed at the end of the stance phase.
- **Clinical presentation:**
  - More in females.
  - Most common cause of adult-acquired flat foot.
  - Tenderness inferior to the medial malleolus with inability to perform a single-limb stance heel rise.

- **Staging**

Stage	Clinical presentation	Treatment
I	PTT tendonitis alone, no collapse of the midfoot. Pain on the medial aspect of the foot.	• Short, articulated ankle foot orthosis (**AFO**) or foot orthosis (**UCBL**), Custom-molded leather and polypropylene orthosis (**Arizona brace**), plantarflexion activities, gastrocnemius tendon stretching and an aggressive high-repetition home exercise. • If this fail, surgical treatment (see stage 2)
II	• Flexible flat foot • 2B is with forefoot abduction and more than 40% of the talar head becomes uncovered.	• Non operative treatment: see stage 1. • **Flexor digitorum longus** (FDL) tendon transfer to the navicular, medializing calcaneal osteotomy and gastrocnemius lengthening. • +/- other procedures (lateral column lengthening (in 2B), spring ligament repair, medial column arthrodesis) (one or more combination of these surgeries as needed)
III	Fixed flat foot	• Triple arthrodesis • If the forefoot supination can be fully corrected (or can be corrected to less than 7°), isolated subtalar arthrodesis can be considered, however, this is not preferred).
IV	stage 2 or 3 with Involvement of the ankle (valgus)	• Pantalar arthrodesis

- Stage I and II PTTD: initial treatment is non operative (see table).
  - Best result of the bracing is achieved in elderly patient with a sedentary lifestyle.
  - Patients with stage II PTTD and fixed forefoot supination: the insert that can be used for non operative treatment: medial heel lift, longitudinal arch support, and medial forefoot posting.
  - None of the braces for PTTD should have lateral wedge.
  - If decided to use brace for stage IV (elderly patient, or refused surgery), cannot use articulated AFO or UCBL as it will not adequately control the ankle (can use Arizona brace).
- Surgical treatment of stage II (see the table) is usually: Achilles tendon lengthening, **FDL** transfer to navicular, and calcaneal osteotomy (or lateral column lengthening).
  - FDL transfer is contraindicated in patients with a fixed hindfoot deformity, hypermobility, or neuromuscular compromise. The results of the technique are worse in obese and elderly patients (>70 years old).

- o Nonunion is the most common problem associated with lateral column lengthening procedures performed through the calcaneocuboid joint.
- o In cases which have a marked collapse at the naviculocuneiform joint, medial column arthordesis should be added to the calcaneal osteotomy or the lateral column lengthening.
- o Stage II PTTD: if there is fixed forefoot supination, Cotton procedure is indicated (first cuneiform osteotomy) to plantar flex the first ray.
- o PTTD stage III (no ankle affection), treated with triple arthrodesis, stage IV (ankle affection) with pantalar arthordesis. (see the table). *(Scenario: 56 years old, 5 years' history of progressive flat foot, failed non operative, stiff hindfoot, normal ankle, XR shows deformity and secondary arthritis of the subtalar, treatment?) (triple fusion)) (Scenario :60 years old female, 30 months' history of progressive valgus foot, cannot perform single heel rise, subtalar fixed in valgus position and cannot be corrected, forefoot had fixed supination, normal ankle XR, treatment?) (triple fusion)). (Scenario: 57 years' female, medial foot pain, foot collapse, initial treatment? (orthosis and structured exercises))*
- Other causes of adult acquired flat foot:
  - o Injury to calcaneonavicular ligament (Spring ligament) can lead to flatfoot deformity.
  - o Arthritis of the mid foot (see mid foot arthirits section).

Tibialis Anterior Rupture

- Can occur without history of trauma (more common with diabetes, inflammatory arthritis, with eccentric contraction).
- Patient will complain of difficulty dorsiflexion the foot (difficulty in stair climbing). Foot-slap gait.
- Treatment: acute ruptures in young patients are treated with primary repair. Chronic injuries are treated by tendon transfer (tibialis posterior transfer).

Achilles tendon pathology:
Anatomy (See Anatomy Chapter):
- The Achilles tendon does not have true tendon sheath; it is surrounded by a paratenon.
- A vascular watershed region in the tendon is located 2 to 6 cm above its calcaneal insertion.

Achilles Tendon Rupture:
- Clinical presentation: weak plantar flexion, decrease resting plantar flexion (compared to the other side), positive Thomas sign.
- Treatment options:

- o Non surgical.
- o Operative: open, minimal invasive, and percutaneous
- Results of treatment:
    - o Early mobilization (after either surgical or non surgical treatment) was found to have better range of motion and functional results with no increase re-rupture rate.
    - o Surgical treatment has less re-rupture rate than non-operative treatment.
        - ▪ Surgical repair with early range of motion in a functional brace preserve motion without increasing the risk or re-rupture.
        - ▪ The most common complication associated with surgical repair of an Achilles tendon rupture is skin healing problems (other less common complications are infection, stiffness and re-rupture).
    - o No difference in re-rupture rate, sural neuropathy, or calf circumference between open technique and minimal invasive technique.
    - o The minimal invasive technique (compared to the open one) has less scarring and stiffness. Open group has greater number of postoperative complications.
    - o Percutaneous Achilles repair (compared to open repair) has decreased incidence of wound complication and infection.
    - o The most common complication of percutaneous repair of an acute Achilles tendon rupture is sural nerve entrapment. *(Question: what nerve at risk with percutaneous repair of Achilles tendon?).*
    - o Perfusion of the Skin overlying the Achilles tendon is maximal in the position of 20° of ankle plantar flexion and it is reduced beyond 20° of plantar flexion. *(Question: what position after surgery maximizes perfusion to the wound?)*
    - o Achilles tendon tension is not affected by knee position when the ankle is in 20° to 25° of plantar flexion (no need to immobilize the knee with Achilles tendon repair).
    - o **Chronic Achilles tendon tears:**
        - ▪ Gap =< 5 cm: a V-Y repair. V-Y advancement will preserve the native muscle tendon unit and will fill a defect of 2 cm to 5 cm
        - ▪ For gaps > 5 cm (especially for cases presenting more than few months): tendon transfer (flexor hallcis longus) with possible added Achilles tendon turndown. *(Scenario: 40 years old, Achilles rupture one year ago, now has difficulty with ambulation and increasing pain, MRI: interval 7 cm, treatment? (FHL transfer plus Achilles tendon turndown)).*

Chronic Achilles Insertional Tendinitis (Tendinosis):

- Pathology:
    - o Occurs at the most distal part of the tendon (insertional).

- o Microscopically: picture of anaerobic degeneration (absence of acute and chronic inflammatory cells) (not real tendinitis).
  - o Risk factors for Achilles tendinopathy: quinolone antibiotics, diabetes mellitus, obesity, steroid exposure, hormone replacement therapy, oral contraceptive.
- XR: **calcification at the insertion**
- Treatment:
  - o Initial treatment is non operative (therapy and heel lifts).
    - ▪ Therapy: by **eccentric strengthening exercise.** In both insertional and non insertional Achilles tendinopathy: physical therapy by **Eccentric** strengthening
  - o Never injection of cortisone.
  - o If fails, Achilles debridement with possible calcaneal ostectomy (exostectomy) (excision of Haglund's exostosis).
    - ▪ This surgery may take 12 months in elderly patients to regain their ankle function.
    - ▪ If more than 50% of the Achilles tendon is affected, **flexor hallucis longus tendon transfer** or reattachment of the Achilles tendon with bone anchors will also be needed (in conjunction with the above procedures). *(Scenario: 40 years male, 9 month history of a painful swelling of the Achilles tendon at its insertion. Failed non operative management. MRI shows degeneration affecting most the tendon, treatment?) (Scenario: 67 years male, 2 years history of swelling and pain of the insertion of Achilles tendon, failure of all non operative methods, XR calcification, treatment?)*

Tendon Ensethopathy:
- Inflammation of Achilles tendon insertion with triad of asymmetric arthritis, urethritis, and uveitis is suggestive of Reiter's syndrome (order HLA-B27).

Non-Insertional Achilles Tendinosis (Tendinitis):
- Can be tendinosis or paratendonosis (peritendinitis)
  - o Achilles tendon does not have a true synovial sheath.
  - o Degeneration of the tendon or the paratenon.
  - o Peritendinitis is similar to tendinosis; but thickening and tenderness is affecting the paratenon tendon sheath (in contrast to tendinosis which refers to the inflammation and degeneration of the tendon itself).
- Occur 2 to 6 cm proximal to the insertion of Achilles tendon (watershed area).
  - o Patient will complain of pain and swelling proximal to the insertion.
- Treatment: main treatment is therapy by eccentric muscle strengthening (see above).

Neurological Foot and Ankle Conditions:

Drop Foot:

- Possible etiologies include peroneal nerve palsy or post compartment syndrome (non functioning antero-lateral compartment with functioning posterior compartment).
- Initial treatment is ankle foot orthosis (AFO) with dorsiflexion assist.
- Surgical treatment:
  - If the drop foot is due to common peroneal nerve palsy with good ROM of the ankle (passive dorsiflexion past neutral) and intact posterior tibial nerve (5/5 ankle planter flexion and inversion): the treatment is posterior tibial tendon transfer to dorsum of foot.
  - Achilles tendon lengthening can be added if it is tight. *(Scenario: 40 years old male, motorcycle accident 2 years ago, examination shows no active dorsiflexion or eversion, can be passively stretched to 5 degrees ankle dorsiflexion, initial treatment? (Brace), if not able to tolerate, treatment? (posterior tibial tendon transfer)) (Scenario: post operative drop foot, no improvement with observation and neurolysis, treatment?) (Scenario: knee dislocation with common peroneal nerve palsy 2 years ago, no improvement, and patient does not want to continue using AFO, treatment?) (Scenario: missed compartment syndrome 3 years ago, non functioning anterolateral compartment, functioning posterior compartment, initial treatment? if not able to tolerate non operative, treatment is?)*
  - As a general rule, for muscle transfer to work: the deformity has to be passively correctable. Contracture cannot be treated with muscle transfer.

Spastic Equino Varus Deformity

- Pathology:
  - Can occur post cerebral stroke.
  - Premature firing and spasticity of the triceps surae muscle.
- Treatment:
  - Achilles tendon lengthening and split tibialis anterior transfer to the lateral cuneiform (transfer of the posterior tibialis to the lateral side may result in overcorrection and planovalgus deformity).

Cavus Foot

- See cavus foot in pediatric chapter. See also Charcot Marie Tooth in systemic conditions chapter.
- If there is subtalar varus with arthritis: triple fusion (to correct the deformity).
- Mild cavus deformity with subtle hind foot varus:
  - Associated with repeated lateral ankle sprains/instability and possible repeated 5th MT stress fractures.

- o May need to be addressed at the time surgical repair of ankle instability (see later).
- o If the deformity is minimal and no instability: can be treated by cavus orthosis (brace with lateral heel wedge and medial recession for the 1st MT head).

Nerve Related Conditions:

Tarsal Tunnel Syndrome:

- Paresthesia and numbness in the plantar surface of the foot. The most reproducible objective finding in the clinical exam is a positive Tinel sign over the compressed nerve.
- Nerve conduction studies and EMG are have good accuracy in establishing the diagnosis (about 85%).
- Can be due to space occupying lesion in the tarsal tunnel. Ganglion cyst is a relatively common cause of tarsal tunnel, excision of the ganglion usually leads to resolution of symptoms.
- Initial treatment: non operative.
- Surgical treatment (after failure of non operative treatment) release of the nerve:
  - o Best results of treatment can be expected in cases in which there is a space-occupying lesion causing compressing of the nerve. *(Scenario: 35 years female, 5 months of numbness in the foot, MRI shows cystic swelling, diagnosis? treatment?)*
  - o If there is an associated heel pain, decompression of the first branch of the lateral plantar nerve should be added.
- **Heel pain triad:**
  - o **Adult**-acquired flatfoot, plantar fasciitis, and tarsal tunnel syndrome.
  - o Failure of the dynamic and static supports of the medial longitudinal arch will result in increase traction on the posterior tibial nerve.

Compression of The First Branch of The Lateral Plantar Nerve (Baxter's Nerve):

- Clinical presentation: patient will present with heel pain (**medial** plantar heal pain).
- Tenderness over the abductor hallucis origin with a positive Tinel's sign radiating to the lateral foot.
- More common in **athletes** (especially runners).
- Anatomy (see also the anatomy chapter) (see Fig 1 anatomy chapter):
  - o The first branch of the lateral plantar nerve changes direction (from vertical to horizontal) on the medial aspect of the heel, then passes under the abductor hallucis and heads laterally to supply to the abductor digiti minimi.

- o It can be compressed between the abductor hallucis fascia on one side and inferomedial margin of the quadratus plantae muscle and plantar fascia on the other side (see Fig 1 in anatomy chapter)).
- Treatment:
  - o Nonsurgical treatment for minimum of 6 months.
  - o If non-surgical treatment fails: release of the deep fascia of the abductor hallucis muscle is needed to achieve release (it requires division of both superficial and deep fascias of the adductor hallucis to reach to the nerve).

Superficial Peroneal Nerve Entrapment:

- Seen in runners, pain over the lateral aspect of the distal leg and paresthesia over the dorsum of the foot.
- Pain increase with plantar flexion/inversion. Examination will reveal tenderness over a defect in the superficial fascia about 10 from joint with positive Tinel's sign.
- Treatment is release of the fascia at the exit of the nerve with nerve neurolysis.

Anterior tarsal tunnel syndrome:

- Compression of the deep peroneal nerve under the **inferior** extensor retinaculum.
- Patient will complain of burning sensation across the dorsum of the foot with paresthesias in the first web space.
- On exam: wasting and weakness of the extensor digitorum brevis.

Morton (Interdigital) Neuroma:

- Clinical presentation:
  - o Clinical examination is the standard method for diagnosis of an interdigital neuroma *(Question: what is the most accurate method of diagnosis?) (Question: what is the gold standard for diagnosis?)*.
  - o Burning sensation on the plantar aspect of the forefoot, distal to the metatarsal heads between two adjacent toes (most commonly third and fourth digits).
  - o Palpation of the web space or compression of the forefoot recreates the symptom.
- Risk factor: females.
- Pathology: perineural fibrosis (not true neuroma).
- Treatment:
  - o Initial treatment: non operative (wide shoes, steroids injection).

o Injections of local anesthetic and corticosteroid can be diagnostic and therapeutic (repeated injections are not recommended as it can cause iatrogenic instability of the MTP joint).

o Surgery: excision of the neuroma, can be done through dorsal or plantar approach:

- Dorsal approach: higher risk of missed neuroma (lumbrical muscle excision instead). Dorsal approach is more commonly used in primary neuroma excision.
- Plantar approach: higher risk of painful scar.
- Revision: should be done through plantar approach

o The most common cause of recurrence of symptoms after excision of the neuroma is inadequate excision:

- The neuroma can become tethered to the plantar skin by plantar directed branches. To avoid this tethering, neuroma excision should extend to at least 4 cm proximal to the transverse metatarsal ligament which is proximal to all plantar branches.

Dorsomedial Cutaneous Nerve to The Hallux:

- This is the termination of the medial branch of the superficial peroneal nerve.
- It can be injured during surgeries on the hallux (see anatomy chapter). *(Scenario: hallux valgus, scarf osteotomy, now has burning sensation, what nerve injured?)*

Sural Nerve Neuroma:

- Due to injury of the sural nerve during lateral approaches of the hindfoot (e.g. fixation of calcaneus fractures).
- Patient will complain of burning pain on the lateral side of his ankle and foot with positive Tinel's sign along the nerve course.
- Temporary relief can be obtained by local cortisone injection at the site of the tenderness.
- Treatment: Excision and burial of the sural nerve.

Heel/ Sole pain

Calcaneal cyst:

- Common accidental finding.
- No need to treat (unless occupying the full width of the bone or more than one third of the length). *(Scenario: child with Sever's disease, XR shows anterior cyst in calcaneus, treatment? (reduced activity (for the Sever's disease) and Observation (for the cyst)).*

Plantar fasciitis:

- Plantar medial heel pain that is more with getting out of bed in the morning (first few steps in the day), then improves after a few steps. The pain then worsens towards the end of the day.
- Commonly associated with tight heel cord.
- Radiograph: 50% of cases will have heel spur (non specific, not sensitive not the etiology of the pain).
- Treatment:
    - Initial treatment: non operative:
        - Plantar fascia stretching, Achilles stretching, toe intrinsic stretching.
        - Night splints
        - Cortisone injection (can lead to rupture of the plantar fascia or heel pad atrophy).
        - Less proven measures: PRP injection, ultrasound-tripsy.
    - Surgical: only after exhaustion of all non operative. Gastrocnemius recession (for tight heal cord). Partial plantar fascia release (open or endoscopic).
- Differential diagnosis:
    - Stress fracture of the calcaneus (pain with medial and lateral compression of the heel).
    - Compression of the first branch of the lateral plantar nerve.

Ankle Sprain Inversion injuries:

- Most commonly affected ligament is anterior talo-fibular ligament (with inversion and plantar flexion).
- Can be associated with subtle cavus deformity and mild hindfoot varus
- The injury can lead to:
    - Osteochondral talar dome lesions.
    - Peroneus tendons tears and/or subluxation.
    - Stretch of the superficial peroneal nerve, leading to pain and paresthesias along its distribution.
    - Soft-tissue impingement lesions in the anterolateral capsule:
        - Anterolateral capsular thickening following ankle sprain.
        - Patient will complain of anterolateral chronic ankle pain for prolonged period after ankle sprain.
        - Clinical presentation: pain with pressure over the anterolateral ankle.
        - Normal XR; MRI will show the lesion.
        - Treatment of anterolateral impingement: therapy and possible cortisone injection; if this fails: arthroscopic debridement of the lesion.

- MRI should be considered if pain persists for more than 8 weeks after an acute ankle sprain (to exclude the above causes).
- Treatment of ankle sprain:
  - Early patient mobilization (weight bearing as tolerated in a cast or controlled ankle movement (CAM) boot) and a guided proprioceptive and strengthening rehabilitation therapy program (early functional rehabilitation).
  - No role for surgery in acute ankle sprain (this had been recently challenged in high level atheles).
  - Return to play: when patient has pain-free ROM of the ankle.
  - Surgical treatment (treatment of ankle instability): failure of non operative treatment with positive signs of instability (positive talar tilt stress exam, see ankle exam).
    - Reconstruction of the anterior talo-fibular ligament (modified Brostrum) (the reconstruction does not cross the subtalar joint).
    - If there generalized ligament laxity or in cases of failure of previous repair, tendon graft should be considered. Tendon graft or tendon rerouting (crossing the subtalar joint) can lead to subtalar stiffness.
    - Correction of underlying pathology (subtle cavus deformity).
    - Chronic lateral instability can be associated with a longitudinal split tear of the peroneus **brevis** tendon which may be a source of persistent pain if not addressed during surgical repair of the instability. _(Scenario: 20 years old, chronic ankle instability, had surgery, still in pain, why?)_

Posttraumatic Tibiofibular Synostosis:
- Follows a high ankle sprain (disruption of the interosseus membrane).
- Ossification of the interosseus membrane develops within 6 to 12 months after the injury.
- Clinical presentation: stiffness with lack of ankle dorsiflexion.
- XR will show the tibio-fibular synostosis.
- Treatment: initial treatment is non operative.
  - Surgical excision (after the lesion is cold in bone scan) is reserved for cases of persistent pain that fails to respond to nonsurgical management.

Peroneal Tendon Tears/ Subluxation:
- Clinical presentation: pain, swelling, ecchymosis and popping in the lateral ankle.
- Common in skiers, usually caused by inversion injuries (inversion injury to a dorsiflexed ankle with rapid reflexive contraction of the PL and PB tendons).
- The subluxation occurs due to disruption of the **superior** peroneal retinaculum.

- Tears commonly affect the brevis tendon at the level of the fibular groove.
- Subluxation is assessed by resisted eversion and dorsiflexion (from the inverted plantar flexed position) (will be able to observe the subluxation of the tendon).
- XR: normal. MRI will show the lesion.
- Treatment of peroneal tears:
  - Chronic peroneal tendon injuries are usually treated with tenodesis to the healthy tendon (tenodesis of the brevis tendon to the longus tendon).
- Treatment of subluxation:
  - Surgical intervention to avoid repeated subluxation and development of longitudinal tear of the peroneus brevis.
  - Surgical treatment is by reconstruction/repair the **superior** peroneal retinaculum (extending from the posterolateral ridge of the fibula to the lateral calcaneus), and/or deepening the fibular groove. *(Scenario: ankle injury 6 months ago; now has pain and popping in the lateral side, MRI shows the peroneal tendon subluxed from the groove, what structure needs to be fixed? (superior peroneal retinaculum)) (Question: what anatomic structure is important in stabilization of personal tendon (superior peroneal retinaculum)).*

Peroneus quartus:
- A supernumerary muscle arising commonly from the peroneus brevis in about 20% of individual).
- May lead to lateral ankle pain and peroneal tendon symptoms due to mass effect within the peroneal tendon sheath. *(Scenario: young adult with lateral ankle pain, clinical picture showing a muscle arising from the peroneus brevis, what is that structure?)*

Posterior Ankle/ Foot Pain in Ballet Dancers:
- Due to landing and the standing on planter flexed ankle and toes.
- Pain can be due to impingement of the os trigonum or focal entrapment of the flexor hallucis longus tendon (see below).
- The most common location for stress fractures in dancers is at the proximal metaphyseal-diaphyseal junction of the second metatarsal. *(Scenario: ballet dancer, mid foot pain for the last month, diagnosis?)*

Flexor Hallucis Longus Tendinitis (See The Anatomy Chapter):
- A common cause of posterior ankle pain in dancers (when in the "en pointe" position).
  - Clinical presentation: tenderness at posteromedial ankle, pain with motion of the hallux with possible clicking or catching sensation. Pain can be elicited with resisted plantar flexion of the hallux IP joint.

- The muscle courses directly behind the talus:
  - Stenosing tenosynovitis commonly occurs in the fibro-sseous tunnel posterior to the talus (can cause triggering).
- Os trigonum syndrome is usually associated with FHL tendinopathy (see below).

Os Trigonum Syndrome
- The os trigonum is an accessory ossification center at the lateral tubercle of the posterior process of the talus.
- Possible pathologies/ pain sources:
  - Traumatic disruption of the synchondrosis between the os trigonum and the talus.
  - Stress fracture can sometimes occur between fused accessory ossicle and the posterior talar process.
  - Impingement of the os trigonum: forced plantar flexion leads to impingement of the os trigonum against the posterior tibial plafond causing pain.
- Common in some athletes (ballet dancers and basketball players).
- Tenderness on the posterolateral aspect of the ankle. Pain increase with plantar flexion of the ankle.
- CT will show the accessory bone. MRI will show fluid surrounding the os with associated marrow edema
- Treatment by excision (either open or arthroscopic) of the inflamed os trigonum. (s*cenario: basketball player, posterior ankle pain for 18 months, CT shows the lesion, treatment?)*
  - FHL lies between os trigonum and posterior tibial nerve. *(Question: what structure protect the nerve during excision of the os trigonum?)*

Foot ulcers:
- Wagner classification
  - Grade 1: Superficial Diabetic Ulcer.
  - Grade 2: Ulcer extension to ligament, tendon, joint capsule or fascia (No abscess or Osteomyelitis).
  - Grade 3: Deep ulcer with abscess or Osteomyelitis.
  - Grade 4: Gangrene to portion of forefoot.
  - Grade 5: Extensive gangrene of foot.
- The best initial test to assess the etiology of failure of healing of a foot ulcer is ankle brachial index (Noninvasive vascular studies). *(Scenario: 60 years old, diabetic, smoker, resistant forefoot ulcer, initial test?)*
- The most predictive factor for development of future ulcer: history of previous foot ulcer.

- All diabetic patients need *foot-specific patient education.* *(Scenario: diabetic patient with small ulcer; cannot feel Semmes-Weinstein 5.07 monofilament. Ulcer healed by wound care, what should be the next step? (Foot-specific patient education, depth inlay shoes with orthosis)).*
- Total-contact casts are effective in treatment of plantar foot ulcers:
  - It is the gold standard for nonsurgical treatment.
  - Mechanism of action by decreasing the pressure and **shear stress**. It leads to even distribution of pressure across the plantar surface of the foot
  - The ulcer recurrence rate after total contact cast is high (about 50%).
  - About 50% of the recurrence occurs within the first month after the patient resumes walking without the cast.
- Forefoot ulcer:
  - Achilles lengthening can improve the healing of **resistant** forefoot plantar ulcers by decreasing the pressure over the forefoot during ambulation, **decreasing the recurrence of the ulcer**. *(Scenario: 65 diabetic patient, 5th MT head ulcer, resistant to all form of treatment, what procedure can help healing?) (Scenario: resistant ulcer over tarso-matetarsal amputation stump, exam limited dorsiflexion, next step?) (Scenario: diabetic male, ulcer over 3rd MT head, multiple recurrence, neuropathy, not communicating with bone, most predictable method for wound healing without recurrence?) (Scenario: ulcer over the second metatarsal head, treated with total contact cast, healed, recurred after 4 weeks, what procedure can be done?)*
- For infected ulcers: deep biopsy is needed to assess the organism (see below). Avoid wound swabs.
- Failure of an ulcer to heal may indicate underlying osteomyelitis.
  - Best clinical indicator for osteomyelitis is an ulcer that probe to bone.
  - The best test to confirm osteomyelitis is bone biopsy (will confirm pathology and determine the causative organism)
    - If a foot ulcer probes to bone, the treatment is surgical debridement (with antibiotic and dressing changes). Probing to bone is associated with osteomyelitis.
- After ulcer healing:
  - Assess the need for Achilles tendon release (if not already done) (see before).
  - Orthopedic shoes with custom-molded soft inserts that accommodate the contours of the feet (especially with partial amputation to avoid shift in a shoe).
- **Markers for potentials of healing:**
  - Trans- cutaneous oxygen level of > 40 mm Hg (best indicator, direct measure of tissue oxygenation).
  - Albumin level >2.5 g/dl, Total lymphocyte count >1500/ml, HgA1C <8, Absolute toe pressures > of 40 mm Hg, ABI >0.45 (ABI not very good

indicator if there is calcification of the vessels). *(Remember the number 40 for TCO2, Toe pressure and ABI)*

- **Ischemic ulcer:**
  - o Assessed first by noninvasive vascular studies such as ABIs and trans-cutaneous oxygen.

Amputation in diabetic patients (See the rehabilitation chapter):

- Multi disciplinary approach of diabetic foot ulcer can decrease the need of future amputation by about 50%.
- Ray amputation can be done for up two rays. If more rays needs to be amputated, trans-metatarsal amputation is needed.
- **Below knee amputation Vs Syme's amputation:**
  - o If patient has low albumin and lymphocyte but with ABI > 0.45, transcutaneus oxygen > 40, the management should include: Local wound care, antibiotic treatment, nutritional and metabolic support, and reevaluation in 1-2 weeks.
    - ▪ If heeling markers (albumin, lymphocyte count) improved: Syme's amputation can be considered, otherwise, below knee (transtibial) amputation should be done.
  - o If blood supply to the foot is not adequate (ABI < 0.45 and transcutaneus oxygen < 40): trans-tibial amputation should be considered from the beginning.
  - o Syme's amputation will not heal without palpable posterior artery pulse.
  - o Syme's amputation has the advantage (over BKA) that it can give full-load-bearing residual limb that is nearly normal in length.

Diabetic Neuropathy of The Foot (see foot ulcers):

- Sensory neuropathy is the most common form of diabetic neuropathy of the lower extremity.
  - o Clinical presentation: burning pain.
  - o Treatment: Gabapentin, antidepressants.
- Motor neuropathy affects the intrinsic muscles of the foot (leading to development of claw toes).

Charcot: Neuropathic Destructive Arthropathy.

- Most common cause of Charcot foot is diabetic neuropathy. *(Scenario: 60 years old male, foot deformity, next step? (check for diabetes)).*
- The pathophysiology of bone destruction is believed to be hypervascularity of bone.
- For insensate foot: the patient should use depth inlay shoes with a custom foot orthosis accommodating the shape of his foot.
- Surgical treatment for Charcot arthropathy:

- o Indications: recurrent ulcers and instability not controlled by a brace. If there is Charcot foot with deformity and ulceration, the ulcer should be treated with wound care and total contact cast with frequent cast change then the management should consist of surgical correction of the deformity to prevent recurrent ulceration and infection, Achilles tendon lengthening, and therapeutic footwear. *(Scenario: 45 diabetic neuropathy, no protective sensation, forefoot abduction, ulcer of talar head, after control of the ulcer by total contact cast, next step is?)*
  - o Surgical options are exostectomy or reconstruction with osteotomy and fusion.
- **Eichenholtz classification:**
  - o Eichenholtz stage 1 (stage of development/ fragmentation):
    - Foot is warm, red, and swollen. Charcot arthropathy causes edema and redness of the foot, which will disappear with elevation of the foot, unlike infection in which the redness and edema will continue even after foot elevation.
    - The infection markers are usually elevated but can be normal.
    - XR: bone destruction and fragmentation, subluxation.
    - Treatment is non-weight-bearing casting (to help prevent deformity) until the swelling resolves and evidence of consolidation is seen on radiographs with frequent cast changes. *(Scenario: 56 years diabetic, swollen red foot, WBCs normal, ESR and CRP mildly elevated, MRI: navicular fracture, treatment?) (Scenario: 50 years old, foot swelling, redness, mild pain, good sensation to light tough, XR: tarso-metatarsal fracture dislocation, diagnosis? Neuropathic arthropathy (light touch sensation can be normal in Charcot)). (Question: what is the preferred treatment for early Charcot ankle?)*
  - o Eichenholtz stage 2 (stage of coalescence):
    - Decreased warmth, erythema and edema.
    - XR: absorption of small bone parts and fusion of large fragments to adjacent bones.
    - Treatment: advance to weight bearing in a cast or cam boot.
  - o Eichenholtz stage 3 (stage of reconstruction or remodeling):
    - Resolution of edema. Persistence of foot deformity (patients with Charcot ankle will usually develop severe varus deformity causing ulcer over their distal fibula).
    - XR: rounding of the bone ends with decrease in sclerosis.
    - Treatment is correction of the deformity with possible calcaneal-tibial fusion (the talus is usually completely destroyed by the Charcot process).
    - Surgery treatment is better done in stage 3.

- Diabetic patients with neuropathy, who sustain trauma or undergo surgery, can develop Charcot arthropathy in adjacent joints. *(Scenario: 65 years male, diabetic, does not feel Semmes-Weinstein 5.07 monofilament, had ankle fracture treated surgically 3 months ago, and now has swelling and redness of the foot, mechanism?)*

Plantar puncture wound:

- The most sensitive imaging modality for detection of wooden foreign body in the plantar aspect of the foot is ultrasound. *(Question: suspecting tooth pick in the sole of the foot, what imaging modality to order?)*
    - For glass foreign body: first test is XR (with soft tissue dosing).
- Most common organism of **infection** after puncture wound is: staph aureus.
- Pseudomonas aeruginosa is the most common organism causing **osteochondritis** (infection of the bone and cartilage) in pediatric puncture wounds of the foot and most common cause of **osteomyelitis** after puncture wound (especially with puncture through the sole of rubber shoes).
- Treatment:
    - Administration of tetanus immunization. In patients with up to date immunization: no need for tetanus toxoid.
    - Patient presenting late (more than 48 hours) after puncture wound with continued pain and swelling: treatment is by exploration of the wound with debridement in the operating room followed by parental antibiotics.
    - For children with plantar puncture wound presenting few days after injury with increased pain and swelling, treatment is surgical debridement. *(Scenario: 8 years old, nail puncture wound, treated with local wound care and antibiotic in the ER, 3 days later presenting with increased pain and swelling, treatment?)*

Cardiac Emboli to Foot After Cardiac Surgery:

- Small gangrenous areas in the foot may rarely occur due to small emboli related to the cardiac surgery. The management is observation.

Frost Bite (See Hand Chapter)

- Pathology: occurs due to development of intracellular ice crystal formation. Re-warming can lead to thrombosis and necrosis of the cells affected by the ice crystals.
- Most reliable method to reduce the risk of cold exposure injury is to reduce thermal heat loss (protective socks and shoes) and reducing moisture in the shoes.
- Acute management: rapid re-warming by using a water bath at 40° to 42°C for 30 minutes. Administration of TPA (tissue plasminogen activator) within 24 hours of injury may be used to decrease necrosis associated with re-warming.

Gunshot Wounds to The Foot:

- Stable fracture, no joint penetration, less than 8 hours: local wound care, no need for antibiotic prophylaxis (tetanus toxoid if no booster dose within 5 years), hard sole shoe.
- If > 8 hours or there is joint penetration: antibiotic prophylaxis and formal debridement is needed
- Unstable fractures (pieces of bone in the wound, multiple bones fractures): surgical stabilization (internal or external) is needed.

Tumors of The Foot And Ankle:

- **Common lesions:**
  - Most common bony sarcoma in the foot: chondrosarcoma.
  - Most common soft tissue sarcoma in the foot: synovial sarcoma. Other common tumors include giant cell tumor of the tendon sheath and neurolimmoma.
  - Most common malignancy in the foot in general is: malignant melanoma.
  - Most common bony lesion in foot: enchondromas.
- **Malignant Melanoma:**
  - All subungual lesions that do not resolve after 6 weeks should undergo biopsy along with removal of the nail.
  - Standard treatment of melanoma is surgical excision.
- **Plantar fibromatosis (Ledderhose Disease).**
  - A benign tumor of the plantar fascia that consists mainly of fibromyoblasts producing excessive amount of collagen (similar to the cells found in the palmar fascia of patients with Dupuytren's contracture of the hand).
  - Patient will complain of painful mass on the bottom of the foot.
  - Clinical examination will show the local nodule in the plantar aspect of the foot.
  - MRI scan show the lesion arising from the plantar fascia.
  - Initial treatment is nonsurgical. Local recurrence after simple surgical excision is high. Wide local excision (the whole plantar fascia) is usually indicated to avoid recurrence. Observation is preferred over excision due to the high local recurrence.
- **Subungual Exostosis**
  - Occurs in young patient, common on the dorsal and the medial aspect of the great toe.
  - Painful slowly growing mass which may produce ulceration of nail
  - Treatment is excision of the exostosis with complete excision of the nail.

Tips:

- "Cardiac surgery few days ago": think in embolus to the foot.
- Causes of adult onset valgus deformity: PTTD and mid foot arthritis (tarsal-metatarsal) (check the XR to see where the collapse in the arch)
- Heel pain: plantar fasciitis, calcaneus stress fracture, impingement of the first branch of the lateral plantar nerve.
  - Dancers with posterlateral ankle pain: think Os trigonum. Dancers with posteromedial ankle pain: think flexor hallucis tendinitis.

Shoulder and Elbow

Examination and Radiographs:

- **Some specific physical exams related to shoulder:**
  - Active external rotation of the shoulder:
    - With the arm 90° abducted: mainly by teres minor (axillary nerve).
    - With the arm adducted: mainly by infra-spinatus (supra scapular nerve).
  - Rotator cuff testing:
    - The dropping sign (very sensitive test for irreparable damage to infraspinatus): with the patient seated the shoulder is placed in 0° of abduction and 45° of external rotation and the elbow in 90° flexion, the examiner holds the patient's forearm in this position and instructs the patient to maintain it when he/she let it go. Positive test (dropping sign) is when the patient's forearm drops back to 0° of external rotation, despite efforts to maintain external rotation.
    - Empty can test (Jobe test): the arm is positioned 90° of forward flexion in the plane of the scapula (approximately 30 degrees of abduction), full internal rotation with the thumb pointing down (emptying a soda can). One hand of the examiner stabilizes the shoulder and the other hand applies downward pressure on the superior aspect of the distal forearm and the patient resists. Positive test result is **significant** pain (tendinopathy) and/or weakness (tear).
  - The drop arm test:
    - Test for rotator cuff tears (mainly the supraspinatus tendon). Controlled lowering of the arm from 90° abduction.
    - Positive test: inability to smoothly control the lowering of the arm.
  - Assessment of subscapularis muscle
    - Bear-hug: Resist internal rotation with the shoulder in 90° flexion. Found by some studies to be more sensitive than (lift-off, belly-press).
  - Jerk and Kim test.
    - For posterior inferior labral tear.
    - **Kim test**: With the patient sitting, and the arm 90° ssof abduction, the examiner holds the elbow and lateral aspect of the proximal arm, and a strong axial and posterior loading force is applied to the shoulder. While maintaining the axial and posterior load, the arm is moved to front of the torso. A sudden onset of posterior shoulder pain indicates a positive test result.
    - **Jerk test**: This test consists of placing an axial load through the humerus, with the shoulder forward flexed to 90 degrees. While stabilizing the patient's scapula with one hand and holding the affected

arm at 90° abduction and internal rotation, the examiner grasps the elbow and axially loads the humerus in a proximal direction. The arm is gradually adducted. A positive result is indicated by a sudden clunk.

- **Some specific radiological exams related to shoulder pathologies:**
  - Stryker notch: to detect Hill Sachs lesion
  - AP - Internal Rotation: to detect Hill Sachs lesion.
  - West point: to detect glenoid deficiency.
  - The axillary view: to detect locked posterior shoulder dislocation.
  - CT shoulder: to detect amount of glenoid bone loss in shoulder instability, glenoid morphology and version in cases of shoulder arthritis.
  - MR arthrogram (intra-articular gadolinium): to detect labral pathology.
  - Both ultrasonography and MRI have same sensitivity in diagnosing full-thickness rotator cuff defects.
  - The normal coraco-clavicular distance on AP radiograph should be >13 mm.

Acute Traumatic Antero-Inferior Shoulder Dislocation:

- Most commonly injured nerve with anterior shoulder dislocation is the **axillary nerve.**
- For older patients, anterior shoulder dislocation may be associated with **rotator cuff tear** *(scenario: 70 years old male, shoulder dislocation, reduction, follow up in clinic, patient unable to abduct, what study to obtain? (MRI (to detect rotator cuff tear))), (same scenario with patient age 17 years old, the answer will be EMG (to detect axillary nerve palsy)).*
- **Acute** re-dislocation after first time dislocation occurs usually in elderly and middle age in cases with fractures of the glenoid rim or the greater tuberosity.
- Management:
  - The initial treatment of the first time dislocator should be **sling immobilization** for 2-3 weeks (no benefit for longer immobilization periods) followed by range of motion and strengthening.
  - Return to play may be possible after 2 weeks of immobilization, provided the patient undergoes appropriate therapy for range of motion, cuff strengthening, and scapular stabilization exercises. The athlete may be allowed to finish the season.
  - Immobilization with the arm in 30 degrees of external rotation was found to reduce of the detached labrum (Bankart lesion) to the glenoid resulting in reduction in recurrence rates.
  - Age at the time of the initial dislocation is the most important prognostic risk factor for recurrent instability following traumatic anterior dislocation.
  - For young patient (especially athletes), surgical repair after the first attack can be considered; this must be discussed with the patient and the family.

Recurrent anterior shoulder instability

- Pathology:
  - Commonly due to separation of **anteroinferior** labrum from the glenoid (**Bankart lesion**).
    - The standard Bankart lesion involves detachment of the labrum along with the middle glenohumeral ligament and inferior glenohumeral ligament.
    - With bony Bankart lesion, the anterior band of the inferior glenohumeral ligmant is usually attached to the avulsed piece.
    - Bony Bankart lesion (avulsion of bony piece from the anterior glenoid) is treated with internal fixation to prevent recurrence (see later) (do not excise the bony piece).
    - ALPSA (Anterior Labroligamentus Periosteal Sleeve Avulsion) (medialized Bankart): The labrum with a periosteal sleeve avulses from glenoid then heals to medial glenoid neck. This has a higher rate of recurrent dislocation. During surgical stabilization, the labrum and periosteal sleeve must be mobilized and repaired laterally to avoid recurrence.
- Less commonly: the antero-inferior dislocation is associated with **h**umeral **a**vulsion of the **g**lenohumeral **l**igament (HAGL) lesion (indication for open surgery) (usually in older patients) (see below).
- The recurrent dislocation can lead to compressive injury of the posterosuperior humeral head (which abuts against the anterior glenoid)
  - This can lead to Hill Sacks injury (bone loss in the posteromedical aspect of the humeral head).
    - This can be radiologically detected by Stryker notch or AP view with internal rotation or better with a CT
- Recurrent dislocation can also lead to bone loss of the anterior glenoid rim which will decrease the effective depth and concavity of the glenoid; this will cause loss of the ability of the rotator cuff to stabilize the joint through production of compression of the humeral head in the glenoid.
  - Glenoid bone loss can be detected by West point view or CT.
- Clinical examination: positive anterior apprehension test and relocation test.
- Imaging:
  - CT or CT arthrogram. CT will show the humeral head deficiency (Hill Sacks) and/or glenoid deficiency. An arthrogram can enhance the ability to evaluate the capsule and ligamentous attachments.

- o MRI scan can show the associated pathology (e.g. Bankart, ALPSA lesion or HAGL lesions).
- **Surgical treatment option for recurrent anterior shoulder instability:**
  - o Bankart injury: treatment is by Bankart repair (open or arthroscopically).
    - Open Vs arthroscopic:
      - Slightly better range of motion of the shoulder after an arthroscopic repair.
      - Recurrent instability not statistically different (may be slightly higher with arthroscopic).
      - Collision athletes (e.g. football) may have a lower recurrence rate with open surgery.
      - Return to work and/or sports has been shown to be equal or slightly better with open procedures.
    - For a small bony Bankart lesion involving less than 15% of the glenoid joint surface, arthroscopic repair incorporating the bone lesion can be done.
  - o HAGL injury: open repair for the ligament avulsion from the humeral end.
  - o If there is deficient glenoid (an anterior inferior glenoid bone defect): bony glenoid augmentation procedure: as coracoid transfer (Bristow-Latarjet procedure).
    - The procedure achieves stability through the increased glenoid surface area that the bone block provides.
    - For collision sports, coracoid process transfer (Latarjet or Bristow) is the preferred surgical treatment over Bankart repair.
  - o Large engaging Hill sack lesion: may require infra spinatus transfer (Remplisssage procedure) (Hill sack lesion >35% of the humeral head usually will require Remplissage procedure).
  - o The middle glenohumeral ligament (MGHL) can sometimes be a cordlike and robust structure (Budford complex). The space between the bony glenoid and the Buford complex is a normal variant and should not be repaired or tightened to the bony glenoid. If this structure is inadvertently repaired, it will result in loss of external rotation with the arm adducted at the side (the position of tightness of this ligament).

HAGL (Humeral Avulstion of Gleno-Humeral Ligament) Lesion:

- Avulsion of the humeral insertion of the inferior glenohumeral ligament.
- Rare cause of anterior stability (much less common than the classic Bankart lesion).
- A possible cause of recurrence if not addressed during surgery.

- Mechanism of injury: abduction, hyperextension, and external rotation (similar to regular joint dislocation pathology).
- The MRI scan will show the lesion as pouch in the infro-medial aspect of the humeral head (obvious in the coronal view)
- Treatment: indication of open repair (repair has to be on the humeral side)

Multidirectional instability (MDI):
- More common in females and with certain sports (e.g. swimming).
- More common in the dominant arm, but it can occur in the non-dominant arm.
- On exam: positive sulcus sign and increased humeral head translation in more than one direction with the load-and-shift test (pathognomonic). Mild weakness of rotator cuff may be seen.
- Treatment: therapy for rotator cuff strengthening/ stabilization and scapulothoracic strengthening.
    - If therapy fails to control patient symptoms: surgery can be considered (only after extensive therapy for long period): rotator interval closure (can eliminate the sulcus sign) and/or capsular shift either open or arthroscopically.
    - Thermal capsulorrhaphy (radio frequency or laser): has been abandoned as it can lead to glenohumeral chondrolysis. Mid-term results have high failure rates. The degree of capsular shrinkage is dependent on the total amount and rate of thermal energy delivered. The capsule typically becomes thin and patulous. It can also cause damage to the axillary nerve. *(Scenario: shoulder surgery for stability 6 months ago, patient is having pain and decreased ROM, XR loss of cartilage, diagnosis? (Chondrolysis)).*

Posterior Shoulder Dislocation/ Posterior Instability:
- If posterior shoulder dislocation is suspected, axillary view should be obtained (lesion can be missed in AP shoulder). *(Scenario: 5 days of shoulder pain after seizure, AP XR normal, next step?)*
- Mechanism of injury:
    - Traumatic: Occurs most often with forward elevation and internal rotation position of the shoulder.
    - Most common cause of posterior shoulder dislocation with no obvious history of trauma is epileptic fit and electrocution (internal rotator muscles are stronger than external rotator).
- The condition is commonly missed (near normal AP radiographs), which will lead to impaction of the anterior part humeral head (reversed Hill Sacks lesion).
- Clinical presentation: shoulder pain with limited external rotation.
- Treatment:

- Acute cases (less than 3 weeks old): closed reduction and assessment of stability. If the arm can be internally rotated to the abdomen while shoulder is still located, then 6 weeks of immobilization in an orthosis that maintains the shoulder in slight external rotation can yield a good result.
- Chronic cases (more than 3 weeks): treatment is open reduction (closed reduction is difficult to obtain), with possible need for bone grafting for the humeral anterior defect (either lesser tuberosity transfer or osteochondral allograft):
  - Reversed Hill Sacks of more than 20% of the head: needs bone graft or lesser tuberosity transfer.
  - If there is loss of 50% or more of the humeral head, treatment is hemi-arthroplasty.
- **Posterior Instability:**
  - Clinical presentation:
    - Patients will have pain and instability sensation with certain shoulder activities that involve internal rotation of the shoulder and adduction (e.g. pushing an object at the level of the shoulder, football player trying to pass-blocking, bench press with heavy weight).
    - Symptoms of posterior labral tears are often vague.
    - Positive Jerk and kim test (see before). A positive jerk test combined with a positive Kim test has a 97% sensitivity for posterior instability.
    - Increased translation and pain with load and shift test
  - Axillary view: posterior subluxation of the humeral head
  - MRI scan may show posterior labral tear.
  - Treatment: physical therapy, if fails, posterior capsule-labral repair (open or arthroscopic).

Glenohumeral Internal Rotation Deficit (GIRD) (Thrower Shoulder):

- Pathology: contracture of the **posteriorinferior** capsule in throwing shoulders (capsular tightness) and scapular dyskinesis.
- Common in baseball pitchers in the dominant hand.
- Patients will complain of **posterior shoulder pain** and difficulty playing (**decrease velocity of pitching**). They may also complain of SICK scapula syndrome (Scapular malposition, Inferior medial border prominence, Coracoid pain and malposition, and dysKinesis of scapular movement). The tenderness over the coracoid has been attributed to a contracture of the pectoralis minor secondary to scapular malposition.
- On exam: with shoulder abducted 90 degrees: decrease internal rotation of the affected side compared to the contra lateral side (more than 20° difference),

increase external rotation in the affected side. *(Question: what rotational differences can be seen in the dominant shoulder of throwing athletes compared to the nondominant side?)*

- Contracture of the posterior-inferior capsule will result in a ***posterosuperior*** shift of the glenohumeral contact, and **will lead to <u>internal impingement</u> and articular sided supra spinatus tendon tear and posterior superior labral tear and SLAP tear (surgery may be needed if the pathology reaches this stage and initial non-operative treatment fails). (See below)**
  - Internal impingement usually causes posterior supraspinatus and anterior infraspinatus tear (in contrast to anterior supraspinatus tear which is more common with external impingement)
- Treatment: **posterior capsular stretching, stretching** of the **pectoralis minor** tendon followed by rotator cuff and scapular stabilization exercises. Rotator cuff repair is not typically required. SLAP repair and rotator cuff debridement may be considered in refractory cases after failure of non-operative treatment. *(Scenario: 18 years collegiate baseball pitcher, decreased velocity and posterior shoulder pain, what finding in clinical exam?) (Scenario: 17 years old, right hand dominant, collegiate baseball pitcher, decreased velocity last few months, exam shows decreased internal rotation of the right shoulder compared to the left one, MRI normal, treatment?) (Scenario: baseball player, pain in the posterior aspect of his throwing arm, decreased internal rotation, MRI scan SLAP lesion and partial-thickness tear of the posterior supraspinatus tendon. treatment? (NSAID, posterior capsular stretching, and rotator cuff strengthening. SLAP repair and rotator cuff debridement or repair can be considered in refractory cases after failure of non-operative treatment)).*
- **Posterior capsular stretching** was found to decrease the possibility of shoulder and elbow injury in high performing athletes.
- Throwers with **anterior shoulder pain** can be due to rotator cuff deconditioning, the pain will increase in severity at the end of the game and resolves the next day. ROM exam will be normal (no GIRD). Treatment is reconditioning of the rotator cuff and scapular stabilizers, combined with a throwing program.
- MR arthrogram of **asymptomatic** throwers, can show posterior labral tear (contrast between the posterior labrum and the glenoid), no treatment is needed in these cases. *(Scenario: thrower has anterior shoulder pain, MR arthrogram shows posterior labral tear, treatment? (Physical therapy, reconditioning of the rotator cuff and scapular stabilizers and a throwing program)).*
- **Internal impingement:**
  - Definition: impingement of the rotator cuff between the humerus and posterior-superior glenoid rim.
  - Occurs in the late cocking phase of throwing with humeral head abduction and maximal external rotation.
  - Articular sided partial posterior supraspinatus and ifraspinatus Tear (PASTA (partial articular supraspinatus tendon avulsion) lesion) + postero superior labral tear+ biceps anchor detachment (SLAP lesion) (see RC tear section

later). *(Scenario: thrower, deep posterior shoulder pain, shoulder arthroscope shows SLAP tear, what is the condition related? (Internal impingement), What stage of throwing?)*

- o Treatment: see above (thrower shoulder). If there is detachment of biceps anchor, arthroscopic repair can be done (see SLAP).

Proximal Biceps Tendon (See Distal Biceps Tendon in The Elbow Section):

- **Dislocated long head of biceps tendon (LHB):**
  - o LHB dislocation (medial displacement of the tendon out of the biceptal groove) is commonly associated with tear of subscapularis tendon.
  - o After failure of non-operative measures, treatment is surgical with either tenotomy or tenodesis. Recentering of the biceps has been found to be unpredictable.
- Tenodesis and tenotomy for proximal biceps pathology (e.g. subluxation with subscauplaris tendon rupture):
  - o No major **functional** difference between tenodesis and tenotomy for biceps tendon pathologies. There is **cosmetic** "Popeye" deformity after tenotomy when compared to tenodesis. Also, tenotomy has been associated with cramping, and fatigue.
    - Tenotomy has been associated with cosmetic deformity, cramping, and fatigue, but no substantial difference in overall outcomes has been demonstrated between tenotomy and tenodesis.
  - o Generally, for patients older than 60 years, tenotomy is the preferred treatment and for those younger than 50, tenodesis is the preferred treatment.
  - o Among tenodesis techniques: The interference screw has proved superior to bone tunnel, suture anchor, and soft-tissue tenodesis techniques.
    - An open subpectoral technique of tenodesis of the long head of the biceps tendon has the advantage (compared to arthroscopic soft-tissue tenodesis techniques) of removal of the biceps tendon from the bicipital groove which may eliminate a possible cause of pain related to the biceps tendon.
    - Subpectoral tendoesis can cause injury musclucuatnaeus nerve

Pectoralis Major Muscle Injury:

- Most common type of injury to the pectoralis major muscle is tendon avulsion (distal tear) of the sternocostal portion of the pectoralis major tendon.
- **Clinical presentations**: loss of the normal contour of the axillary fold, extensive ecchymosis down the arm, **weakness to adduction and internal rotation.**
- **Treatment:**

- Proximal tears, partial tears or tears in elderly or sedentary patients: nonsurgical management.
- Distal tear (at the insertion of the muscle in the humerus): surgical treatment is indicated (open repair of the pectoralis major tendon avulsion)
- Chronic rupture (if causing symptoms): Allograft reconstruction weaved to the humerus.

Impingement Syndrome of The Shoulder:

- A broad spectrum of pathology ranging from tendinopathy, to partial or complete tear of the rotator cuff.
- **Subacromial bursitis.**
  - Inflammatory mediatros responsible for pain with subacromial bursitis include metalloproteases, tumor necrosis factors, and cyclooxygenase 1 and 2.
- Tendinopathy:
  - Disorganized collagen fibers with mucoid degeneration on the microscopic level.
- **Rotator cuff tear (RCT):**
  - Clinical presentation (see examination session):
    - Jobe empty can test: for supraspinatus assessment.
    - Assessment of infraspinatus: active external rotation in adduction and dropping sign.
  - Imaging:
    - A rotator cuff tear allows the dye (arthrography or MRI arthrogram) to leak into the subacromial space.
    - MRI can show the amount of proximal muscle retraction and fatty degeneration in cases of chronic RC tears.
  - **Operative repair:**
    - Relative Indication:
      - Full-thickness and partial-thickness rotator cuff acute traumatic tears (<12 weeks from the time of injury), in patients younger than age 65 years old that failed nonsurgical treatment.
      - Acute complete RCT in young patient: surgical repair can be considered even without trial of non-operative treatment.
      - Young (>65) patients with acute single small tear treated surgically has about 95% success rate.
    - Relative contraindications:
      - Advanced fatty infiltration and muscle atrophy, delamination of the subscapularis and/or the infraspinatus, significant glenohumeral arthritis.

- Patients older than sixty-five years (have significantly lower rates of healing).
- Work related injuries (with workers compensation status) have lower results after repair of RCT.
  - Arthroscopy:
    - If during scoping from lateral subacromial portal, gleno-humeral intra-articular structures are visualized, this indicates a rotator cuff tear with retraction.
    - Tears > 3 cm have higher rate of tear recurrence and/or failure of healing when repaired arthroscopically versus a standard open approach.
    - Tissue failure (suture pulls through the tendon) is the most common cause of early failure of arthroscopic rotator cuff repair. Other causes include failure of the suture anchor, suture, or knot.
  - Double-row anchor fixation of rotator cuff tears has initial higher ultimate tensile load compared to single-row anchor fixation (but no clinical advantage proven).
  - Bone anchor drilling enhances vascularity following rotator cuff repair which stimulate healing. Shoulder motion (post operatively) also enhances blood flow to the repaired rotator cuff.
  - In overhead athlete, the rotator cuff is most susceptible to tensile failure during the deceleration phase of throwing due to eccentric loading as the rotator cuff is the principal decelerator of the arm. It will lead to articular sided tear of the posterior supraspinatus or the infraspinatus, leading to posterior shoulder pain.
  - Age of patient and size of the tear are the most important factors for healing potential.
  - Anterior supraspinatus tendon is the portion which is the most biomechanically prone to gap formation following rotator cuff repair.
- **Partial RTC:**
  - Can be articular sided or bursal sided. Partial-thickness RCT often progresses to full tears.
- **Partial Articular-sided supraspinatus tendon tear (PASTA: partial articular-sided supraspinatus tendon avulsion)**
  - Most commonly involves the supraspinatus tendon, this part has scanty blood supply.
  - More related to GIRD and repetitive microtrauma (throwing), internal impingement and shoulder instability (less often related to acute trauma).

- o Can be better seen in MRI arthrogram with abduction external rotation (ABER): this position allows intra-articular contrast to flow into the defect and increases the sensitivity.
- o 7 mm of exposed bone lateral to the articular margin (arthroscopic measurement) should be considered a significant tear approximating 50% of the tendon substance.
- o Initial treatment is conservative: activity cessation (stopping of all throwing for 6 weeks), a rotator cuff and peri scapular strengthening program, teaching appropriate pitching techniques followed by a slow return to throwing.
- o If conservative treatment options fail:
    - If the tear is >50% (exposure of more than 6 mm of footprint) (see later) are treated with completion of the tear and repair of the tendon.
    - If the tear is <50% (6 mm or less) then treatment consists of debridement of the tuberosity and the undersurface of the tendon.
    (Scenario 18 years old pitcher has right shoulder pain for 4 months MRI scan shows PASTA, treatment? (conservative, stopping all throwing activities for 6 weeks))
    (Scenario: 55 years old, shoulder pain, positive Howkin test, failed conservative, arthroscope done partial-thickness articular-sided supraspinatus tear with 3 mm of supraspinatus footprint exposed, treatment?)

- **Bursal side tear:**
    - o Initial treatment is conservative.
    - o If fail: surgery is indicated:
        - If the depth of the tear > 3mm: repair of the tendon, if 3mm or less: debridement can be done.

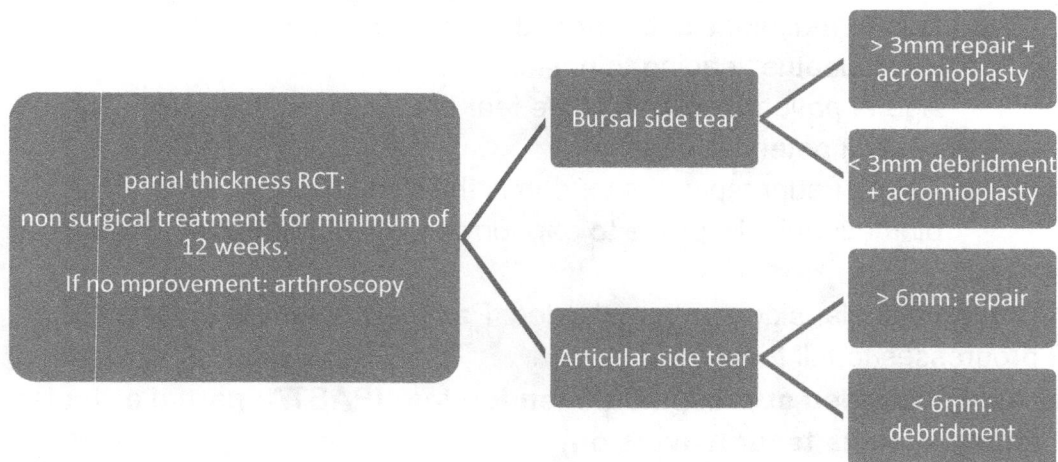

```
                                          ┌─ > 3mm repair +
                          ┌─ Bursal side ─┤   acromioplasty
                          │     tear      └─ < 3mm debridment
parial thickness RCT:     │                  + acromioplasty
non surgical treatment    │
for minimum of 12 weeks. ─┤               ┌─ > 6mm: repair
If no mprovement:         └─ Articular ───┤
arthroscopy                   side tear   └─ < 6mm:
                                             debridment
```

- **Irreparable tear:**
    - o Chronic tears are usually retracted and cannot be repaired.

o Occasionally, patients with chronic massive RCT can be very functional. In these cases, no intervention is needed. Examination will reveal atrophy of supraspinatus and infraspinatus. *(Scenario: 60 years old, had injury while playing tennis one week ago, not able to move his shoulder, exam: atrophy of supra and infra spinatus, MR: fatty infiltration and atrophy, next step? (lidocaine injection and re-assessment, if pain is relieved and motion is restored, can do shoulder (not RC) strengthening (pain and inability to move the shoulder is not related to his underlying chronic massive tear))) (70-year-old female, left massive RCT, good ROM, no advanced degenerative changes in the shoulder joint. Treatment?)*

o Superior humeral migration on upright XR indicates rotator cuff tear arthropathy, repair cannot be done at that advanced stage.

o Fatty infiltration on MRI and atrophy of the supraspinatus and infraspinatus in the physical exam indicate chronic nature of the tears, repair will most probably result in bad outcome.

o Acute massive tear (e.g. following shoulder dislocation) has more chance of being tension-free repaired.

o Treatment:
  - If rotator cuff repair is not possible, a partial rotator cuff repair (e.g. repair of infraspinatus) should still be considered as it can balance the kinematics of the joint.
  - Other options including acromioplasty, reverse acromioplasty (tuberoplasty), and tenotomy of the biceps tendon (to improve shoulder pain).
  - If these procedures fail, then a muscle transfer procedure (latissimus dorsi) can also be considered in select patients (See later).
  - Biceps tenotomy is an effective treatment option for patients with irrepairable RCT if pain is the main symptom.
  - In all cases of irreparable tears, the integrity of the coracoacromial ligament should be preserved to prevent proximal migration of the humeral head (anterosuperior escape). Resection of the coracoacromial ligament can result in increased glenohumeral joint translation

o **Latissimus dorsi tendon transfer:**
  - Indication: younger adult patient (50s) with an irreparable posterosuperior rotator cuff tear (supraspinatus and infraspinatus), **lack of advanced glenohumeral arthritis**, an intact subscapularis function (stabilize the humeral head after latissimus transfer), with some active forward elevation (more than 90°).
  - Worse clinical outcome: deficiency of the deltoid (axillay nerve palsy) (absolute contraindication) or subscapularis (Positive lift-off test), advanced fatty infiltration of the posterosuperior cuff, advance arthritis

or condrolysis, complete loss of external rotator function or forward flexion, female patients, presence of antero-superior escape of the humeral head.

- Absence of the CA ligament may allow anterosuperior escape in RC deficient shoulders but has not been shown to lead to worse outcomes after a tendon transfer. Prior surgery was not shown to affect transfer results either.

- **Subscapularis tears**
  - The typical mechanism of injury is a fall while the patient grasps something to prevent the fall. This maneuver forces the arm into external rotation against resistance.
  - On exam: positive bear hug, belly push test and lift off test, increased external rotation of the affected shoulder compared to the other shoulder. *(Scenario: 45 years old, injury to the shoulder few months ago, exam shows the clinical picture seen (picture of positive belly push or lift off test), diagnosis?) (Question: what muscle is examined by belly push/ lift off test?)*
  - Arthroscopy: Uncovered lesser tuberosity, comma sign (retracted tendon with the two ligaments, see below), subluxation of the biceps tendon.
  - The coracohumeral and superior glenohumeral ligaments (content of rotator interval) form a complex that marks the superolateral margin of the subscapularis tendon. With chronic tears of subscapularis the tendon retract medially together with the both these ligament. The tendon and the two ligaments detach from the humerus but continue to be attached together forming the "**comma sign**" that marks the superolateral border of subscapularis.
  - Treatment:
    - Chronic symptomtic rupture of the subscapularis tendon is treated by sub-coracoid pectoralis major transfer.
    - The biceps should either be tenodesed or tenotomized since it is unstable in the vast majority of cases. This prevents biceps related symptoms.

- **Rehabilitation after rotator cuff repair:**
  - NO active movement for at least 6 weeks (8 weeks for large tears). Only passive ROM exercises are allowed.
  - Early passive range of motion exercises are initiated to prevent adhesive capsulitis.
  - Technique of repair (double row vs. single row) does not affect the post-operative rehab.
  - Cannot isolate deltoid rehab (cannot rehab the deltoid without activating the RC), so cannot start deltoid muscle rehab before 6-8 weeks.

- **Asymptomatic RCT**
  - The percentage of asymptomatic RCT in MRI for patient > 60 years old is about 55% (with about half full thickness and half partial thickness)
  - The percentage asymptomatic RCT in US for patient > 60 years is about 30%. (*Scenario: 75 years old, referred to you after PCP performed MRI for shoulder lipoma showing 8-mm full-thickness tear of the supraspinatus tendon, exam showing mild limitation of the ROM, treatment? (observation)*))
- **Rotator cuff arthropathy:**
  - It occurs in cases of chronic massive RC tears with proximal (antero-superior) migration of the humerus and severe arthritis of the joint.
  - XR will show superior migration of the head with extensive degeneration sclerosis, subchondral cysts.
  - Initial treatment is non-operative (anti-inflammatory medication and/or steroid injection). If non-surgical treatment fails, treatment is reverse shoulder arthroplasty (RSA) (preferred) or hemi-arthroplasty. *(Scenario: elderly, shoulder pain, XR proximal migration, failed non-operative, treatment? (RSA)) (Scenario: shoulder pain, inability to raise the shoulder, proximal migration in XR, local injection lead to pain relief but still cannot raise arm, treatment? (RFA)) (Scenario: 85 years old, shoulder pain, XR shows proximal migration, treatment? (NSAID, steroid injection)).*
    - TSA is contraindicated in the treatment of Rotator cuff arthorpathy as it will lead to glenoid failure by the "rocking horse" phenomenon.

SLAP Tear (Superior Labral Tear From Anterior to Posterior):

- Associated with overhead throwing and internal impingement and posterosuperior rotator cuff tear (see before).
- Can be associated with paralabral ganglion cysts (spinoglenoid notch cysts) which can cause compression over the supra scapular nerve (see below).
- Classification:
  - Type II: the tear will involve biceps origin
- O'Brien test:
  - The shoulder is in 90° of flexion and about 10° of adduction and internal rotation, the forearm is pronated. The examiner pushes down distally on the arm while the patient resists with an upward force. Positive result is when there is pain and/or clicking when the arm is in internal rotation but not when the arm is in neutral rotation.
  - Low sensitivity and specificity (false positive with rotator cuff tear).
- MRI arthrogram: dye underneath the labrum (between labrum and glenoid).
- Treatment:
  - Initial treatment: physical therapy (effective in most cases).

- o If conservative treatment fails, surgery may be needed.
  - ▪ Type two: labral repair and reattachment and fixation the biceps tendon origin (or tenodesis/tenotomy).
  - ▪ Other types: debridement of the lesion. *(Scenario: 25 years old, tennis player, deep shoulder pain, got better with therapy but still not able to play, positive O'Brien test, MR arthrogram shows dye under biceps anchor, next step? (Arthroscopic repair)) (Scenario: 30 years football coach, shoulder pain, failed conservative management, shoulder scope shows type II SLAP, what treatment will give the highest satisfaction?)*

Distal Clavicle Excision:

- Arthroscopic technique has the advantage (compared to open technique) of the ability to evaluate the glenohumeral joint and can persevere the superior AC ligament while removing the inferior AC ligament and distal clavicle.
- Do not resect more than 1 cm to preserve the CC ligament

Accessory Acromion (Os Acromiale):

- Present in about 8% of the population.
- Types (Fig 1):
  - o Failure of fusion of physis between the pre acromion and meso acromion.
  - o Failure of fusion of physis between meso acromion and metaacromion
  - o Failure of fusion of physis between meta acromion and base of spine.
- The condition is usually asymptomatic, occasionally can cause pain and tenderness over the acromion.
  - o The most commonly symptomatic type is failure of fusion between mesoacroiom and metaacroion (called meso os acromiale).
  - o Patients with a symptomatic os acromiale often report impingement-type symptoms with pain over the superior acromion, especially with overhead activities or sleeping. XR will show the failure of fusion.
- If causing symptoms: most patients can be treated nonsurgically. If this fails; surgery can be done.
  - o Internal fixation and bone grafting for the mesoacromion type or excision for the preacromion type.

Most common symptomatic o Os
Acromiale (Meso Os Acromiale)

Pre acromion

Meso acromion

Meta acromion

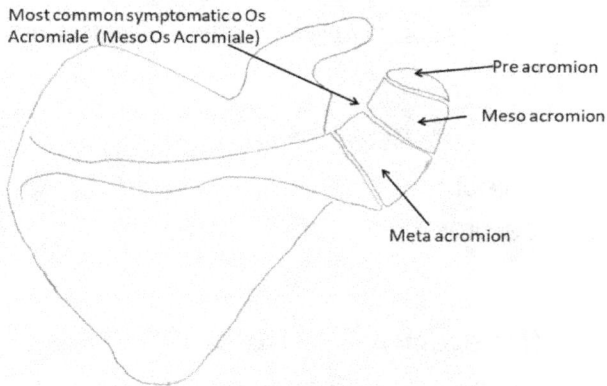

Fig 1: Types os accessory acromion.

Phases of Throwing:

- 5 stages: wind up, cocking (early and late), acceleration, deceleration, follow-through.
  - ○ Late cocking phase creates maximum stresses on medial collateral ligament of the elbow.
- The leg and trunk provide a stable base for arm motion, supply rotational momentum for force generation, and generate 50% to 55% of the total force and kinetic energy in overhead athletic activities.
- The scapula has an important role in the overhead throwing motion. It must rotate during cocking and acceleration to clear the acromion and to prevent impingement on the rotator cuff.

Scapular Winging:

- Medial winging: (prominent medial border of the scapula) (the inferior angle points medially):
  - ○ The scapula retracts, and the inferior pole rotates medially. Winging increases with attempts to elevate the arm.
  - ○ **Injury to serratus anterior muscle** (which is innervated by long thoracic nerve from C5,6,7).
  - ○ Treatment is physical therapy for 3-6 months, if no improvement, surgical reconstruction (transfer of pectoralis major to the scapula).
- Lateral winging: (prominent lateral border of the scapula) (the inferior angle point lateral):
  - ○ Injury to trapezius muscle (innervated by spinal accessory nerve (cranial nerve XI)).
  - ○ Initial treatment is non-operative; if no improvement, surgical reconstruction (lateral transfer of the levator scapulae and rhomboid minor and major.

(Scenario: patient undergoes lymph node removal from the posterior neck, post op: patient has weak elevation of the shoulder with prominent lateral border, no improvement after 4 months, treatment?)

Scapular Crepitus:
- Initial treatment is non-operative (therapy, injection).
- If this fail: arthroscopic resection of the superomedial part of scapula

Suprascapular Nerve Compression (Posterior Scapular Atrophy):
- Two common sites of compression: suprascapular notch and spino glenoid notch.
  - At the spinoglenoid notch:
    - Due to cyst associated with posterior superior labral tears (as in overhead thrower) (see thrower shoulder and SLAP lesion).
    - Will cause weakness of the infra-spinatus muscle (external rotation with the arm adducted). Supraspinatus will not be affected
    - MRI will show the spinoglenoid cyst with associated posterior superior labral tear.
    - Treatment is arthroscopic repair of the labral tear and decompression
      (Scenario: 24 years volleyball old presenting with posterior shoulder pain and weakness, MRI show cyst and atrophy of the infraspinatus, treatment?) (Same scenario, what will be the exam of the patient?)
  - At the suprascapular notch by the transverse scapular ligament.
    - Weakness of both supraspinatus and infraspinatus muscles (weak abduction and external rotation).
    - Treatment by release of the ligament. *(Scenario: 30 years old, posterior shoulder pain, normal exam except weak external rotation, MRI no cyst at the spinoglenoid notch, next step? (EMG and nerve conduction study to assess level/ location of compression)).*

Quadrangular Space Syndrome (See Anatomy Chapter):
- Compression of the axillary nerve and posterior circumflex humeral vessel.
- Usually caused by muscle hypertrophy (weight lifting).
- Patient will complain of weakness of the external rotation with 90 abduction (teres minor muscle weakness). MRI will show atrophy of the muscle.

Subclavian Vein Thrombosis:
- Clinical presentation: upper extremity pain, swelling, bluish/mottled appearance, sense of coolness in the extremity and/or paresthesias.
- Imaging:

- o   Initial: Doppler ultrasound.
- o   Definitive diagnosis: venography.

Brachial Neuritis (Parsonage-Turner Syndrome):
- Pain and/or weakness of the shoulder and upper extremity. Normal passive ROM. Normal MRI.
- May be associated with viral illness or flu vaccine.

Shoulder Osteoarthritis:
- Pathology:
  - o   Contracture of the anterior capsule and subscapularis is common finding in primary OA.
    - Patient will usually have limited external rotation.
  - o   The wear pattern in most cases of shoulder OA is **posterior** glenoid wear with posterior subluxation of the humeral head.
  - o   RC tears are rarely associated with primary OA (about 15% of cases only)
- Initial treatment is non-operative (NSAIDs, cortisone injection, and physical therapy). If this fails, arthroplasty:
  - o   The option of arthroplasty is Total Shoulder Arthroplasty (TSA) unless there is RC pathology (in this case, Reverse Shoulder Arthroplasty (RSA) should be used). *(Scenario: 65 years old, long history of shoulder pain, failure of extensive nonsurgical management, examination shows painful limitation of ROM, good RC strength, treatment?)*
  - o   Patients with repairable rotator cuff tears should undergo repair at the time of surgery (TSA). RSA is not indicated with rotator cuff tears that are repairable.

Inflammatory Arthritis
- Pathological difference from OA:
  - o   Most cases have associated RC tears.
  - o   Concentric joint space narrowing and medial glenoid wear (compared to posterior glenoid wear in OA).

Adhesive Capsulitis:
- Pathology: fibroblastic infiltration process (of the rotator interval and axillary fold).
- Clinical presentation:
  - o   Limited ROM (active and passive) especially external rotation, pain with shoulder motion, XR: relatively normal.

- o More common in women between the ages of 40 and 60, and most cases are idiopathic.
- **Risk factors:**
  - o Previous involvement of the contra-lateral shoulder, **diabetes**, thyroid disease, cardiac surgery, cervical spine pathology.
    - ▪ Smoking is not a risk factor.
  - o Can occur post traumatic and post-surgical (post-surgical adhesive capsulitis has generally a worse prognosis)
- **Treatment:**
  - o Initial: gentle stretching therapy program (stress more on motion rather than strengthening).
    - ▪ Home exercise program were found to be as effective as organized therapy.
  - o Intra-articular steroid injection to decrease inflammation.
  - o Manipulation under anesthesia and arthroscopic surgical treatment are used when symptoms remain refractory despite initial nonsurgical management. *(Scenario: 45 years old female, diabetic, 5 months shoulder pain, exam shows limited ROM (active and passive) especially external rotation, treatment?) (same previous scenario with MRI showing partial tear of the RC? (same treatment as previous)) (Scenario: 50 years old female, mild pain with positive Neer's, Hawkins and empty can test. External rotation is 10° (with the arm to the side) compared to 65° on the other side, limited internal rotation (affected side reach to the L5, contra lateral side reach to T8), XR normal, treatment? (Same treatment)).*

Osteonecrosis of The Humeral Head:

- Pathology: AVN with collapse of the humeral head.
- Risk factor: steroids intake, fracture proximal humerus.
- MRI can delineate the area of necrosis.
- Initial treatment is non-surgical. If fails, shoulder hemiarthroplasty (no need for TSA due to lack of involvement of glenoid).

Calcific Tendinitis:

- Deposition of calcium carbonate apatite crystals into the structure of the rotator cuff tendons.
  - o The deposit is usually in **supraspinatus** tendon.
- Plain radiograph is the gold standard for diagnosis. MRI can be difficult to interpret because the signal of the calcific lesion is frequently similar to that seen in normal supraspinatus tendon.
- **Stages of the disease:**

- o Formation stage: radiographs will show a well-circumscribed mass. **The calcific deposit in this phase is granular, hard to aspirate**
- o Resorptive phase: more intense pain, the Ca deposition will be similar to toothpaste.
- **Treatment:**
  - o Non-operative treatment: physical therapy and NSAIDs. Extracorporeal shock wave therapy has mixed results in literature.
  - o Operative treatment: (if no response to non-surgical treatment): arthroscopic or open debridement of the calcific deposit.

Shoulder Arthroplasty:

- Deltopectoral approach (see anatomy chapter):
  - o Requires detaching the subscpularis tendon to gain access then repair at the end of the procedure. To avoid failure of repair, passive excessive external rotation and active internal rotation in the post-operative rehab should be avoided. *(Question: the limiting factor in the postoperative rehabilitation of a total shoulder arthroplasty?) (Scenario: 75 years old, 5 weeks after TSA, fall, tried to protect himself with the affected shoulder, shoulder pain, good forward flexion and external rotation, limitation of internal rotation, XR normal: diagnosis? (Subscapularis repair rupture)).*
- Post-operative protocol:
  - o Begin immediately (do not wait for 3 weeks) with an active assisted range-of-motion program for forward elevation and external rotation to the side (can reach to 60° external rotation if the subscapularis tendon repair was adequate).
  - o Active strengthening after about 6 weeks (to allow subscapularis muscle to heal).
- Rotator cuff tear arthroplasty can be treated by hemi-arthroplasty or RTA (see RC tear section).
  - o RC deficiency is a contra indication for standard arthroplasty (can use hemi or reversed).
  - o For patient with large external rotation lag sign: use hemiarthroplasty (RSA can decrease active external rotation).
  - o For patient with anterior superior escape: use RSA.
    - Hemi-arthroplasty for rotator cuff tear arthropathy can fail due to **anterosuperior escape**, treatment is conversion to RSA. *(Scenario:75 years old had hemiarthroplasty for RC arthropathy 3 years ago, patient continued to have pain, limited foreword flexion with anteriosuperior bulge of the shoulder with trial elevation, treatment?).*
- **Hemiarthroplasty:**

- Tuberosity mal-position will result in loss of ROM of the shoulder and poor functional results. The most significant factor associated with poor postoperative functional results is malposition of the tuberosities.
- After hemiarthroplasty, if the patient develops erosion of the glenoid (as a possible complication) with pain and decreased function, the treatment is conversion to total shoulder arthroplasty.
- Hemiarthroplasty for proximal humerus fracture:
  - **Tuberosity healing** (after 3 or 4 parts fracture) is important for good function results after hemiarthroplasty.
  - Failure of tuberosity healing is related to poor position of the implant (higher position or in adequate version), mal position of the tuberosity, females, older age (>75 years).
- **Total shoulder arthroplasty**
  - For retroverted glenoid (common pathology with shoulder OA (see before)): CT to assess the version.
    - If the version is > 15°: posterior glenoid bone grafting (allograft).
    - If the version is < 15°: **eccentric reaming** without excessively compromising glenoid bone stock and risking glenoid vault penetration by the glenoid component.
    - Eccentric reaming to correction excessive retroversion (>20°): may lead to glenoid vault perforation.
  - TSA is associated with more pain relief (compared to hemiarthroplasty).
  - Metal-backed glenoid components have higher rates of loosening than cemented all polyethylene glenoid components.
  - Cemented curve-backed pegged PE components have lower radiolucent lines than cemented keeled/flat backed PE.
  - Glenoid loosening after TSA is relatively common, and can result in failure of component and need for revision.
  - Common causes for revision surgeries include RC tears, glenohumeral instability, and periprosthetic humeral fractures.
    - Loosening of the glenoid component can lead to pain after TSA. XR will show loosening of the glenoid component and possible superior humeral migration (indicating rotator cuff dysfunction which can lead to progressive failure of the glenoid component due to rocking horse phenomenon that results in premature loosening and failure of the glenoid component.). *(Scenario: 70 years old, TSA 5 years ago, having shoulder pain in the last 6 months, XR shows loosening of the glenoid component and superior humeral migration, diagnosis?)*
  - Patient with TSA can develop RC tears (with or without shoulder injuries) and will complain of pain, weakness and limited ROM. *(Scenario: 70 years male, TSA 5*

years ago, fall yesterday, pain, examination normal except weak rotator muscles, diagnosis? (RC tear))

- **Reverse Shoulder Arthroplasty (RSA):**
  - Biomechanical advantages:
    - **Medialization** of center of rotation (larger moment arm for abduction by deltoid).
    - Lowering of the humerus (increasing deltoid tension).
    - Large articulation surface (stability and increase ROM).
  - The classic indications for a RSA is an **elderly** patient with advanced arthritis and **advanced RC pathology** (however, recently the use of RSA is expanding with more cases of RSA is performed in younger patients with shoulder arthritis).
    - Axillary nerve palsy is a contraindication to the use of a RSA.
  - Scapular notching: a complication of RSA, thought to be due to impingement of the humerus component with the inferior scapular neck.
    - To reduce incidence of notching: inferior position of the glenoid base plate component, inferior inclination of the glenoid base plate, increased lateral offset, and increased glenoid sphere size.
    - Asymptomatic notching: management is observation.
  - RSA anterior dislocation occurs with the arm in the position of extension, adduction, and internal rotation (pushing out of a chair).
    - Dislocation is more common with delto-pectoral approach than superior approach.
  - Complications following RSA are highest when performed for failed shoulder arthroplasty.

Infected Shoulder Arthroplasty:

- Similar principles to THA and TKA (please refer to these two sections in their respective chapters).
- Classification: acute post-operative infection, chronic infection, acute hematogenous.
- **Male** gender and younger patients are the most predictive risk factors of deep infection following shoulder arthroplasty.
- **Chronic infection:**
  - Clinical presentation: pain and stiffness in the shoulder. XR: lucent lines surrounding the implant. Lab: increase ESR and C-RP.
  - If there is suspicious of infected arthroplasty: aspiration of the shoulder (see hip joint). *(Scenario: hemi-arthroplasty of the shoulder few years ago, now has shoulder pain, XR bone changes (lucent lines), next step?)*

- Cultures can take longer time (to be able to show infection with Propionibacterium acnes).
  - Low-virulence organism.
  - If there is persistent discharge with negative culture, think in Propionibacterium acnes, as it needs cultures for 3 weeks.
- **Preferred treatment is** two-stage revision. *(Scenario: hemiarthroplasty of the shoulder few years ago, now has shoulder pain, XR some bone changes, aspiration shows positive growth, what is the best option to allow eradication the infection and maintain function?)*
- It the aspiration is negative, with high clinical, radiologic and lab results likelihood for infection; the next step should be open irrigation and debridement with implant removal and possible two stage exchange arthroplasty. *(Scenario: 74 years old, TSA 4 years ago, white blood cell count of 13000/mm3, an ESR 80 mm/h, and a c-reactive protein of 3.8. The shoulder is aspirated, and cultures are negative at one week, what is the next step?)*
- **Hematogenous infection:**
  - Occurs after bacteremia. Patient will complain of shoulder pain. Elevated lab results. Diagnosis by aspiration. Treatment according to the time of since bacteremia (see THA infection). *(Scenario: TSA 7 years ago, patient has pneumonia one week ago, now has shoulder pain, next step? (XR and aspiration)).*

Shoulder Arthrodesis:
- Position of fusion: 30-30-30 (30°forward flexion, 30° abduction, 30° internal rotation).
  - Indications: paralysis of the deltoid, tumors, resistant joint infection). *(Scenario: 40 years old male, axillary nerve paralysis, failed muscle transfer, treatment?)*

Amputation (Glenohumeral Disarticulation):
- When the arm is amputated at the level of glenohumeral joint, the shoulder girdle muscles are unopposed, resulting in upward movement of the glenoid (referred to as "hiking" of the shoulder girdle)
- In a growing child, removal of the entire upper limb can result in scoliosis of the spine due to muscle imbalance.

Neuropathic Arthropathy:
- Due to neuropathy affecting the shoulder joint.
  - Most common cause is cervical intra-thecal anomaly (e.g. syringomyelia).
- Pathology: marked destruction of the shoulder joint.

- XR will show the bone destruction and possible joint dislocation. *(Scenario: 50 years old with mild shoulder joint pain, deformity and loss of motion, XR showing bone destruction, what is the next diagnostic test? (MRI cervical spine)).*

Sternoclavicular Septic Arthritis/ Osteomyelitis:

- Predisposing factors: rheumatoid arthritis, alcoholism, intravenous drug use, HIV, DM, end stage renal disease and chronic debilitating diseases.
- Clinical presentation: pain, swelling and hotness over the SC joint.
- Infection can spread to the chest cavity (retrosternal area and pericardium), CT is recommended before debridement
- Treatment: I&D, may require excision of the joint. *(Scenario: 35 years, HIV, pain and swelling on the SC joint, diagnosis?)*

Acromioclavicular Joint (See Anatomy And Trauma Upper Extremity Chapters):

- Acomioclavicluar arthritis: pain with cross arm movement.
- Mumford procedure: excision of the lateral part of the clavicle articulating in the AC joint.
    - Excision should be for less than 8-10 mm to avoid injury to CC ligament
- The posterior and superior acromioclavicular ligaments (postero-superior part of the capsule) provide the most restraint to posterior translation of the acromioclavicular joint (displacement in the horizontal plane) and must be preserved during a Mumford procedure.
- Conoid and trapezoid ligaments (parts of the CC ligament) provide the most restrain against superior migration of the clavicle (vertical plane).
- Anatomic AC joint reconstructions techniques are biomechanically superior to nonanatomic techniques (e.g. Weaver-Dunn procedure):
    - Anatomic repair has less risk of horizontal instability. Persistent antero-posterior instability may cause persistent symptoms following reconstruction by modified Weaver-Dunn.
- Osteolysis of the distal clavicle:
    - Common in **Weight lifter**.
    - Treatment is distal clavicle resection.

Shoulder Surgery General Consideration:

- Shoulder surgery has an increased risk of infection with Propionibacterium acnes, a slow-growing anaerobic gram-positive rod.

- o Cultures may take 7-21 days to become positive.
  - o The most common organism to cause late infection in shoulder arthroplasty is Propionibacterium acnes.
- Worker's compensation patients undergoing shoulder surgery (e.g. arthroscopic subacromial decompression with acromioplasty) have been shown to have less functional improvement and lower patient satisfaction than non-worker's compensation patients (however, work related injuries are not contra indication for performing surgeries).
- Inter-scalene brachial plexus regional block for shoulder surgery:
  - o Sensory neuropathy (temporary paresthesia to the arm and hand which can last for up to 6 months) is the most common complication after inter-scalene block for shoulder surgery.
  - o Can cause difficulty breathing due to affection of the phrenic nerve which lies in close proximity to the site of anesthetic injection causing unilateral diaphragmatic paralysis, the condition can be easily compensated in a healthy patient.
    - Hemidiaphragm paralysis after inter-scalene regional anesthesia has been reported to occur in nearly all cases.
    - Respiratory insufficiency is a contra indication for inter scalene block.
    - Management is continued observation and monitoring.
- Postoperative stiff shoulder: can occur after any surgery (fracture repair, arthroplasty): decrease ROM in all direction. Initial treatment is physical therapy for range-of-motion exercises. *(Scenario: 76 years old, ORIF of proximal humerus 4 weeks ago, coming with UE in the sling, exam shows decrease ROM, treatment?).*

Elbow:

Elbow Dislocation (See Trauma-Upper Extremity Chapter)
- Simple (no associated fracture).
- Complex dislocation (associated fracture).

Elbow Instability:
- Posterolateral instability: injury to the lateral ulnar collateral ligament (see below).
- Valgus instability: mainly due to injury to anterior band of medical collateral ligament (see below).
- Varus postero medial instability: mainly due to coronoid fractures (see below).
- **Posterolateral Rotatory Instability:**
  - o Due to injury of **the lateral ulnar collateral ligament**.

- Can occur with lateral elbow approaches (e.g. treatment of chronic lateral epicondylitis).
- Recurrent instability after elbow dislocation is commonly due to injury to the lateral ulnar collateral ligament. *(Scenario: 35 years old, postero lateral elbow dislocation 6 months ago, complain of pain and instability, what anatomical structure is responsible for the lesion?)*
- Most common pattern of injury of lateral collateral ligament is proximal ligamentous avulsion (from its humeral attachment).
  - The mechanism of injury is a combination of axial load, external rotation of the forearm (supination), and valgus force
  - Positive lateral pivot shift test:
    - Valgus and axial loading of the elbow to extended supinated forearm while the elbow is gradually flexed. Radius will subluxate posteriorly on the capitellum (painful clunk) or apprehension by the patient (at about 40°).
    - Lateral elbow pain when rising from a chair is equivalent to a positive pivot shift test.
  - Treatment:
    - Chronic lesions are treated by lateral collateral ligament **reconstruction (not repair)** with possible plication of the capsulo-ligamentous structures. *(Scenario: 38 years old, elbow dislocation 5 months ago, pain with rising from chair, treatment?)*
- **Valgus instability of the Elbow (See elbow pain in throwers) (See MCL injury):**
  - Stability is by both the medial collateral ligament and the bony structures.
    - The medial collateral ligament is the primary restraint to valgus instability in cases of radial head resection.
  - The moving valgus stress test: is performed by applying a valgus stress to a maximally flexed elbow, then passively extending the elbow *(Question: what test is used to diagnose medial instability of the elbow?)*.
    - If symptoms develop in the mid arc of flexion: MCL insufficiency.
    - Pain at the end of extension suggests posterior compartment symptoms (olecranon impingement, see below).
- **Varus postero medial instability**
  - Due to coronoid (anteromedial facet) fracture (with possible lateral ulnar collateral ligament tear).
    - CT can better delineate of the coronoid fracture.
  - Management: surgical fixation of anteromedial facet fracture (possible repair of the lateral ulnar collateral ligament).

Elbow Pain in Thrower (See Phases of Throwing Before):

- **Late cocking/early acceleration** is the position of maximal stress upon the medial collateral ligament complex of the elbow in the overhead throwing motion.
- In skeletally immature children the injury is usually avulsion fracture of the medial epicondyle at the **physeal level**, which can occur in response to the valgus load placed on the elbow while throwing (acute injury on top of chronic stress overuse injury).
    - o Diagnosis by XR (may require views of the uninjured elbow to evaluate for physeal anatomy).
- In older pitchers (after fusion of the medial epicondyle physis), the ulnar collateral ligament is usually the affected structure rather than the bone of the medial epicondyle.
- Medial epicodyle appear at the age of 5 years (girls)/ years 6 (boys) and it is the last physis to fuse at the 15-16 years old.
- Flexor carpi ulnaris and flexor digitorum superficialis are dynamic stabilizers for the elbow during cocking and acceleration phases of the overhead throw.
- **MCL injury:**
    - o Repetitive valgus stress on the medial aspect of the elbow joint during throwing or racquet sports.
        - ▪ Injury is usually to the **anterior** bundle of the MCL.
    - o Clinical presentation: pain at the medial aspect of the elbow (during early acceleration phase) and decrease velocity of throwing.
        - ▪ "Pop" sensation at the elbow during throwing can sometime indicate an MCL injury.
        - ▪ Partial tears of the MCL of the elbow: positive moving valgus stress (see before) and milking tests
        - ▪ The milking maneuver:
            - • Pull on the patient's thumb with the forearm supinated, shoulder extended, and the elbow flexed to 90 degrees.
            - • A positive result when there is a localized medial elbow pain and a subjective feeling of apprehension and instability.
        - ▪ Moving valgus stress test: see before.
    - o Management:
        - ▪ Rest and physical therapy is the initial treatment for MCL injuries.
        - ▪ If conservative management fails, **reconstruction** of the **anterior band** of the ulnar collateral ligament (MCL) may be needed.
        - ▪ Athletes who want to return to a high level of throwing will require surgical reconstruction. Allograft reconstruction gives the best results.
        - ▪ If there are concomitant ulnar nerve symptoms: ulnar nerve transposition should be added to the reconstruction of the MCL.

(Scenario: Javelin thrower, complain of elbow pain and decreased velocity, pain with valgus stress at the range from 40-100, what anatomic structure is responsible? what is the treatment?)

Posterior Impingement:
- Impingement by olecranon osteophytes against the olecranon fossa.
- Initial treatment is non-operative. If this fail, resection of the osteophytes.
  - Excessive olecranon resection increases the stresses on the medial collateral ligament during throwing.

Distal Biceps Rupture:
- Clinical presentation: "hook test" the examiner's finger is inserted beneath the distal biceps tendon. Failure to "hook" indicates distal biceps rupture.
- Surgical repair of complete distal biceps rupture is mainly indicated to restore full supination strength.
  - Failure to repair the distal biceps tendon will result in loss of about 40% of the supination strength and about 10% of flexion strength.
- One incision surgical repair:
  - Most common complication associated with the treatment of the distal biceps ruptures is lateral antebrachial cutaneous nerve injury, second most common is PIN injury. Keeping the forearm supinated helps to protect the PIN by keeping the nerve further away from the tendon insertion.
- Two incisions surgical repair:
  - Most common complication is development of HO.
- Partial distal biceps rupture:
  - Clinical presentation: occurs in manual workers in the dominant arm. No history of trauma, pain in the forearm with weak supination, painful with resisted supination.
  - Initial treatment: rest and therapy. If fail: detachment of the tendon, debridement and re attachment.

Lateral Epicondylitis:
- Pathology: angiofibroblastic tendinosis and degeneration of extensor carpi radialis brevis **(ERCB)**.
- Clinical presentation is lateral-sided elbow pain. Symptoms exacerbated with resisted wrist extension.

- o 10 % of cases are associated with radial tunnel syndrome. *(Scenario: patient with lateral epicondylitis, no improvement with conservative treatment, surgery done, no improvements, what is the reason for not improving?)*
- Treatment is mainly non-operative:
  - o Initial treatment is physical therapy (**eccentric** conditioning and strengthening program).
  - o Surgical treatment is only after **exhaustion of all non-operative methods**.

Osteochondral Lesion (Osteochondritis Dissecans) of The Capitellum (See pediatric Orthopedic):

- Clinical presentation:
  - o Occurs in children older than 13 years (younger children will have Panner's disease).
  - o Common in gymnastics. May be related to repeated micro trauma.
  - o Elbow pain, locking of the elbow, loss of terminal degrees of extension.
- MRI will show the lesion (lucency around the lesion, possible separation).
- Treatment:
  - o Stable lesion in skeletal immature patient can heal with nonsurgical management (no sport activity). Surgical procedures are generally not necessary for the treatment of these lesions.
  - o Unstable lesion (separated): requires surgical treatment (fixation or excision). *(Scenario: gymnast, 13 years old, elbow pain, no instability, 10 degrees loss of elbow extension. Radiographs OCD of capitellum 4mm. MRI scan reveals a single solitary lesion, with no signal around the lesion. There are no intra-articular loose bodies, treatment?) (Same scenario, but MRI shows separated lesion, treatment?)*

Post Traumatic Elbow Stiffness:

- Functional range of motion: Most activities of daily living require elbow ROM from 30° to 130° (flexion extension) and 50° in each direction of pronation and supination.
- Can occur after fractures (even non displaced ones) treated with immobilization.
- Flexion deformity can cause ulnar neuropathy and ulnar nerve symptoms (numbness of the ulnar two fingers).
- Initial treatment is physical therapy and stretching and/or serial casting.
  - o If this fails: capsular release can be done (anterior capsule for flexion deformity and posterior capsule for extension deformity). Ulnar nerve transposition can be added if there is ulnar neuropathy.
  - o Arthroscopic release of the capsule of the elbow anterior to the radial head and neck can lead to injury to the radial nerve, located along the anterolateral capsule just distal to the radiocapitellar joint.

- It is safer to release the elbow capsule from its proximal insertion than from its distal insertion.
- **Heterotrophic ossification (HO) of the elbow:**
  - Defined as the inappropriate formation of mature lamellar bone in non-osseous locations.
  - Clinical presentation: swelling with progressive loss of elbow range of motion.
  - Simple elbow dislocation can be complicated by the development of anterior heterotrophic ossification and loss of elbow motion.
    - Brachilais muscle is prone to develop HO after contusion.
  - Treatment:
    - Surgical resection and capsulectomy (NSAIDs and irradiation are prophylaxis measures and not treatment modalities).
    - Combined lateral and medical approaches offer exposure both anterior as well as posterior HO. Anterior approach allows anterior exposure but cannot be used for posterior HO.
    - If there is extension contracture (limited elbow flexion), release of the posteromedial band of the MCL and the posterior capsule should be done (through medial approach).
    - Release of the ulnar nerve is needed in most cases of elbow surgical release.
    - Prophylaxis for post-operative recurrence should be given: indomethacin or low-dose radiotherapy (see hip chapter).

Elbow Rheumatoid Arthritis:

- For early stage arthritis (soft tissue swelling or mild narrowing of the joint): synovectomy with possible radial head resection.
- For patient with limited elbow flexion (<90): synovectomy can be done to improve ROM.
- The preferred treatment for end stage rheumatoid with involvement of the ulnohumeral and radiocapitellar joint is total elbow arthroplasty.
  - Semiconstrained total elbow arthroplasty is a better option than unconstrained arthroplsasty in rheumatoid patients due to ligamentous instability in those patients.
- Elbow arthrodesis or resection arthroplasty are considered salvage techniques and are generally not considered as a primary treatment method for elbow rheumatoid arthritis.

Elbow Osteoarthritis

- More common in manual workers (e.g. carpenter).
- Clinical presentation: painful mechanical locking of the elbow in the mid-range of elbow movement.
- Treatment:
  - Initially nonsurgical options (NSAIDs, therapy, injection).
  - If failed: surgical treatment options include: ulnohumeral arthroplasty (Outerbridge procedure), interpositional arthroplasty, open/arthroscopic debridement with capsular release, loose body removal, osteophyte decompression, and/or total elbow arthroplasty (TEA).
  - For a young manual worker, surgical treatment (after failure of non-surgical options) should **start** with **open/arthroscopic debridement with** capsular **release**, loose body removal, and osteophyte decompression.
    - Arthritis in young patients can be treated by interposition arthroplasty if bone stock is preserved and the elbow maintains inherent stability. Contraindications for soft-tissue interposition arthroplasty include elbow instability, active infection, or pain without motion loss. *(Question: elbow arthritis with instability, treatment? (TEA)).*
    - Failed interposition arthroplasty (with ligamentous instability) is treated with **constrained** total elbow arthroplasty.

Cubital Tunnel Syndrome:

- Anatomy: see anatomy chapter.
- Clinical presentation: numbness of the ulnar two fingers, intrinsic muscle weakness.
  - Advanced cases will show ulnar nerve motor neuropathy: an ulnar clawhand, wasting of the interosseus muscles, Wartenberg's sign, and Froment's sign (see anatomy chapter, nerve section).
- Initial treatment is night time elbow extension bracing. *(Scenario: athlete, postereomedial elbow pain, decreased grip power, numbeness of the ulnar fingers, elbow exam and XR normal, initial treatment?).*
- Surgical treatment:
  - No differences in outcome between simple ulnar nerve decompression and anterior transposition of the nerve.
  - **The presence of subluxation of the ulnar nerve is not a contraindication to in situ decompression.** However, ulnar nerve instability may be best treated by transposition rather than simple decompression.
  - Submuscular transposition (with or without medial epicondylectomy): mainly for revision surgery or patients who are thin.
  - Adequate nerve decompression is the most important predictor of outcome.

- Branches of the medial antebrachial cutaneous nerve can be injured during the approach to ulnar nerve (can result in the development of painful neuroma and paraesthesia).

Elbow Arthroplasty:
- Most commonly used type is semi-constrained version.
  - Semi constrained allows flexion/ extension and 10° varus/ valgus movement.
  - Fully constrained type allows only flexion/ extension movement and has high failure rate due stress transmission to the bone cement interface.
  - Unlinked (unconstrained) prosthesis has high failure rate due to subluxation and dislocation.
    - The most common mode of failure following unconstrained total elbow arthroplasty is **instability** which can also occur from component malpositioning that leads to undue stress to the collateral ligaments
    - Loosening, polyethylene wear and bushing wear are more common complications in constrained and semiconstrained elbow arthroplasty.
- Following total elbow arthroplasty, patients should be instructed to permanently limit the load bearing to 5 pounds or less.
- If using Bryan-Morrey approach (the triceps is dissected free from its ulnar insertion and reflected laterally then at the end of the procedure, the triceps tendon is reattached to the ulna through drill holes), the surgical wound should be splinted for 7-10 days in 60-90° flexion to allow for soft tissue healing.
  - Prolonged immobilization (4-6 weeks) can lead to stiffness.
  - Following the short immobilization period, the patient can start active flexion and gravity-assisted passive extension. Active resisted extension is delayed (6-8 weeks) to protect the triceps tendon repair. *(Scenario: TEA, at 4 weeks during resisted active movement felt a pop, now pain and weak extension, diagnosis?)*
  - Loss of elbow extensor power can be a complication of this approach.
- Complications:
  - Aseptic component, bushing wear.

Elbow Arthroscopy (See Anatomy Chapter)
- Neurovascular complications are the most common complications reported with elbow arthroscopy.
- Ulnar neuropathy with prior submuscular ulnar nerve transposition is a contraindication to elbow arthroscopy.
- Portals (see anatomy chapter)

Tips:

- Surgical treatment for shoulder pathology is usually after therapy and injection.
  - If reasonable time of therapy did not achieve healing, more therapy will most probably not help
- Weight lifter:
  - Osteolysis of distal clavicle.
  - Quadrangular space syndrome
  - Tearing sensation during bench pressing: pectoralis major rupture (loss of normal anterior axillary contour).
- Lateral elbow pain when rising from a chair is equivalent to a positive pivot shift test.

Chapter 11: The Hand

Arthritis of the hand

Rheumatoid Hand Affection (See RA in Systemic Conditions Chapter):

- Disease-modifying anti-rheumatic drugs (DMARD) had resulted in dramatic decrease is surgical interventions for rheumatoid hand patients.
- Rheumatoid arthritis can result in severe MCP joint involvement with dislocation/subluxation and fixed deformities of the fingers:
  - MCP joint arthroplasty is the procedure of choice (fusion of the MCP of fingers 2-5 is not well tolerated).
    - Arthroplasty for MCP joint can improve the extensor lag and partially improve of the ulnar drift.
  - Thumb MCP joint involvement is usually treated with arthrodesis.
  - Reasons for inability to extend the MCP in rheumatoid arthiris: PIN palsy (as a result of nerve affection due to radio-capitillar joint synovitis), tendon rupture, dislocation of the MCP joint, or subluxed tendon (rupture of the radial sagittal band with ulnar subluxation of the tendon).
    - PIN palsy: patient will retain the tenodesis effect by the intact tendons (the diagnosis can be confirmed by nerve conduction test). _(Scenario: rheumatoid arthritis patient, inability to extend the ulnar 4 digits; with passive wrist flexion the digits are extended, how can the diagnosis can be confirmed?)_
    - Rupture of extensor digitorum communis (EDC): loss of active MCP extension.
      - Treated with flexor digitorum sublimis (FDS) of the middle and ring finger transfer to EDC. The FDS is routed radially, around the radius in a dorsal direction (rather than through the interosseous membrane) (technically easier, avoid synovitis on the dorsum of the wrist, and correct ulnar deviation of the fingers through the line of pull from the radial side of the forearm).
      - Another option in case of rupture of EDC to 4th and 5th is to transfer extensor indicis proprius (EIP) (no functional deficit as a result of the transfer)
- Rupture of the small finger extensor (The extensor digiti quinti/minimi):
  - Small finger extensors (EDQ and EDC tendon to the small finger) are the most prone tendons to rupture in a patient with rheumatoid arthritis due to: DRUJ synovitis and pressure by dorsally dislocated ulna
    - **Vaughan-Jackson syndrome** is the rupture of the digital extensor tendons on the ulnar side of the hand and wrist (the extensor digiti minimi and EDC tendon of the small finger). Ring and little fingers extensors are the most likely tendons to rupture in RA.

- o Extensor tenosynovitis that remains refractory after 6 months of medical treatment and splinting should be treated by tenosynovectomy.
  - o Treatment is tendon reconstruction and excision of the distal ulna
  - o Injury to EDQ can be masked by EDC (which can provide extension to the fifth finger). The EDQ is at high risk since it is overlying the ulnar head where it is prone to attritional rupture.
- Mannerfelt:
  - o Rupture of the FPL (inability to flex the IP of the thumb) due to synovitis and/ or bony osteophytes.
  - o Treatment is tendon reconstruction with either Palmaris longus or FDP of the index (direct repair cannot be done due to attrition of the tendon).
- As a general rule, in tendon attritional rupture in rheumatoid arthritis, avoid primary repair.
- In cases of concomitant wrist, elbow and shoulder affection: start first with more proximal joints (rather than reconstruction of the hand) as the hand therapy will usually require shoulder/elbow movement.
- Fusion (arthrodesis) Vs Total wrist arthroplasty for wrist arthritis is RA patients:
  - o For bilateral wrist fusion: one in mild extension and one in mild flexion for ADL.
  - o Fusion: more for active individual; total wrist arthroplasty: more for low demand individual.
  - o Fusion: more for the non dominant hand; total wrist arthroplasty: more for dominant hand.
  - o The primary indication for performing a total wrist arthroplasty in a patient with painful rheumatoid arthritis is the presence of contralateral wrist fusion.
- Trigger finger in RA:
  - o Pathology is true tenosynovitis (in contrast to the tendovaginitis present in the idiopathic trigger digit).
  - o Treatment is open tenosynovectomy of the flexor tendon.
  - o Release of the A1 pulley is not recommended in rheumatoid arthritis patients due to the potential for worsening deformity.
- Swan-neck deformity
  - o Etiology: associated with volar plate and collateral ligament laxity
  - o Treatment:
    - Flexible deformity: initial treatment is splinting; if this fail, FDS tenodesis or Fowler central slip tenotomy.
    - Rigid deformity: dorsal capsular release, lateral band mobilization, collateral ligament release, and extensor tenolysis.

Gout Affection of The Hand (See Gout in General Condition Chapter):

- Can cause acute wrist arthritis (with similar presentation to septic arthritis), aspiration will be needed to assess the joint fluid (looking for crystals).
- XR will show Joint destruction (both sides of the joint) with bunched out osteolytic lesions (See Fig 1)

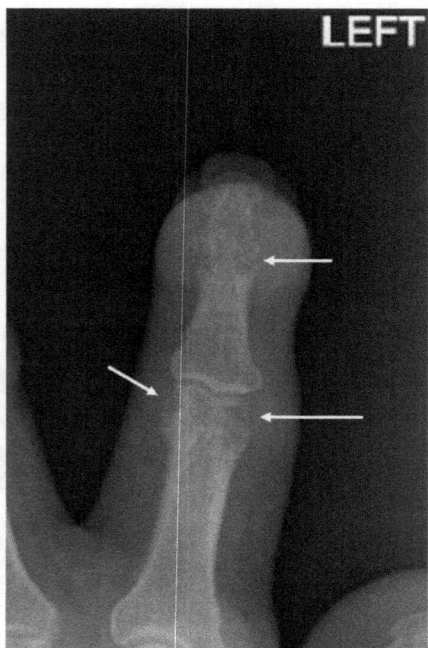

Fig 1: 56 years old male with long history of bilateral hand pain and swelling. XR AP of the hand shows osteolytic bunched out lesions on both sides of the PIP and DIP of the index. The patient was found to have gout which was confirmed with crystal exam of the joint fluid.

Psoriasis of The Hand:

- Severe erosion and destruction of the distal IP producing cup in pencil deformity.

Basilar Joint (Trapezial-First Metacarpal Joint) (1st CMC) Arthritis:

- Proposed etiology is attenuation of the volar (Beak) ligament of the 1st CMC joint.
- Up to 50% of the patients with 1st CMC arthritis has associated carpal tunnel syndrome.
- If operative treatment is needed:
  - Necessary element of the procedure is **excision of trapezium**, with possible ligament reconstruction and possible interposition of muscle (FCR or abductor pollicis longus). _(Question: surgical management of 1st CMC arthritis should always include what procedure?)._
  - Hyperextension of the metacarpo-phalangeal joint should be corrected if more than > 30° by arthrodesis. If hyperextension is less than 30°: pinning of the

joint or capulodesis can be performed. (Failure to correct hyperextension will lead to adduction contracture and collapse of the basilar joint).
- o Subsidence of the thumb is expected, but does not seem to have a clinical implication.

IP Arthritis:
- For patients with OA: DIP is more affected than PIP.
- Mucus cyst (on the dorsum of the DIP) is related to arthritis of the DIP.
  - o Initial treatment by observation. If this fails or there is impending rupture through the skin, treatment by excision and **removal of the underlying osteophytes** (to prevent recurrence).
    - ▪ Fusion of the IP is not needed in most cases (reserved for patients with severe pain and advanced arthritis).
    - ▪ DIP fusion: the angle of fusion increase ulnarly (from 20°to 40° going from index to small finger) to allow for gripping by ulnar digits.

Radiocarpal Arthritis:
- The severity of post-traumatic radiocarpal arthritis following distal radius fracture does not correlate with the presence of symptoms.
- Treatment options:
  - o Radio carpal fusion.
  - o Total wrist arthroplasty.
  - o Radioscapholunate fusion can be performed for posttraumatic (distal radius fracture) arthritis in conjunction with excision of the triquetrum and distal pole of the scaphoid (for improving radial deviation and the flexion-extension arc of motion of the wrist).
  - o Anterior interosseous neurectomy: can decrease the pain sensation of wrist arthritis.

DRUJ arthritis:
- DRUJ arthritis in a manual worker (after failure of conservative treatment) can be treated by the Sauve-Kapandji procedure (fusion of the DRUJ with creation of pseudoarthrosis of the ulna proximal to it).

Triangular Fibro-Cartilage Complex (TFCC) Injury:
- Most common mechanism of injury is falling while in the position of extension/ pronation of the wrist.
- Central tear:

- o If there is ulnar positive and patient is young: ulnar shortening; if there is no ulna positive and patient is older: debridement of the tear
- Traumatic Peripheral tear:
  - o Repair can be considered.
- Longitudinal radio-ulnar dissociation: reconstruction of the **central band** of the interosseous membrane (IOM) will best restore load transfer characteristics.

Kienbock's disease:

- Avascular necrosis of the lunate bone.
- Associated with increased stress transfer across the radio carpal joint which may be related to relative ulna minus (ulnar shortening).
- Stage I:
  - o XR: Normal picture of the lunate with possible ulna minus wrist.
  - o MRI: hypovascularity (decreased signal intensity) on T1 weighted image of the lunate. _(Question what the confirmatory test if suspecting Kienbock's disease is?)_
- Stage II:
  - o Radiographs will show increases lunate density.
- Stage III:
  - o A: Collapse of the lunate with no carpal instability (no rotation of scaphoid).
  - o B: Collapse of the lunate with scaphoid rotation.
- Stage IV:
  - o Degenerative changes in the wrist around the lunate.
- Treatment:
  - o Initial treatment (especially for stage I) is NSAIDs and immobilization.
  - o Most patients with Kienbock's disease will require surgical intervention.
  - o Stage I/II/III A:
    - Radial shortening osteotomy (especially in cases of ulna negative patients).
    - Other options include capitate shortening (especially if there no ulna minus) or radial core decompression (thought to work by stimulation of local vascular healing response).
  - o III B: Proximal raw carpectomy (PRC) or limted carpal fusion (S-T-T fusion or S-C fusion)
  - o IV: PRC or wrist fusion.

Hand and Wrist Trauma:
Distal Phalanx Fracture:

- Most of these fractures can be treated non surgical.
- If unstable fracture: closed reduction and percutaneous pinning.
- Distal phalanx non union: if symptomatic (pain with grip), treated with open reduction, internal fixation and bone grafting

Proximal Metacarpal Fracture of The Thumb (See Fig 2):

- 3 types: extra-articular, partial articular (Bennett's fracture), complete articular.
- **Bennett's Fracture:**
  - There is displacement of the thumb metacarpal shaft from the volar ulnar portion of the metacarpal base (which remains congruent within the 1st CMC joint).
  - The thumb metacarpal is displaced radially, dorsally and proximally (by the combined pull of the APL, EPL, and EPB) and adducted and supinated by the adductor pollicis. _(Question: what nerves are responsible for the deformity? (PIN and deep ulnar))_
  - Treatment by CRPP (the reduction maneuver is traction, pronation, abduction, with direct dorsal and radial push on the proximal part of the MC). The 1st metacarpal can be pinned to the second metacarpal or the carpal bones.

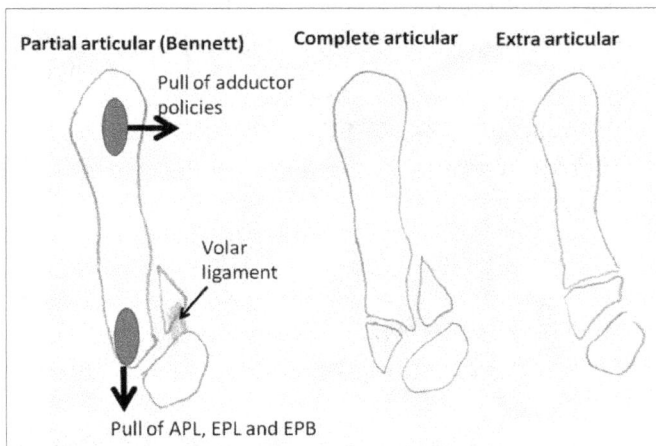

Fig 2: Types of fractures of the base of the 1st Metacarpal. Bennett's fracture has APL, EPL, EPB and adductor policies deforming the distal fragment while the proximal ulnar fragment is fixed by the volar ligament.

Traumatic Dislocation of The Thumb CMC Joint:

- The volar oblique ligament usually tears off the first metacarpal in a subperiosteal fashion.
- Treatment options are either closed reduction with pinning or ligament reconstruction. The reconstruction leads to better abduction and pinch strength (preferred in young patients).

Fracture of the Proximal/Middle Phalanx:

- Most of these fractures can be treated non operative; apply splint with MCP joint in flexion.
- Transverse fractures of the phalanges are stable fracture that can be treated in a splint.
    - Angulated transverse shaft fractures can usually be treated with closed reduction and splint (especially non comminuted fractures)
- Indications for internal fixation: open fractures, long spiral fracture with mal-rotation, distal condylar intra-articular fracture (fracture with extension into the joint), proximal fracture with sagittal angulation (relative indication). *(Scenario: elderly female, proximal phalanx proximal end comminuted fracture with dorsal angulation, treatment? (closed reduction and percutaneous pinning)) (Scenario: displaced long spiral fracture with joint extension, treatment? (open reduction and rigid fixation)).*

Metacarpal Shaft Fractures

- Most of these fractures are stable fractures and can be treated with splint in the intrinsic plus position (flexion of the MCP joints and extension of the IP joints). This will decrease the deforming forces by intrinsic muscles and will avoid extension contracture of the MCP joints.
- Shortening of metacarpal should be avoided as it will lead to extensor lag of about 7° for every 2 mm of shortening, decease in grip strength. This effect is not digit-specific.
- Indication for fixation: multiple metacarpal fractures (loss of support from adjacent intact metacarpal, treatment is ORIF for all fractured metacarpal), fractures with rotational deformity and open fracture.

Hook of Hamate Fracture:

- Common in baseball and golf players; frequently missed injury, and can progress to develop non union.
- Patients will complain of ulnar-sided wrist pain, ulnar nerve irritation (numbness and tingling in the fourth and fifth digits), and irritation of flexor tendons to the ulnar fingers (grating sensation in the ulnar fingers with motion) and possibly attritional ruptures of the flexor tendons (inability to flex the ulnar fingers).
- Carpal tunnel view can show the fracture but CT is most sensitive imaging modality.
- Treatment consists of excision of the hook of the hamate
    - Excision of the fragment is more predictable than fixation of the broken segment.

- o   If there is tendon rupture: tendon repair. *(Scenario: Golf player, ulnar sided wrist pain for 6 months, now unable to flex the small finger. Diagnosis and treatment?) (Scenario: golfer, 6 months of ulnar sided pain, hook of hamate fracture, treatment?)*

Pisiform Fracture:

- Pain over the ulnar side of the wrist and the hypothenar eminence.
- Most cases are initially missed on routine radiographic views. An oblique or carpal tunnel view can be helpful in visualizing the fracture and the pisotriquetral joint. CT can show the fracture more obvious.
- Treated by excision.

Scaphoid Fracture:

- Imaging:
    - o   For non displaced fracture, initial plain radiographs can be falsely negative.
    - o   If XR is negative and there is high suspicions of the diagnosis, either casting and repeat XR after 2 weeks or obtain MRI (if the patient prefer not to have a cast (e.g. a surgeon who wants to continue working).
- Treatment:
    - o   Non displaced waist fracture can be treated by cast immobilization or percutaneous fixation:
        - ▪ Non-displaced scaphoid fracture: percutaneous screw fixation (compared to cast immobilization) allows faster return to activities.
        - ▪ Long arm cast has been associated in some studies with decrease time to healing (controversial).
    - o   Non-displaced (or minimal displaced) fracture of the proximal pole: treatment is by percutaneous fixation through dorsal approach by cannulated screws (Internal fixation with a compression screw).
        - ▪ Proximal pole fracture has higher incidence of delayed union, nonunion, and/or osteonecrosis with nonsurgical management (see anatomy chapter).
    - o   Displaced scaphoid fractures are treated with open reduction and compression by screw.
        - ▪ Displaced proximal pole fracture is treated with open reduction and screws using dorsal approach while fractures of the scaphoid waist can be approached either by volar or dorsal approaches.
        - ▪ Correction of flexion deformity is better achieved through volar approach.

- The optimal biomechanical screw placement position to treat a waist-level scaphoid fracture is the central axis of the distal and proximal fragments.

- **Scaphoid non union:**
  - Treated with ORIF and bone grafting.
    - The graft is needed to correct the flexion deformity of the fracture that develops in cases of scaphoid non union. Tri-cortical bone graft can give better correction of the deformity (better support).
    - Flexion deformity (humpback deformity) is better corrected by a tricortical graft applied from volar approach.
    - If no AVN, regular non vascularized bone graft can be used.
    - Indication for vascularized bone graft: AVN or failure of previous non vascularized bone graft.
  - Non union with AVN: Pedicled vascularized bone graft (e.g. 1,2 inter-compartmental supraretinacular artery (1,2 ICSRA)vascularized bone graft from distal radius).
    - Non union of the proximal pole: pedicled vascularized bone graft (1,2 ICSRA vascularized bone graft). *(Scenario: 25 years, baseball player, 6 months of wrist pain, CT proximal pole non union, treatment?)*
  - Non union with AVN and humpback deformity: free vascularized bone graft from the medial femoral condyle is preferred (1,2 ICSRA vascularized graft less effective in correction of flexion deformity of the scaphoid).

- **SNAC (Scaphoid Nonunion Advanced Collapse) Wrist**
  - Classification
    - Stage I: Arthritis affecting the radial styloid (localized to the distal scaphoid and radial styloid).
    - Stage II: Radioscaphoid plus scaphocapitate arthritis, but preservation of the capitolunate joint.
    - Stage III: Periscaphoid affection with scaphocapitate and capitolunate joints arthritis (midcarpal joints).
  - Treatment:
    - Stage I: radial styloid excision with bone graft of scaphoid nonunion.
    - Stage II and III: Scaphoid excision and 4-corner fusion (with added excision of the radial styloid to increase the ROM).
    - Other options:
      - Stage II: Proximal raw carpectomy (contra-indicated if there arthritis of the capitolunate joint (stage III)).
      - Stage III: wrist arthrodesis.

Perilunate Injuries:

- **Trans-Scaphoid Peri-Lunate Carpal Dislocation (Fig 3):**
    - In perilunate fracture dislocation the lunate bone will remain in the lunate fossa while the rest of the carpal bones will dislocate in relation to the lunate (in contrast to lunate dislocations where the lunate is dislocated in a volar direction and no longer has normal radiolunate articulation).
    - Sequence of events (progressive perilunar instability):
        - Scaphoid extension (with opening of the space of Poirer), scaphoid fracture, and distal row dissociation, hyperextension of the triquetrum, lunotriquetral ligament rupture, and dorsal dislocation of the carpus.
        - The short radiolunate typically remains intact.
- **Lunate dislocation:**
    - Dislocation of the lunate from the lunate fossa.
        - The space of Poirier: lies around the proximal pole of the capitate. Lack of ligaments allows dislocation of the lunate through this area.
    - Compression of the median nerve by the lunate will lead to numbness of the radial 3-3.5 fingers (direct compression over the nerve and not compartment syndrome from local swelling).
        - This will need urgent reduction. Release of the transverse carpal ligament may also be needed if closed reduction does not result in resolution of symptoms.
    - Treatment: urgent Closed reduction (to avoid prolonged compression on the median nerve) followed by ligament repair via dorsal (or combined dorsal/volar approaches) on a semi-elective basis.
        - Transverse carpal ligament release should be added for cases with acute carpal tunnel syndrome that does not improve by closed reduction. *(Question: what is the urgent treatment for lunate dislocation?). (Scenario: 40 years old, work injury, numbness of the finger, XR shows perilunate dislocation, what is the nuerological exam? (Numbness of the volar aspect of the radial 3 fingers))*

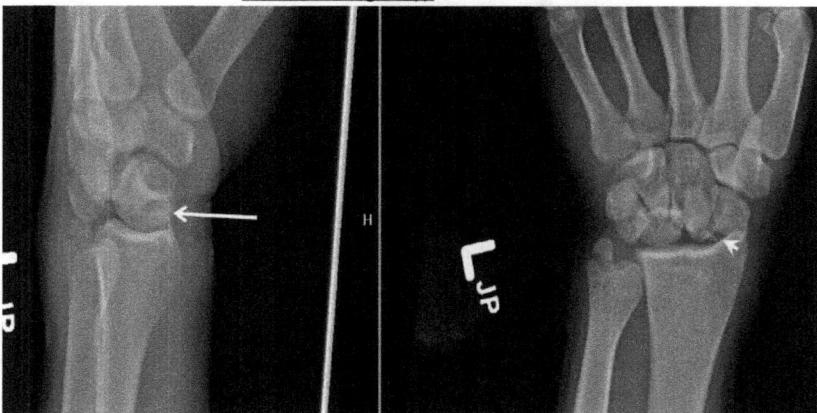

Fig 3 perilunate trans-scaphoid fracture dislocation: Lateral view shows lunate bone in the lunate fossa (arrow) with the rest of the carpal bone dislocated dorsally. AP shows scaphoid fracture (arrow head).

Carpo-Metacarpal Dislocation (Fig 4):

- Occurs at the 4th and 5th CMC joints. The lesion can be better seen in the oblique view. It is usually associated with coronal fracture of the hamate
- Treatment is reduction (closed or open) and internal fixation with Kirschner wires which are removed at about 6 weeks.

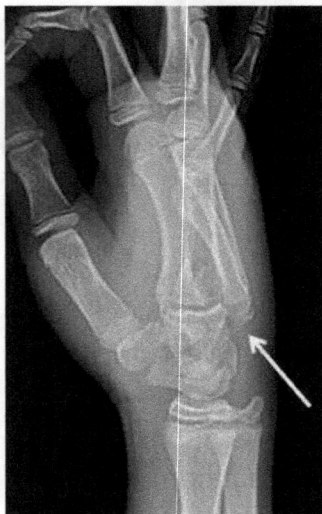

Fig 4: Dislocation of the 4th and 5th CMC joint with coronal fracture of the hamate (arrow).

Dorsal Metacarpophalangeal (MCP) Joint Dislocation:

- Can be simple or coplex dislocation (irreducible by closed means):
  - Structure most likely preventing the joint from being closed reduced is the volar plate. Open reduction will be needed (this can be through dorsal or volar approach).

PIP Dislocation:

- **PIP Dorsal Dislocation:**
  - Dislocation with no associated fracture:
    - Treatment is by closed reduction and buddy tapping.
  - Fracture dislocation:
    - Occurs with fracture of the volar proximal part of the middle phalanx
    - If it involves more than 50% of the articular surface, fixation (internal/external) is needed.
      - For comminuted fracture, internal fixation may not be possible; dynamic external fixation will achieve joint reduction and avoid stiffness.
    - If there is fracture of small fragment (less than 20%): extension block splint.

- Between 20-50%: assessment of the stability. For unstable injuries, fixation is needed.
  - Most important to factor determining outcome is **concentric reduction of the PIP in the lateral view** (i.e. maintaining reduction of the base of the middle phalanx on the condyles of the proximal phalanx) (not anatomic reduction of the fracture).
  - Volar plate arthroplasty can be used for treatment of acute unstable (as a last resort) and chronic cases.
    - The volar fragments of the middle phalanx are excised and a trough in the metaphysis is created for advancement of the volar plate which is released from the collateral ligaments.
    - Chronic dorsal dislocation: the treatment is open reduction with volar plate arthroplasty.
    - Collateral ligament must be excised when performing a volar plate arthroplasty of the PIP joint to allow gliding of the middle phalanx on the articular surface of the proximal phalanx.
- **PIP Volar Rotatory Dislocation.**
  - Can be irreducible due to entrapment of the one side of the middle phalanx between the central slip and lateral band.
- **Palmar dislocation of the PIP:**
  - Treatment: closed reduction in acute cases.
  - In late chronic cases, the treatment is open reduction and central slip repair.

Mallet Finger (Baseball Finger):

- Etiology: avulsion of the terminal extensor tendon from the distal phalanx, or bony avulsion of the dorsal proximal part of the distal phalanx.
  - Due to forcible flexion of the DIP joint (e.g. trying to catch a ball) while the finger extended.
- The treatment:
  - Soft tissue mallet: continuous extension splinting of the DIP joint for 6 weeks, followed by night splinting for an additional 6 weeks. No need to include the PIP in the immobilization.
  - For bony avulsion:
    - If there is no volar subluxation: can be treated as soft tissue mallet.
    - If there is volar subluxation: extension block pinning of the DIP joint (Fig 5).
    - The fragment size, amount of displacement, and degree of articular incongruity usually do not affect final outcome, as long as the joint is reduced.

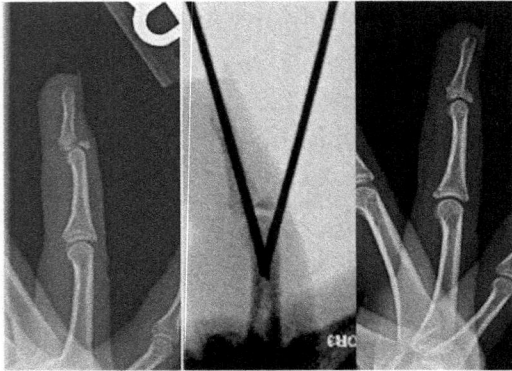

Fig 5: left: ring finger bony mallet injury with mild volar subluxation of the distal fragment. Middle: extension block pinning of the DIP was done with one pin blocking the small doral fragment form migrating proximally and a second pin to better the aling the distal and middle phalanges. Right: two months follow up shows healing of the bony mallet and better alignment of the DIP joint

Distal Radius Fracture:

- Pathology: about 30% of intra-articular distal radius fractures have an associated intercarpal (predominantly scapho-lunate) ligament injuries.
- **Treatment:**
    - Both surgical and nonsurgical management of distal radius fractures in **elderly patients** produce identical functional outcomes at 1 year follow up.
        - Surgery can give better early ROM; however, at one year follow up the grip strength was the only parameter which was significantly better in the operatively treated group.
        - Extra-articular fracture with dorsal angulation: In elderly patients (older than 65-70 years): closed reduction and splinting is the first line of treatment.
        - Low-demand elderly patients can be treated by closed reduction with accepted minor mal-reduction.
    - Acceptable criteria after closed reduction:
        - Less than 20° of dorsal tilt from the anatomical 14° volar tilt (less than 5-10° dorsal angulation from neutral), less than 3-5 mm shortening, less 3mm step off at the joint.
        - To restore the volar tilt: palmar directed force over the carpus.
        - If there is progressive loss of reduction after distal radius fracture treated by closed reduction, surgical treatment is warranted. _(Scenario: 60 years old female, distal radius fracture, good reduction, followed up in clinic, progressive loss of reduction, treatment?)_
    - Comminuted angulated intra articular distal radius fracture **in young age** is better to be treated with open reduction and internal fixation using volar plating (better maintenance of reduction and early ROM).
    - Surgsical treatment:
        - The best approach to reduce and stabilize a displaced volar lunate facet fracture of the distal radius is through extended carpal tunnel

incision (the disadvantage of this approach is not being less able to visualize the radial styloid fragment). The lunate facet should be reduced and well fixed (or well buttressed) in these types of fractures.

- Volar plate should be applied proximal to the watershed area to avoid flexor tendon irritation.
- Most common tendon rupture with volar plating is FPL.
- For volar fracture dislocations (volar Barton fractures), the treatment is open reduction through a volar approach and stabilization with a volar buttress plate.
- For dorsal Barton (partial articular fracture), the treatment should be ORIF through dorsal approach.
  - o If there is an associated distal ulna (ulnar styloid) fracture, after surgical stabilization of the radius, the DRUJ should be assessed.
    - In the vast majority of cases, the ulnar styloid does not have to be fixed (even if displaced). If there is instability of DRUJ, pinning of the joint in the reduced position can be done.
- **Complications:**
  - o Distal radius fracture can be complicated by rupture of EPL, this occur at about 1-2 months after injury.
    - The mechanism is not exactly known but it can be related to affection of blood supply, compartment syndrome within the muscle, compression by callus, sharp ends of fracture, nonunion of Lister's tubercle, or compression by cast.
    - Treatment by extensor indicis proprius (EIP) transfer to the extensor pollicis longus tendon (NOT repair of EPL) (EIP is ulnar to the index branch of EDC, see anatomy chapter). *(Scenario: 45 years, non-displaced distal radius fracture, cast treatment, two months later not able to extend the thumb, what structure affected?)).*
  - o Vitamin C reduces the prevalence of complex regional pain syndrome after distal radius fracture fractures. A daily dose of 500 mg for fifty days is recommended.
  - o The most common complication of dorsal plating is extensor tenosynovitis, (can cause pain and will require hardware removal).
  - o The proximal pins of distal radius external fixators can injure the branches of the superficial radial nerve (when the sensory branch of the radial nerve penetrates the fascia dorsal to the brachioradialis tendon to become a subcutaneous structure).
    - Sensory radian nerve injury is the most common complication of external fixation for distal radius fractures.

Boutonniere Deformity

- Pathoogy: PIP joint flexion with hyperextension at the DIP joint.
- Rupture of the central slip of the extensor tendon (acute closed boutonniere injury):
  - Usually occurs with PIP volar dislocation (see before): History of trauma to the finger (with possible reduction of dislocation). Patient will present few weeks later with boutonniere deformity (due to lateral band volar migration)
    - Closed injury is treated by splinting (static splint in full extension of the PIP) for 6 weeks, followed by night splinting (the DIP can be left free to avoid contracture).
- Chronic boutonniere deformity:
  - Can be treated by the Dolphin tenotomy (devision of the terminal extensor mechanism). The patients will still be able to achieve near normal extension of the DIP joint as the result of the intact oblique retinacular ligament of Landsmeer.
  - The steps for a PIP flexion contracture release are: retract the flexor tendons; release check rein ligaments; then release accessory collateral ligament and volar plate; and finally, the proper collateral ligament (check extension after each step, if adequate, no need to release more structures).
  - Rigid contractures can be treated with PIP joint arthrodesis or arthroplasty.

Sagittal Band Rupture:

- The diagnosis of sagittal band rupture is made based on inability to actively extend the MCP joint with the ability to maintain MCP joint extended after passive extension
- Most common sagittal band rupture is radial band of the long finger (the finger will deviate ulnarly).

The Thumb MCP Joint Ulnar Collateral Ligament Injury (Game Keeper/ Skiers thumb):

- Pathology:
  - Injury to the ulnar collateral ligament (relatively common injury).
  - Stener's lesion: retraction of the collateral ligament proximal to the adductor aponeurosis. This happens when the ligament is completely torn. This lesion will need surgical repair.
  - Occasionally (especially in adolescent) the injury is due to fracture of the ulnar proximal base of the proximal phalanx (Salter Harris type III injury).
- Assessment of the stability of the joint:
  - At 30° of flexion to test the proper collateral ligament.
  - At full extension to test the volar accessory collateral ligament and the volar plate.

- o Instability is defined as > 35° angulation or > 20° difference from the contralateral side when the thumb is radially stressed.
- Treatment:
  - o For a complete tear of the ligament complex to occur, there will be laxity in full extension and full flexion: these injuries are better treated with surgical repair.
  - o Incomplete tears respond well to thumb spica casting for 3 weeks followed by gradual resumption of range of motion.
  - o Prolonged immobilization of incomplete injuries leads to higher rates of MCP joint stiffness.
  - o Indication to fix avulsion fracture: is the presence of unstable joint.

FDP Tendon Injuries:

- Tendon nutrition is through the vincula, the intra-tendinous vessels, and perfusion at the insertion site; avascular regions are nourished by imbibition.
- **Quadrigia effect**:
  - o Excessive advancement of the FDP during repair may lead to "quadrigia effect" (shortening of an FDP tendon decreases the excursion of the neighboring FDP tendons because they all originate from a common muscle belly)
  - o If the FDP is advanced more than 1.5 cm, there is a risk of development of quadriga effect. *(Scenario: 40 years old, FDP rupture from 2 weeks, surgical repair, complain now of weak grip, mechanism?)*
- **Lumbrical plus:**
  - o When patient tries to flex the DIP, the joint will be extended.
  - o Due to rupture of FDP with intact lumbrical muscle.
  - o Treatment is by tenotomy of the radial lateral band (to prevent the action of the lumbrical muscle). *(Scenario: Amputation of the index finger at the distal phalanx, patient extends the DIP when he tries to flex it, treatment?)*
- **Flexor digitorum profundus (FDP) rupture/ avulsion (rugby finger/ jersey finger):**
  - o Often occurs after the player catches the shirt of the opposing player.
  - o Leddy classification (the smaller the numbers, the worse):
    - ▪ Grade I: retract to the palm, must be done ASAP (within one week). Pulleys will collapse and the vinculae will be stripped from the tendon affecting its blood supply; repair is needed as soon as possible.
      - ▪ If presenting late (> 2 weeks), options include: 2 stage tendon graft, fuse the DIP or observe (see below).
    - ▪ Grade II: retract to A2 pulley at the PIP (stopped by the vincula) (can be done within 2 months).

- Grade III: bony avulsion: retract to the A4 pulley. *(Scenario: football player, finger caught while tackling, cannot move the DIP, XR shows avulsion of the volar proximal segment of the P3, what structure is affected?) (FDP))*
- Occasionally, there may be both bony avulsion fracture of FDP and the tendon can avulse from the avulsed fragment (double avulsion).

- **FDP lacerations:**
  - Acute lacerations: see below
  - Chronic cases of FDP injury: Treatment options:
    - If the patient wants near normal function: two-stage tendon graft. First stage involves silicone rod (to create pathway) then the second stage for tendon graft.
    - DIP fusion (especially in the presence of DIP hyperextension).
    - Observation: If FDS is intact with good ROM of the finger, it may be better not to do the reconstruction of the FDP and leave the patient with a sublimis finger (for fear of worse outcome after reconstruction).

Pulley Rupture:

- Disruption of the annular pulley system of the finger.
- Mostly seen in rock climbers, will result in obvious bowstringing of the flexor tendon. Diagnosis is confirmed by MRI.

Repair of Tendon Laceration:

- Strength of the repair is proportional to the number and the caliber of the core suture used for the repair.
- Preferred suture technique for flexor tendon laceration is 4-strand core suture repair with epitendinous augmentation (this will allow immediate postoperative protocols of controlled active flexion).
- In children: post-operative immobilization (in mitten cast) for 4 weeks is the standard post-operative protocol.
- Zone II flexor tendon injuries can involve both FDP and FDS and can be associated with a higher risk of adhesion formation and poorer outcomes.
  - Zone II: the preferred treatment is repair of both FDP and FDS (only if the surgeon thinks he/she can perform the repair and still the tendons can slide adequately). Other options are: repair of FDP and one slip of FDS or FDP only repair and sacrifice the FDS.
- Flexor and extensor tendon lacerations with ≤ 50% affection: no need to repair the tendon, if there is triggering in the sheath, trimming of the edges can be done.

- Awake anesthesia (surgery done under local anesthesia; after the repair is done, surgeon will ask the patient to move the fingers and assess the repair) is the best method of assessment of the quality/ tension of the repair.
- Risk of re-rupture is greatest at first 3 weeks post repair (usually fail at the knots).
- Chronic flexor tendon injuries in young patients are better treated by two staged reconstruction (using temporary rod) (see above for chronic FDP injuries).
  - Two-stage reconstruction is also the preferred method in cases of segmental loss of tendon, disruption of the pulley system, or extensive tendon scarring.
- Chronic FPL tear: A transfer of the flexor digitorum superficialis of the ring finger to the insertion of the flexor pollicis longus on the distal phalanx provides good results with a one-stage operation.
- Tendon laceration with late presentation:
  - Zone II: two stage reconstruction (silicon rod followed by tendon graft) (see before).
  - Zone III: Possible one stage tendon graft (less concerns for adhesions)
- Zone V extensor tendon injuries resulting from fight bites can be associated with traumatic arthrotomy of the MCP joint. These will require joint inspection, debridement, and the administration of antibiotics.

Carpal Instability

- **DISI** (Dorsal intercalated segment instability):
  - The lunate is dorsiflexed, the angle between lunate and scaphoid increases.
  - Seen with the SL ligament disruption or with scaphoid fractures.
- **VISI** (Volar intercalated segment instability)
  - The lunate is flexed, and angle between lunate and scaphoid decreases.
  - Seen with lunotriquetral ligament incompetence.
- **Scapholunate Dissociation (Scapho-Lunate Ligament Injury):**
  - Pathology: disruption of **dorsal** scapho-lunate interosseous ligament is required for scapho-lunate dissociation to occur.
  - Clinical presentation: often there is a history of injury (e.g. falling) with continued wrist pain for few days/weeks. On examination there will be dorsal tenderness. No tenderness over the snuff box or the ulnar side for the wrist.
  - Scaphoid shift test:
    - Used to diagnose scapholunate instability.
    - Dorsally-directed pressure on the scaphoid distal pole as the wrist is moved from ulnar deviation to radial deviation.
    - If there is instability: subluxation the scaphoid dorsally over the dorsal ridge of the distal radius will occur. A painful "clunk" will occur when pressure is released and the scaphoid reduces.

- XR may show increased distance between the scaphoid and the lunate and ring sign of the scaphoid (the distal pole of the scaphoid viewed end-on due to flexed position) (Fig 6).
    - If routine XR wrist is (normal) and the surgeon has high suspicious for the diagnosis, diagnosis can be confirmed by PA wrist with clenched fist (will give more accurate identification of SL ligament disruption because the proximally migrated capitate forces the two proximal row bones apart).
    - *(Scenario: 18 years old, fall down, XR normal , dorsal tenderness, next step?)*.
    - Can be associated with distal radius fracture (see distal radius session (Fig 6)).

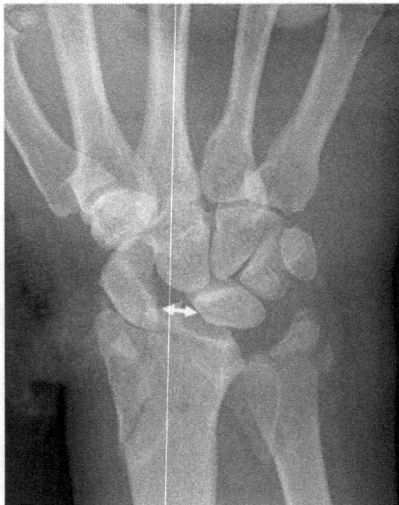

Fig 6: distal radius fracture associated with scapholunate dissociation. Notice the increased distance between the lunate and the scaphoid (double sided arrow).

- **SLAC**:
    - The end stage of chronic scapholunate instability.
    - Follows a pattern similar to SNAC (see before).
    - Stage I: disease arthritis between scaphoid waist and the radial styloid.
    - Stage II: the arthritis progresses to the proximal pole of the scaphoid and the scaphoid fossa of the radius.
    - Stage III: arthritis of the capitolunate joint (degenerative changes spare the radiolunate facet).
- Treatment:
    - For acute cases: open repair of the scapho-lunate joint (through dorsal incision) and percutaneous pinning.
    - Dorsal capsulodesis can be performed for chronic missed cases.
    (Scenario: 60 years, MVC, wrist pain for 4 weeks, XR shows SL widening, what structure is affected?) (Scenario: 45 years old, fall from height, distal radius fracture,

repaired surgery, intra-operative C-arm picture showing increased SL distance, next step?)
- In chronic cases with SLAC:
  - Stage I and II proximal row carpectomy or scaphoid excision with 4 corner fusion.
  - Stage III: scaphoid excision with 4 corner fusion, or wrist fusion.
  - The radioscaphocapitate ligament is the prime stabilizer of the radio-carpal joint (preventing ulnar translocation of the carpus by its oblique orientation). This ligament should be protected during scaphoid excision and proximal row carpectomy.
- **Mid-carpal instability:**
  - Test of instability: wrist in neutral with pronated forearm then palmar directed force is applied at the level of the distal capitate. The wrist is axially loaded and ulnarly deviated. If this reproduces the patient's symptoms, the test is considered positive.
  - Midcarpal injuries are usually considered nondissociative.
    - Radiographs are usually normal (apart from mild VISI)
  - Treatment is usually conservative.

Infections of the Hand:
- Felon (pulp space infection):
  - Most common organism is staph aureus.
  - Drain by incision at the lateral border (avoid fish mouth incision)
- Paronychia:
  - Candida albicans is the most common organism in chronic cases.
  - Treatment by eponychial marsupialization (with removal of a crescent shaped full-thickness dermal layer at the germinal matrix).
- Flexor tenosynovitis:
  - Kanavel signs (diffuse fusiform swelling, tenderness along the flexor sheath, pain with extension, flexed position)
  - The flexor sheaths are in continuity with the deep spaces of the hand.
    - Flexor sheath of the little finger communicates with the ulnar bursa.
    - Flexor sheath of the thumb communicates with the thenar space of the palm and the radial bursa.
    - Both the ulnar and radial bursae communicate with each other in most cases.
    - The central digits do not communicate with deep spaces of the hand.
- Human bite (e.g. fist bunch in the face):

- o Most common organism is Staph aureus, most characteristic is Eikenella corrodens.
  - o Treatment: irrigation and debridement with exploration of the MCP joint (see tendon laceration session before).
- Cat and dog bites:
  - o Most common organism is Pasterella.
    - ▪ Pasteurella canis is the most common pathogen of dog bites (50%).
    - ▪ Pasteurella multocida is the most common pathogen of cat bites (75%).
- Myocobacterium marinum:
  - o History of water relate injury (e.g. fish hook) with diffuse dactylitis.
  - o Will require Ziehl–Neelsen stain or LJ medium (see microbiology).
  - o Treatment: surgical debridement with 12-18 month of 2 or 3 anti mycobacterium antibiotic (clarithromycin, sulfonamides, rifampin, ethambutol, and trimethopriam sulfamethoxazole).
- Vibrio infection
  - o Brackish water can cause infection by Vibrio vulnificus infections.
  - o Patients may have a severe invasive infection, with mortality rates of up to 50% in cases of Vibrio septicemia.
  - o Treatment by third-generation cephalosporin.
- High speed spray gun injury (even if they look very benign) is treated by immediate surgical intervention for irrigation and debridment.
- Diabetic hand infection
  - o Risk factors for amputation in patients with diabetes mellitus: end stage renal disease and infections with gram-negative organisms or polymicrobial infection.
- Herptic Whitlow:
  - o Viral infection, common in dental health workers. NO surgery is needed.

Tendinitis:
Extensor Carpi Ulnaris Tendinitis/subluxation:
- Common in tennis player and other racquet games.
- Tenderness at the dorsoulnar aspect of the wrist
- The pain is recreated with ulnar deviation and wrist flexion/extension.
- Treatment is usually non-surgically with immobilization in rest brace. Subluxation of the tendon may require long arm cast in pronation and radial deviation.

Intersection Syndrome (Squeakers Wrist) (Crossover Tendinitis):

- It occurs where the first compartment (abductor pollicis longus and extensor pollicis brevis) pass over the second compartment (ECRB and ECRL), resulting in fibrosis, and inflammation of the bursa in this area which is approximately 4 to 5 cm proximal to the proximal dorsal wrist crease (more proximal to the pain of de Quervain).
- Clinical presentation: Pain, tenderness (5 cm from the tip of the radial styloid) and possible audible sound at the intersection point.

De Quervain:

- Tenovaginits of 1st compartment tendons (APL and EPB).
    - Certain positions (eg carrying the infant (new mothers)) are risk factors for this disease. *(Scenario: mother of 4 months old boy with wrist pain, diagnosis?)*
- Treatment:
    - Non-operative: NSAIDs, steroid injection, splint.
    - If non-operative fails: surgical release all compartments involving the EPB or APL has to be done (in more than 50% of cases there is separate compartments for EBP and APL). *(Scenario: release of De Quervain 3 months ago, patient still complaining of similar symptoms, explanation? (failure to release all compartments)).* EPB release can be confirmed by traction on the tendon which will result in MCP joint extension and a visible muscle belly.

Trigger Fingers:

- Thickening of A1 pulley over the flexor tendons resulting in constriction and triggering of the digits at the level of the pulley.
- Treatment:
    - Steroid injection (about 80% of non-diabetic patient can expect to obtain relief of symptoms with one or two injections). If this fail: surgical release of A1 pulley
    - In diabetics, the success of injection is limited, surgery is preferred.
    - Trigger thumb: there is risk of injury to the radial digital nerve.
    - Avoid releasing the A2 pulley (the oblique) during A1 release, as it will result in bowstring of FDP (if this happen, the treatment is reconstruction of the oblique pulley).
    - The radial digital nerve of the thumb is at risk during trigger thumb release.

Dupuytren's contracture:

- Pathology:
    - The main predominant cells in this pathology are myofibroblast, with increase in type III collagen.

- Risk factors include alcoholism, diabetes mellitus, HIV, and anti-epilepsy medications.
- Normal fascial bands changes into pathologic cords resulting in contractures:
  - Central cord: contracture of the MCP.
  - Spiral cord: contracture of the PIP (resistant contracture).
  - MCP joint contractures are easier to correct (and more likely to stay corrected) than the PIP joint (PIP are more resistant).
- Spiral cord: involves pre-tendinous band, spiral band, lateral digital sheet and Grayson ligament.
  - Cleland ligament is NOT part of it (Cleland's ligament is generally not involved in the Dupuytren's contracture)
- Spiral cords displace nerves superficially (palmarly) (there may be no overlying fascial cover) toward the center of the digit (eg radial digital nerve will be pushed ulnarly).
  - This displacement is typically seen at the level of the MCP joint.
  - The presence of dense adhesion at the level of the MCP joint (palmodigital crease) between the dermis and the pretendinous cord/central cord indicates absence of spiral cords. This indicates that the neurovascular bundle is not displaced superficially and centrally in the digit (not at a higher chance of injury during surgery)

- Indication for surgery: PIP contracture (of any degree) or MCP contracture >30°.
- Treatment:
  - Medical treatment: Collagenase enzyme (from Clostridium) which is a metalloprotease enzyme that lyses collagen (the effect on collagen types is least against type IV collagen which is main collagen component in the basement membranes of nerves and blood vessels). Complications include tendon rupture, reflex sympathetic dystrophy and pulley ruptures.
  - Surgical treatment included fasciectomy, aponeurotomy or dermatofasciectomy.
    - Dermatofasciectomy with full-thickness skin grafting offers NO advantage over conventional fasciectomy.
    - Aponeurotomy is less effective than fasciectomy in contracture release with higher recurrence rate.

Flaps, Grafts, Finger Tip Injuries and Replantation:

- **Replantation:**
  - Indication of replantation:
    - Multiple digit amputation.
    - Thumb amputation.

- Single digit amputation in a child (replantation is always attempted in children).
- Wrist and forearm amputation.
- Relative indication: single digit distal to FDS insertion (zone I).
- Contraindication to a single digit replantation is an amputation at the level of the proximal phalanx or PIP joint (proximal to the level of insertion FDS) (Zone II).
  - o Timing limits of replantation:
    - At the level of the wrist: 6 hours of warm ischemia or 12 hours for cold ischemia.
    - At the level of the digit: 12 hours of warm ischemia or 24 hours for cold ischemia.
  - o Failure of replantation.
    - Early: arterial occlusion (may need possible revision).
    - After 12 hours: venous occlusion, can be treated by leeches (secret hirudin), (leeches can cause of infection by aeromonus hydrophilia).
  - o Order of repair: debridement, fracture fixation, extensor tendon repair, one artery anastomosis (to restore blood flow to the segment), venous anastomosis, flexor tendon repair, second artery anastomosis, nerves repair, possible fasciotomy and skin closure.
  - o Sharp nature of the trauma and laceration is an important factor in the decision to replant. Crush injuries have worse outcome.
- **Fingertip amputations:**
  - o Finger tip amputation with non-exposed bone (soft tissues covering the bone): allow healing by secondary intention.
  - o Most crush or avulsion fingertip amputations in children (particularly those younger than age 2 years), can be treated with serial dressing changes, even with bone exposed (children have a greater capacity to heal soft-tissue injuries than adults). Also, the amputated tip in children can be sutured back to the finger.
  - o Wounds with more tissue loss dorsally (oblique dorsally) or transverse wounds: A V-Y flap. Volar V-Y for dorsal loss, can give good sensation (important for certain jobs).
  - o Wounds with more tissue loss volarly (oblique volar): cross finger flap.
  - o Amputation of the tip of thumb with exposure of tuft of the distal phalanx: coverage could be achieved by volar advancement (Moberg) flap closure (by bilateral, longitudinal, midlateral incisions, with a advancement on the two neurovascular pedicles). This option (Moberg) option is only for thumb.

- o Transverse amputation of the index: can use thenar flap or V-Y advancement flap.
- o Dorsal metacarpal artery flap (DMCA) (neurovascular island flap) is most popular flap for coverage of dorsal finger defects.
- o Skin defect on the dorsum of the hand with exposed tendons can be covered by radial forearm rotational flap (local flap).
- o Thenar flap can be used for volar defect for index or middle finger mainly for children or young adults (less than 35 years old) as it can lead to stiffness of the digit.
- Ring avulsions: carry bad prognosis (compared to lacerations).
- STSG cannot be used alone if there are exposed tendons, bones or joints.
- **Flaps:**
  - o Blood supply:
    - ▪ Posterior branch of the radial collateral artery is the pedicle supply to the lateral arm flap.
    - ▪ Radial artery (passes between flexor carpi radialis and brachioradialis) and perforators from the radial artery to the overlying skin are the pedicle for radial forearm free flap
    - ▪ Medial femoral circumflex artery is the arterial supply for gracilis flap.
    - ▪ Thoracodorsal artery (branch from subscapular artery) is the arterial supply latissimus dorsi flap.
    - ▪ Inferior epigastric artery (branch from the external iliac artery) is the arterial supply for rectus abdominis flap.
    - ▪ The superficial circumflex iliac artery is the arterial supply for groin flap.
- Z- plasty: all limbs of the incision must
- be same length.
  - o 60° angles between limbs with give 75% increase in the length of scar.

Nerve Palsies and Compression Neuropathy:

- See also Neurology section in basic science chapter and Nerve supply in Anatomy chapter.
- Preganglionic lesions (e.g. root avulsion) cannot be surgically repaired. Postganglionic injuries (peripheral nerve ruptures or stretch injuries) can be repaired surgically.
- The radial, musculocutaneous, and femoral nerves have the best recovery potential followed by median, ulnar, and tibial nerves which have moderate potential. The peroneal nerve has the worst prognosis for motor recovery

- If after nerve repair, the motor recovery is not functional: proceed with tendon transfer. *(Scenario: low median nerve laceration, what surgery can be done few months after repair to enhance function? (opponensplasty using exentsor indices as full motor recovery is usually not expected)).*
- **Radial nerve injury:**
  - Wrist drop.
  - Most commonly performed tendon transfer for radial nerve palsy is Brand transfer:
    - Pronator teres to ECRB (wrist extension).
    - Palmaris longus to EPL (thumb extension).
    - FCR or FCU to the EDC (finger extension) (FCR is preferred for maintaining throwing activity to allow patient to keep FCU for wrist flexion/ ulnar deviation movement)
- **Posterior interosseus nerve (PIN) injury:**
  - The injury is usually at level of the proximal forearm.
  - Inability to extend the fingers at the level of the MCP or thumb IP.
  - Weak wrist extension with radial deviation (ECRL is innervated by radial nerve proximal to PIN).
  - Tenodesis effect of the extensor tendon will remain intact (passive finger extension with flexion of the wrist, see rheumatoid hand).
  - Post-operative nerve injury: if the surgeon is sure that nerve was not lacerated, not entrapped in the fracture or underneath the hardware: treatment is observation for recovery. EMG studies can be done after 6 weeks from the insult.
  - Treatment (if not spontaneous improvement): FCR to EDC (finger extension) and PL to EPL (thumb extensor).
- **Cubital Tunnel: see shoulder/elbow chapter**
- **PIN palsy:**
  - Treated with observation, if no improvement, release of the nerve at the radial tunnel.
- **Carpal tunnel syndrome:**
  - Diagnosis:
    - Clinical (pain and numbness of the radial 3 fingers) and by nerve conduction test (distal motor latency > 4.5 msec).
  - Treatment:
    - Non-surgical: Night time wrist brace (to prevent wrist flexion).
      - The carpal tunnel/carpal canal pressure varies with wrist position. The pressure is lowest with the wrist in neutral position. For this reason, nocturnal wrist splints should hold the wrist in neutral position.

- Carpal tunnel release (open or endoscopically).
  - Main advantage of the endoscopic technique: decreased postoperative pain (6-12 weeks).
  - Nerve, vascular injury and infection rates complications are not statistically significant.
- Adding flexor tenosynovectomy with an open carpal tunnel release (versus open carpal tunnel release alone) for idiopathic carpal tunnel syndrome does not lead to long-term clinical benefit.
- Symptoms severity (not duration) has negative correlation with the degree of post-operative symptom relief after surgery.

- **Acute carpal tunnel syndrome:**
  - Can occur after trauma or surgery of the wrist.
  - Patient will complain numbness in the palmar aspect of the thumb, index, and middle fingers with severe wrist pain.
  - Treatment by urgent open carpal tunnel release. _(Scenario: surgery for distal radius, few hours later patient complains of numbness in the radial 3 finger, treatment?)_

- **Radial tunnel syndrome:**
  - Posterior interosseus nerve compression with pain in the forearm (no motor weakness).
  - Possible compression sites: the proximal fibrous edge of the supinator (arcade of Frohse) (the most common site of compression), the distal edge of the supinator; fibrous bands superficial to the radiocapitellar joint; tendinous medial margin of the extensor carpi radialis brevis (ECRB); radial recurrent artery (leash of Henry).

- **PIN syndrome:**
  - Presents with motor deficits only, in contrast to radial tunnel syndrome which presents with pain only.

- **Cubital tunnel syndrome: see shoulder/ elbow chapter.**

- **Ulnar tunnel syndrome (Guyon's canal syndrome) (see anatomy chapter):**
  - Guyons canal (Fig 7):
    - Zone I: sensory and motor deficits (including hypothenar muscles)
    - Zone II: motor deficit (compression of the deep motor branch of the ulnar nerve)
    - Zone III: sensory (the deep motor branch is preserved as it moves away deep in the palm)
  - Ulnar artery thrombosis: zone III affection (sensory only).
  - Non union of hook of hamate: can lead to zone I or zone II compression.
  - Ganglions are the most common cause of ulnar nerve entrapment in the wrist.

- Numbness of the dorsal hand indicates that the lesion is more proximal in the elbow (proximal to the ulnar canal).
- **Anterior interosseus nerve palsy (AIN syndrome):**
  - Inability to flex the IP of the thumb and DIP of index finger (failure to do OK sign).
  - EMG can help to diagnosis AIN syndrome.
  - Spontaneous atraumatic AIN palsy spontaneously recover in most cases.
  - Initial treatment by observation.
- **Median nerve Palsy:**
  - Tendon transfers for low median nerve injury require the restoration of thumb opposition.
    - The four types of opponensplasties are: the palmaris longus (Camitz), extensor indicis proprius, abductor digiti minimi (Huber, the most common in children), and the ring finger flexor digitorum superficialis.
- **Volkmann's Contracture:**
  - Due to missed compartment syndrome in the forearm. The necrotic muscles will replaced with fibrotic tissue, resulting in contractures with possible irreversible nerve palsy.
  - Inability to extend the finger IPs with the wrist extended
  - Flexor pollicis longus and the flexor digitorum profundus are the most commonly affected muschle.

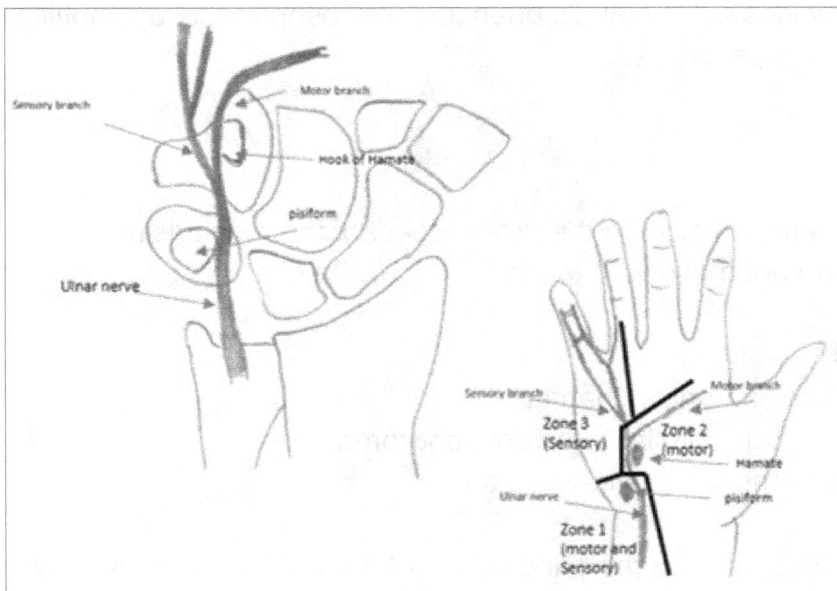

Fig 7: Ulnar nerve compression in Guyon's canal. Zone one is both motor and sensory affection, zone two is motor and zone three is sensory.

Congenital Hand deformity (See pediatric chapter).

Vascular conditions:

- Anatomical considerations (see anatomy chapter):
    - Radial artery: provides the main contribution for the deep arch.
    - Ulnar artery: provides the main contribution for the superficial arch.
    - Ulnar artery is the main contributing vessel to the hand (in about 80% of the patients):
        - Allen's test should be used to assess which artery is the dominant artery for the hand in the patient before any surgery on the arteries.
- **Hypothenar Hammer syndrome:**
    - Vaso-occlusive disorder due to repetitive blunt micro trauma affecting ulnar artery at the proximal palm.
    - Treatment: vein graft.
- **Buerger's diseasae:**
    - Small vessel disease in heavy smoker males.
    - Treatment: medical (cessation of smoking, Calcium channel blockers). If this fails: surgery (sympathectomy).
- **Raynaud's syndrome (phenomenon):**
    - Color changes that occur with cold exposure (or less commonly with stress).
    - The affected part turns white and then blue. As blood flow returns there is numbness and pain and the area turns red.
    - Raynaud's disease: idiopathic Raynaud syndrome.
    - CREST: chondrocalcinosis, Raynaud's phenomenon, esophageal dysmotility, sclerodactyly and telangiectasias.

Hand tumors:

- Retinacular cyst:
    - Firm round cysts 2-4 mm in size on the volar aspect of the digit arising from the pulley system (do not move with tendon motion). Painful with gripping activities
    - Treatment by needle aspiration.
- Sunungal exostosis (see foot and ankle chapter):
    - Occur under the nail, looks similar to osteochondroma.
    - Treatment: removal of the nail plate, excision
- Enchondromas:
    - Pathology: all chondral lesion in the hand behave benign (the histology may show atypia).
    - Most common bone tumor of the hand.

- o May cause expansion and pathological fracture.
- o Treatment: curettage and bone graft.
- Glomus tumor:
  - o Very painful tumor at the tip of the finger, with cold intolerance.
  - o Usually occurz in a subungual location.
- Epithelioid sarcoma:
  - o Most common soft tissue sarcoma in the hand and wrist region.
- Squamus cell carcinoma:
  - o Most common cancer (malignancy) in the hand.

General:
- Inability to fully flex the digits:
  - o Can be due to extrinsic or intrinsic tightness.
  - o Intrinsic tightness:
    - Due to tight intrinsic muscles (interossei and lumbrical muscles).
    - With the MCP joints flexed: the IP joints can flex fully. When the MP joints are extended: IP joints cannot be fully flexed (**with extension of the MP joint, there will be less IP joints flexion**).
  - o Extrinsic tightness:
    - Due to scarring of long extensor tendons (EDC) (eg ORIF of proximal phalanx and post compartment syndrome).
    - With MP flexion, there will be less IP flexion. With MP extension, IP can flex more (**with extension of MP joint, there will be more flexion of the IPs**).
- Hand-grip strength tests assess both the extrinsic and intrinsic muscles. The intrinsic muscles contribute about 50% of hand-grip strength.
  - o Laceration of the ulnar nerve that innervates the intrinsic muscles decrease hand grip by about 50%.
- Wrist arthroscopy:
  - o A useful technique for evaluation and treatment of radiocarpal and midcarpal pathologies.
  - o Extra-articular structures as extensor carpi ulnaris tendon cannot be seen during standard radiocarpal arthroscopy.
- The outcome of treatment (as assessed by DASH scores) of most hand/ wrist conditions (e.g. CTS, trigger finger, de Quervain, non surgical distal radius fracture) has direct correlation with depression.
- **Tendon transfer (upper and lower extremity):**

- The intended joint to be move should be passively corrected to its neutral position (absence of contracture). Transferred muscle cannot move a contracted stiff joint.

Tips:

- Palmar PIP dislocation will lead to injury to central slip while dorsal dislocations can result in distal rupture of the volar plate.
- The lunate remains in the lunate fossa in a perilunate fracture-dislocation but is dislocated in a lunate dislocation.
- Lytic lesion in the hand:
  - Think in gout (well demarcated) (medical treatment), enchondroma, giant cell tumor (both are treated by curettage and bone grafting)
- Toddler or dental hygienist with papules in the finger: think in herpetic whitlow
- Rock climber: think in pulley rupture.

Chapter 12:   The Spine

Pathological Anatomy (See Also Cervical/Thoracic/Lumbar Anatomy in The Anatomy Chapter):

- Root compression with prolapsed disc:
    - Cervical disc prolapse will compress the **exiting** root which carries the same number as the lower vertebra of the disc (eg C5,**6** disc compress C**6** root)
    - Posterolateral lumbar discs prolapse (the most common variant) will compress the **traversing** root which carries the same number as the lower vertebra of the disc (eg L4,**5** disc compress L**5** root).
        - Both cervical disc and posterolateral lumbar disc will compress the nerve root which carries the same number as the lower vertebra of the disc (but each for different reason).
        - Most common disc prolapse: C5,6 disc compress C6 root; L4,5 disc compress L5 root.
    - C5,6 disc will affect C6 nerve root (C6: wrist extension, elbow flexion, brachioradilis reflex, sensation to index and thumb).
    - C6,7 disc will affect C7 nerve root (numbness of the middle finger, elbow extension, wrist flexion, and finger extensors, triceps reflex)
    - L4-5 postero-lateral disc, will compress L5 root, sensation to the dorsum of the foot, motor to EHL and gluteus medius, and no reflexes (normal knee and ankle reflexes).
    - Far lateral lumbar disc and foraminal lumbar disc herniation will compress the exiting root (the nerve root that has the same number as the upper vertebra of the disc; eg. L4-5 left foraminal disc herniation will compress L4 root)
        - L4-5 far lateral disc or foraminal herniation: will compress the exiting root (L4). L4 root: Motor: tibialis anterior, quadriceps (difficulty climbing stairs); knee reflex; sensation: anterior thigh, anterior and medial lower leg, medial aspect of the foot (but not the toes)).
- Root compression with spondylolithesis:
    - Isthmic spondylolisthesis L5-S1 (most common level): compression of L5.
    - Degenerative spondylolisthesis L4-L5 (most common level): compression of L5
    - The most common sites of both degenerative (L4-5) and isthmic (L5-S1) spondylolisthesis will both compress L5 root.
- Foraminal stenosis (due to various etiologies) will compress the exiting root. _(scenario: L3-4 spondylolithesis with foraminal stenosis, what muscle affected? (hip flexor), sensory? (anterior thigh))_
    - The superior facet of the caudal vertebra is the major causative factor in lumbar foraminal stenosis.

- The root in the lumbar spine exits the foramen by passing medial then inferior to the pedicle of the vertebra (e.g. L4 root will exit the L4-5 inter-verterbral foramina underneath L4 vertebra pedicle). *(Scenario: screw violated the inferior cortex of the left L4 pedicle, what are neurological consequence?) (Question: what structure will be injured with medial screw break out?) (Question: neurological injury of L4 root, what screw is responsible? (L4 pedicle screw penetrating medial and/or inferior)).*
- Unilateral sacralization: L5 is fused with the sacrum on one side. It can cause low back pain due to transfer of the stresses from S1-L5 disc to L4-5 disc.
- Cervical stenosis (assessment of the cervical canal diameter in lateral XR):
  - Absolute cervical stenosis: AP diameter of less than 10 mm.
  - Relative cervical stenosis: AP diameter 10-13 mm.
- In case of injury to the vertebral artery during screw insertion, screw placement (or packing by bone wax) is usually sufficient to control bleeding.
- Pedicles of the thoracic spine has highest ratio of cortical to cancellous bone followed by lumbar spine pedicles followed by vertebral bodies.
- The internal carotid artery lies anteriorly within 1 mm of the exit point of a bicortical C1 lateral mass screw or C1-2 transarticular screw.
  - The most common structure at risk with anterior penetration of C1 lateral mass screws is the internal carotid artery.
- At the level of L1-L2, the liver and the vena cava lie to the right. The aorta lies in the midline just in front of the vertebral body. *(Scenario: pedicle finder plunges at L1, what structure can injury).*
- The lumbar pedicle screw starting point is the intersection a horizontal line through the midpoint of the transverse process and a vertical line across lateral edge of the pars interarticularis.

Imaging:

- Plain radiographs are useful for assessing the alignment of the spine, bone destruction by tumors and infections, degenerative intervertebral discs and instability patterns (flexion-extension views).
  - Pavlov (Torg) ratio is the ratio of the width of cervical canal to the width of the cervical body on the lateral view (a ratio less than 0.8 is an indication of cervical stenosis)
- 90-93% percent of asymptomatic individuals older than 60 years have MRI evidence of disc degeneration.
- 60% of normal individual older than 40 years (and 25% in individual younger than 40 years) will have abnormal MRI changes in cervical spine (degenerative disc).
- Discography has a high false-positive rate in patients with abnormal psychometric testing results and can increase disc degeneration.

- SPECT is the best modality to detect isthmic spondylolysis.
- Imaging for non-union of surgical fusion:
  - CT scan is the best modality to assess nonunion in instrumented cases (less affected by metal components than the MRI).
  - XR is not sensitive in detecting nonunion in instrumented cases.
- Retropharyngeal space should be less than 7-6 mm, and the retrotracheal space should be less than 14 mm (see spine chapter).

Spine Exam:

- Progressive weakness:
  - Progressive weakness is usually an indication for surgery. Weakness by itself (so long not progressive) is not indication for surgery.
- Tenderness over the spinous process is indicative for acute/subacute vertebral fracture.
- Lhermitte sign:
  - Elicited by bending the head forward.
  - A positive test: an electrical sensation that runs down the back and into the limbs.
  - Associated with cervical spinal cord pathology (involvement of the dorsal columns of the cervical cord).
- Spurling's sign:
  - The examiner turns the patient's head to the affected side while applying axial compression and extension.
  - Positive test: neck pain radiating to corresponding dermatome (radicular pain), highly specific for ipsilateral cervical nerve-root compression.
- Lasegue sign:
  - Raising the leg straight with dorsiflexion of the ankle.
  - Positive test: pain radiating distal to the knee.
  - Associated with lumbar radiculopathy (disc herniation).
- Hoffmann sign:
  - Tapping the nail or flicking the terminal phalanx of the middle or ring finger.
  - Positive response: flexion of the terminal phalanx of the thumb (pathologic reflex).
  - Associated with cervical myelopathy.
- The inverted brachioradialis reflex:
  - By tapping brachioradialis tendon.
  - Positive response: reflex contraction of the finger flexors with diminished brachioradialis reflex (no elbow flexion) (pathological reflex).

- o Associated with cervical myelopathy.
- Straight leg raising:
  - o Highly sensitive for ipsilateral nerve-root compression.
  - o A positive crossed straight leg raise test result (straight leg raising causing pain in the contralateral side) is highly specific for a contralaterally herniated nucleus pulposus (the side of the pain).

Biomechanics:

- Sagittal balance: the axis from C7 should fall just anterior to the S1.
- The pressure in the disc increase from supine to standing to sitting, to sitting leaning forward, to sitting leaning forward holding weight in the hands.
- The Instant Axis of Rotation (IAR):
  - o With flexion and extension, IAR is normally within the anterior half of the vertebral body, close to the anterior aspect of the intervertebral disc.
  - o With posterior pedicle screw instrumentation, the IAR moves toward the instrumentation with flexion and extension.

Spinal Cord Injury:

- Prognosis after cervical spinal cord complete injuries:
  - o C4 injury: puffer control.
  - o C5 injury: hand controls/ mobility in an electric wheelchair.
  - o C6 injury: manual wheelchair and sliding board transfers.
  - o C7 injury: manual wheelchair and independent transfers.
  - o C8 injury: Independence with bowel and bladder care; bathing and dressing can be performed without assistive devices.
  - o Complete cervical cord injury cannot ambulate with crutches and leg braces (needs wheel chair).
- Complete spinal cord injury:
  - o No sensory or motor function below certain level with presence of bulbocavernosus reflex.
    - ▪ Presence of bulbocavernosus reflex indicates that the patient is **not** in spinal shock stage.
- Early cervical spine decompression in recommended for cervical spine injury associated with cord injuries.
- If you suspect that a patient with traumatic spinal cord injury started to develop symptoms of depression and suicidal ideation, screen the patient for major depression and consult for psychological care
- The MRI finding that is most consistently with a complete spinal injury is a hematoma within the cord.

- Spinal shock stage:
  - Occurs in some cases with the onset of spinal cord injury during which all the reflexes are lost and the patient will have flaccid paralysis. It usually lasts for 24-72 hours. **The bulbocavernosus reflex (S3) will be absent.**
  - The level or the extent of injury cannot be adequately determined during the shock stage.
  - In addition, the patient may have neurogenic shock manifestation (Bradycardia, hypotension) (see below). *(Scenario: 50 years old, T2 fracture dislocation, no sensation or motor function below nipple, bulbocavernosus reflex present, diagnosis? (complete spinal cord injury.)) (Scenario: 40 years old female, MVC, C7-T1 flexion distraction injury, no motor or sensory function distal to the manubrium, absent bulbocavernosus reflex, prognosis? (Cannot be determined), How to assess neurological recovery in the last scenario?? (Repeated exam)).*
- Neurogenic shock:
  - Characterized by systemic hypotension with bradycardia following spinal cord injury due to loss of sympathetic tone and widespread vasodilatation (injury to descending sympathetic system).
  - Neurogenic shock should be treated with judicious use of fluids and **vasopressors.** *(Scenario: 45 years old, C7-T1 fracture dislocation, open femur fracture, abdomen clear, pulse 50, blood pressure 80/43, diagnosis? Treatment?)*
- Autonomic dysreflexia:
  - Occurs with complete spinal cord injury.
  - Due to sympathetic overdrive associated with certain triggers (eg impacted bowl, obstructed urinary catheter, orthopedic injury).
  - Clinical presentation: sudden malignant hypertension, profuse sweating.
- Incomplete cord injuries:
  - Definition: spinal cord injury with any neurological function (eg sensation) distal to injury (eg sacral sparing).
  - Types include: Brown-Sequard syndrome, central cord syndrome, anterior cord syndrome, posterior cord syndrome.
  - Brown-Sequard syndrome:
    - Hemi section of the spinal cord (eg penetrating trauma).
    - Clinical presentation: Ipsilateral motor deficit, loss of ipsilateral deep sensation (eg vibration and sense of position) and light touch sensation, contra lateral loss of pain and temperature.
    - The motor tracks and deep sensation tracks cross at the level of the brainstem (medulla oblingata) while the pain and temperature cross at (or near) the corresponding spinal level (see anatomy chapter, section of spinal cord anatomy).
  - Central cord syndrome:

- More in elderly patient.
- Mechanism is usually hyperextension of the spine (e.g. falling and hitting the forehead against hard object).
- Upper extremity affection more than lower extremity, motor deficit more than sensory deficit, distal affection more than proximal.
- About 40% of patients with central cord syndrome will regain ambulation.
  - Anterior cord syndrome:
    - May be related to vascular injury.
    - Motor paralysis (loss of anterior corticospinal tract) (lower extremity affected more upper extremity), loss of pain and temperature sensation (loss of lateral and anterior spinothalamic tracts), and preservation of vibration and touch sensation (preservation of dorsal columns).
    - Prognosis is generally poor
  - Posterior cord syndrome:
    - Loss of deep sensation.
    - Classically had been described with 3rd stage syphilis.
- Steroid administration in SCI:
  - Methylprednisolone, 30 mg/kg followed by 5.4 mg/kg per hour for 24 hours if initiated within 3 hours of injury and for 48 hours if initiated between 3-8 hours of injury.
    - Spinal cord injury more than 8 hours, no pharmacological treatment should be given
  - Indicated for spinal cord injuries.
    - Not indicated for GSW, root injuries (lumbar injuries or quada equina lesion).
  - Has been falling out of favor due to lack of proven clinical efficacy and high complications rate.
    - MRI shows that it only decreases the extent of cord hemorrhage.
  - Proposed mechanism of action of steroids: prevent neurologic deterioration after traumatic spinal cord injury by limiting secondary insult by:
    - Reduction of TNF-alpha expression, reduction of free radical oxidation.
    - Stabilization of cell membranes, and reduction of the influx of calcium into the injured cells, thus reducing cord edema.
- In cases of SCI, the mean arterial blood pressure should be maintained at above 85 mmHg to prevent secondary SCI.
- **AISA classification of spinal cord injury:**
  - A: complete.
  - B: some sensory preservation.

- o C: motor function incomplete (more than 50% of muscle groups has 1/5 or 2/5 motor function).
- o D: motor incomplete (more than 50% of muscle groups has 3/5 or more).
  - 3/5 is muscle contraction against gravity, 4/5 muscle contraction against gravity and mild resistance.
- o E: normal (only a follow up classification, cannot be used in the beginning as it signifies no injury)
  - *Multiple Scenarios can be made, examples: C7 burst fracture. Motor examination reveals normal strength in bilateral UE, and diminished strength (movement with gravity in ankle dorsiflexors) in the bilateral LE. Rectal tone is absent. The patient's neurologic condition according to AISA?)*
- The level of neurologic injury is the most caudal (distal) level at which motor and sensory levels are intact bilaterally:
  - o Intact motor level is when the key muscle strength is 3 or above while the segment above is normal
  - o Intact sensory level is intact sensation for both pinprick and light touch. *(Scenario: spinal cord injury due to bilateral facet dislocation, one-week exam shows presence of bulbocavernosus reflex, he has intact deltoid function bilateral, intact C6 (elbow flexor, wrist extensor) on the right, and no C6 function on the left, no C7 function (elbow extensor, wrist flexor) bilateral, no motor, sensory on lower extremities, no bowel or bladder control, no sacral sensation, what is the type and level of injury? (Complete, C5)*

Cervical Myelopathy:

- Compression on the spinal cord (NOT roots) at the cervical level.
- Most common causes are cervical stenosis, cervical spondylosis, cervical disc herniation, and OPLL.
- Clinical presentation:
  - o Myelopathy hand:
    - Weakness of hand intrinsic, intrinsic wasting, the small finger abducted by the EDM).
    - Diffuse numbness in both hands, with decreased grip strength and hand clumsiness (e.g. inability to button clothes).
  - o Positive Hoffmann's sign (80% of cases) (see before).
  - o Possible weakness of the lower extremity (upper motor lesion).
    - Wide- based gait (abnormal tandem gait test).
    - Sustained clonus and Babinski signs (one third of the cases).
    - Hyperreflexia and spasticity (not common).
  - o Possible radicular symptoms in the upper extremities.
- Imaging:
  - o MRI: will show compression on the cord by various etiologies associated with changes within the cord. *(Scenario: 45 years old, cervical spine pain, weakness,*

hyperreflexia, next step? (Cervical MRI to assess myelopathy)). (Scenario: 70 years with LE weakness with abnormal gait, MRI of the lumbar spine in within normal for age, next step? (MRI cervical and thoracic spine)).

- Treatment:
    - Nonsurgical management:
        - Only for mild cases with no functional impairment.
        - More successful in elderly patients with higher Pavlov's ratio.
    - Surgical treatment: most cases will need surgical treatment by **decompression**:
        - **Progressive** myelopathy has to be surgically decompressed.
        - Decompression can be posterior (laminectomy or laminoplasty) or anterior.
        - If there is loss of lordosis: the decompression should be anterior (posterior decompression will not be effective in kyphotic patient with cervical myelopathy). *(Scenario: patient has cervical myelopathy with hyperreflexia, what is contra indication for laminoplasty?)*
        - Multilevel involvement (three or more disc spaces) is easier to be managed by posterior approach (if there is no fixed kyphosis)
- Cervical spondylotic disease:
    - Can cause myelopathy (cervical spondylotic myelopathy).
    - If associated with cervical kyphosis: treated by anterior decompression (corpectomy) and fusion.
        - Fixed cervical kyphosiss is a contraindication to laminoplasty or laminectomy in a patient with cervical spondylotic myelopathy.
- Ossification of Posterior Longitudinal Ligament (OPLL):
    - One of the etiologies for cervical myelopathy.
    - Common in Asians.
    - C4-6 is most frequently involved levela.
    - Can be obviously seen in CT scans of cervical spine.
- Laminoplasty:
    - Decompression of the cervical spine by widening of the spinal canal.
    - Laminoplasty can be complicated by root palsy. Most commonly affected root is C5.
- Posterior cervical decompression:
    - Removal of more than 50% of a facet joint can lead to segmental instability and compromises the overall strength of the joint. This will increase the risk of post laminectomy kyphosis:
        - Post laminectomy kyphosis: commonly follows laminectomy without fusion for the treatment of cervical spondylotic myelopathy.
        - It can result in recurrent myelopathy and neck pain and deformity.

- Differential diagnosis for cervical myelopathy:
  - Amyotrophic lateral sclerosis (ALS): Motor neuron disease affecting upper and lower motor neurons which will lead to progressive weakness, muscle atrophy, fasciculation, spasticity, dysarthria, dysphagia, and respiratory compromise.

Rheumatoid arthritis:
- Preoperative evaluations for patients with rheumatoid arthritis should include cervical spine radiographs to assess for possible instability.
- **Ranawat classification:**
  - Surgical intervention has better results for patients with less affection (less than Ranawat stage IIIB myelopathy) as neurologic improvement is minimal for patients with more advanced disease.
  - Patients with more advanced pathology (non-ambulatory patients with objective weakness) will have worse outcome (better to avoid surgery).
- The upper cervical vertebrae (C1-C2) are the most commonly involved spinal segments in rheumatoid arthritis.
  - Normal Anterior Atlanto Dens Interval (AADI) in adults is less than 3.5mm.
  - The change in AADI more than 3mm in lateral flexion extension views indicates spinal instability.
  - AADI more than 9mm requires surgery for stabilization even in asymptomatic patients.
  - C1-C2 affection can be associated with basilar invagination.
- Sub-axial subluxation:
  - Subuaxial subluxation can occur in conjunction with C1-C2 instability and it will make reconstruction more complicated (fixation has to extend to the affected distal level).
- Indication for surgery in patient with Rheumatoid arthritis:
  - Myelopathy in rheumatoid patients with C1-C2 instability.
  - AADI more than 10.
  - Posterior ADI less than 14mm (has more prognostic value than AADI).
    - Posterior ADI (space available for the cord) of greater than 14 mm is the most important preoperative predictor for full neurologic recovery of myelopathy with surgical stabilization.

Anterior Cervical Discectomy and Fusion (ACDF):
- See anatomy section for complication associated with the approach.
- Neurological complications:

- o The most common neurologic injury following ACDF is injury to the recurrent laryngeal nerve (the nerve can be compressed between the retractor and an inflated endotracheal tube balloon).
- o Approaches for lower level fusion have higher rate of recurrent laryngeal nerve injury, the upper level fusions have higher rate of dysphagia.
- o If during surgery there is ipsilateral loss of amplitude in the cortical somatosensory evoked potential with preservation of all other waves, this may be related to carotid compression with focal cortical ischemia:
  - This may be associated with poor collateral flow from the opposite hemisphere due to an incomplete circle of Willis.
- Airway complications:
  - o Risk factors for post-operative dyspnea: multilevel fusion (requiring long period intubation and prolonged soft-tissue retraction), preexisting co morbidities (eg chronic bronchitis), surgical times greater than 5 hours, blood loss greater than 300 mL, discs at or above C3-4.
    - For patients with these risk factors, patients can be left intubated for one or two days after surgery to avoid possible need for urgent re-intubation.
- Long-term dysphagia:
  - o Risk factors: more levels operated, revision surgeries, increased operative time, female gender and older age (however, use of instrumentation, the level of fusion, or type of procedure (corpectomy versus discectomy) are not risk factors).
  - o Incidence of this complication after one year is about 10% to 15%.
- Single level ACDF is not contra indication to return to play contact sports.
- Pseudarthrosis
  - o Risk factors: history of smoking, diabetes mellitus.
  - o Allograft versus autograft: no difference (especially for single level)
  - o The level and sagittal alignment are not risk factors.
  - o Treatment of pseudoarthrosis: posterior fusion (rather that revision anterior fusion). *(Scenario: 45 years old, ACDF for radicular symptoms, one year later has neck pain, CT shows pseudoarthrosis, treatment?)*

Cervical Radiculopathy:
- C5-6 is the most commonly affected disc (will compress on C6) (see before in the section of pathological anatomy).
- Cervical radiculopathy is generally treated non operatively (in contrast to cervical myelopathy).
- **Epidural steroids injection**

    o Relief of radicular symptoms for periods longer than 1 year can be expected in about two thirds (50% to 70%) of patient.

C1-C2 Fusion Techniques:

- Techniques for C1-2 fusion include: Gallie, Brooks, triple wiring, trans-articular screw fixation across the C1-2 articulation, C1 lateral mass-C2 pedicle screw construct.
- Transarticular screw provides the most rigid means of fixation and the highest arthrodesis rates but is technically demanding.
  - o If the surgeon is considering C1-C2 trans-articular screw, MR angiogram or angiography should be done to make sure that patient has no aberrant vertebral artery

Cervical Spine Trauma:

- With cervical trauma, additional CT imaging of the thoracic and lumbar spine is required to rule out concomitant injuries (which may be present in 10% to 15% of patients). (*Scenario: 30 fall from height, neck pain, lower extremity weakness, MRI shows C5 bust fracture, no compression over the cord, next step (CT thorax and lumbar spine)).*
- **Occipital cervical subluxation:**
  - o The definitive treatment is occipital cervical fusion
  - o Power ratio (see Fig 1): can be used to diagnose anterior occipito-cervical dislocation.

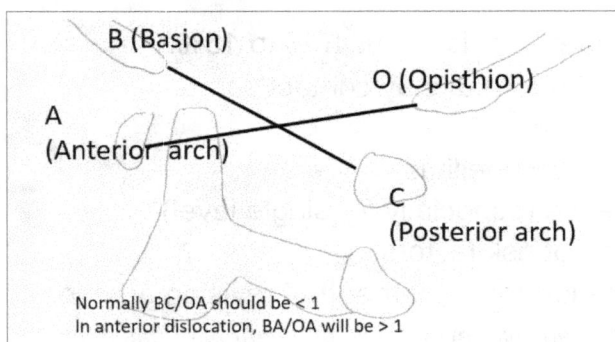

B (Basion)

O (Opisthion)

A (Anterior arch)

C (Posterior arch)

Normally BC/OA should be < 1
In anterior dislocation, BA/OA will be > 1

Fig 1: Power ration to detect anterior accipito-cervical dislocation.

- **Atlas fracture and transverse ligament injury:**
  - o **Fracture C1:**
    - ▪ If there is more than 6.9mm increase of the width of C1 compared to C2 (combined width on both sides as seen in open mouth view) this will indicate unstable injury and incompetent transverse ligament; treatment is the use of a halo vest for 3 months or C1-C2 fusion (due to complication of halo vest especially in elderly, there is tendency toward treating this injury with surgical fusion).
  - o **Transverse ligament injury:**

- Bone avulsion: trial of non-operativetreatment; if this fail: C1-C2 fusion.
- Mid-substance rupture:
  - Normal Anterior ADI is > 3.5 mm in an adult and 4 mm in a child (see before).
  - Increase ADI after trauma in the absence of a bony injury, represents rupture of the transverse atlas ligament.
  - Treatment is surgical by C1-C2 fusion. *(Scenario: MVC, upper cervical pain, XR: increased ADI, MRI: edema posterior to odontoid, treatment?)*

- **Odontoid fracture (See Fig 2):**
  - Type I: at the tip, treatment is collar immobilization for comfort.
  - Type II: through the base of odontoid.
    - Susceptible to nonunion (see risk factors).
    - Non displaced (or reduced with traction): treatment is halo vest or a hard collar immoblization.
    - Nonunion risk factor: displacement more than 5 mm (most important risk factor), angulation >10°, age more 65 years, smoking, diabetes
    - Treatment: young patient (less than 50 years) with no nonunion risk: non operative treatment. If there are risk factors for nonunion: operative treatment is recommended.
    - Operative options include: anterior screw fixation (if the fracture pattern allow), C1-C2 fusion (C1 lateral mass and C2 with pedicle screw or trans-articular screw).
  - Type III odontoid fractures (below the waist, involves the body) is treated with external immobilization (hard collar or halo vest).
  - Elderly patient with odontoid fractures have greater rates of morbidity and mortality. Treatment is non operative in a rigid cervical orthosis for 6-8 weeks (NOT halo vest due to high complication rate). *(Scenario: 82 years old, fell down, neck pain, type III odontoid fracture, treatment?)*

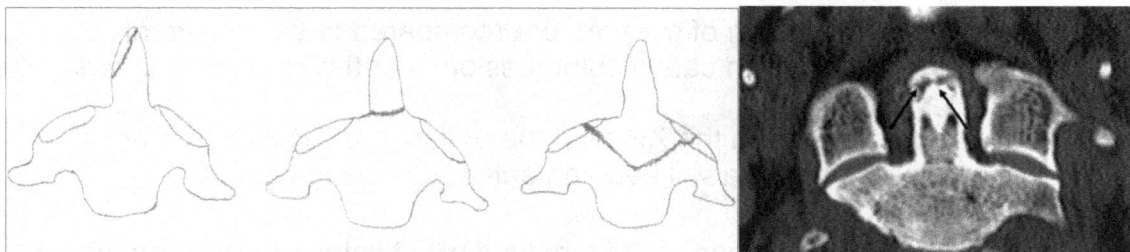

Fig 2: Classification of odontoid fractures. Type I: at the tip, Type II: at base of the odontoid and type III exists at the C1-C2 articulation. Coronal CT showing example of type I odontoid fracture (arrows).

- **C2 Isthmus Fracture (Hangman's) (Traumatic Spondylolisthesis of Axis)**
  - Classification (see Fig. 3)

- Type I: non displaced, non-angulated. Stable injury.
- Type II: displaced > 3mm with vertical fracture line. Treatment is by traction to obtain reduction (acceptable reduction is <3 mm translation and 10° angulation) then halo immobilization for 6-12 weeks.
- Type IIA: marked angulation (flexion) with minimal horizontal displacement (fracture line is more oblique). Traction is contra indicated (very unstable with axial loading, can become easily over distracted with minimal traction). Reduction with hyperextension then halo immobilization for 6-12 weeks.
- Type III: C2-C3 facet dislocation. Needs surgical reduction.

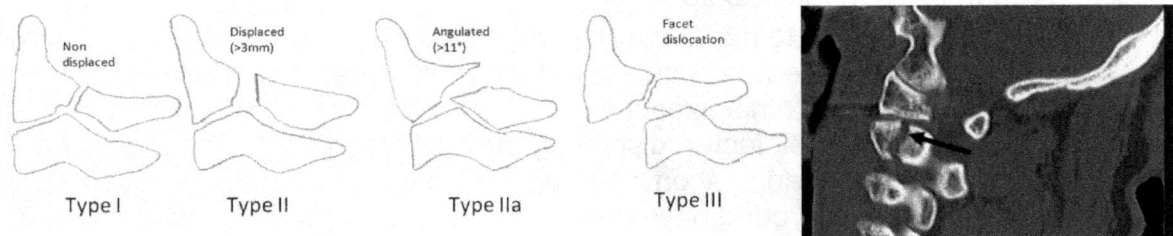

Fig 3: Classification of C2 isthmus fracture. Sagittal CT scan shows 4mm displaced type II fracture.

- **Facet dislocation:**
  o Unilateral and bilateral facet dislocations occur due to flexion-distraction injuries
  o Unilateral facet dislocation:
    - Small amount of translation (minimal encroachment over the cord)
    - Clinical presentation: neck pain, neurological exam is usually normal.
    - The facets are not parallel to each other on plain radiographs.
  o Bilateral facet dislocation:
    - More translation of the vertebra (compared to the unilateral dislocation), can cause compression over the cord (by narrowing the canal).
    - More obvious in the XR than the unifacet dislocation; the upper cervical vertebra will become anterior to the lower one.
  o Treatment:
    - An awake and cooperative patient with bilateral or unilateral facet dislocations: treatment is by awake closed reduction by traction (Gardner-Wells) and repeated neurologic examination, **followed by MRI then fixation and fusion.** _(Scenario: C5-6 unilateral facet dislocation, right-sided C6 nerve root palsy, awake and cooperative, treatment?)_
    - In intubated patient, urgent MRI is needed (to assess if there is associated disc herniation) followed by closed reduction (if no disc herniation).

- If closed reduction by traction fails, open reduction will be needed.
- Open reduction is performed through posterior approach (if there is no disc herniation). If there is disc herniation: anterior decompression, followed by posterior fusion.
- More than 100 pounds' traction can be safely applied to the cervical spine in cases of reduction of facet dislocation.

- **Cervical Vertebral Body Fracture:**
    - Tear drop flexion compression fracture:
        - Large anterior-inferior piece with retrolithesis, unstable injury, needs surgical fixation.
    - Tear drop extension injury:
        - Small anterior inferior fleck, no retrolithesis, stable injury.
    - Compression fracture:
        - Posterior body intact, usually stable injury.
    - Burst fracture:
        - Posterior body disruption, potentially unstable.

- **Whip Lashes Injury:**
    - Treated by early active ROM, NSAIDs, and physical therapy (avoid immobilization). *(Scenario: 35 years old female, had low speed rear-end motor vehicle accident 3 weeks ago, complains of neck pain that sometimes referred to paraspinal muscles and bilateral trapezius region, no weakness, no radicular symptoms, no loss of motion, full flexion extension, cervical spine radiographs normal, diagnosis? next step?)*

- **Halo traction:**
    - Most commonly nerve to be affected with traction is cranial nerve IV (abducent).
    - Anterior pin should be over the lateral half of the orbit (eye brow) to avoid injury to the supra orbital nerve.
    - Pins should be applied 1 cm above the ear line (1 cm above the superior orbital rim), 1 cm below the widest skull circumference with an 8-inch torque.
    - The most common complication is pin loosening. If there is no infection, a loose pin can be re-tightened.
    - Pin site infection is the second most common complication. Superficial infection can be treated with antibiotics, deep infections require pin removal and possible drainage.

- **Halo Vest Immobilization:**
    - Used in cases C2 pars fractures, non-displaced odontoind type II fracture, and C1 lateral mass fractures and burst fractures.
    - Has limited control of sub axial cervical spine (poor control of facet dislocations)

- **Multi-trauma intubated patient:**

- o The cervical spine should be cleared by CT or MRI and the cervical collar removed.
- o Keeping the cervical collar for long periods can cause ulcers in the occipital area.

Thoraco-Lumbar Fractures:

- Types: compression (no affection the middle column), burst (affection of middle column and possible affection of the posterior column), flexion distraction, fracture dislocation (table 1).

	Anterior column	Middle column	Posterior column
Compression	+	-	+/- (distraction)
Burst	+	+	+/-
Flexion-distraction	+/-	+	+
Fracture dislocation	+	+	+

- Compression and burst fractures occur most frequently at the thoracolumbar junction (between T12 and L2) (a transition from the stiff thoracic spine to the more flexible lumbar spine).
- Thoracolumbar injury classification and severity (TLICS):
    - o Scoring system that can help the surgeon decided operative versus non-operative treatment.
    - o Affection of the posterior ligamentous complex (Supraspinous ligament, interspinous ligament, ligamentum flavum, and the facet joint capsules) is one of the parameters of this scoring system.
- **Compression fracture:**
    - o If the loss of height is less than 50% (weight bearing XR): non-operative treatment.
    - o Compression fracture with posterior ligamentous injury are potentially unstable. MRI will show discontinuity of the posterior ligaments (interspinous and supraspinous ligaments and ligamentum flavum) and region of hyperintensity in the posterior region at the level of the injury. These injuries will need posterior spinal fusion with instrumentation (see TLICS above).
- **Burst Fracture:**
    - o XR: affection of the posterior cortex of the vertebral body with retropulsion of bone into the spinal canal, widening of the interpedicular distance in the AP view, possible fracture of the lamina.
    - o For stable thoraco-lumbar (T11-L1) and lumbar burst fracture (no neurological compromise and less than 50 loss of height in the standing XR): non operative treatment is preferred.

- Lumbo-sacral orthosis (LSO) (or body cast) for 3 to 6 months with mobilization when comfortable (***no need for pre-brace bed rest***).
- Non operative treatment gives the same results (neurological outcomes, alignment, back pain and return to function) as operative treatment with less cost and less complications.
- Most lumbar and thoracolumbar fractures can be managed non operatively.

  o Indication for surgery:
  - Neurological injury, 50% or more of loss of height or 30° junctional kyphosis, disruption of the posterior ligamnetous complex.
  - Lumbar burst fracture with fracture lamina and entrapment of the cauda equina roots (in this case, the surgery will include laminectomy, release of the entrapped roots, posterior spinal fusion with instrumentation). *(Scenario: 40 years old, fall down, burst fracture, 20° loss of height, retro pulsed fragment in the canal, no neurologic injury, no palpable spinal step off or increased inter spinous distance, treatment?) (Scenario: 25 years. MVC, burst fracture L1, neurologically intact and has minimal posterior tenderness without increased spinous process separation on examination. XR shows kyphosis of 20 degrees between T12 and L2 with 30% vertebral height loss. A CT scan shows 55% canal compromise, treatment?)*
  - For neurological deficit: anterior decompression (corpectomy with possible strut graft) with possible posterior spinal fusion with instrumentation (this will allow the best chance for neurological recovery after incomplete spinal cord injury due to burst fracture with retropulsed fragment).

  o Flexion distraction injury
  o Flexion distraction mechanism (e.g. lap seat belt without shoulder strap).
  o Can be associated with abdominal injury (about 50% of cases).
  o Common in children.
  o The center of rotation for this injury is anterior to the spine (in the abdomen).
  - The posterior injury is due to distraction.
  o The injury can be ligamentous or bone.
  o Ligamentous injury: surgical treatment.
  - The surgical treatment will be reconstruction of the tension constraint posteriorly.
  o Chance fracture:
  - Single level bony injury due to flexion distraction
  - Can be treated non operative (cast immobilization in hyperextension for 6 weeks, followed by a thoracolumbosacral orthosis) *(scenario: 20 years old, MVC, back seat with lap seat belt, Sagittal CT shows the lesion through one vertebra, treatment?)*
- **Fracture dislocation:**
  o Surgical treatment is needed.
  o Treatment:

- With complete neurological injury: posterior reduction, fusion and instrumentation. Stabilization should include two segment above and below.
- With incomplete neurological affection: anterior decompression and stabilization.

Osteoporotic Vertebral Compression Fractures:

- Most common fragility fractures in elderly patients, can also occur with other etiologies of osteoporosis (eg steroid induced).
- Associated with deteriorating gait, early satiety, further future fracture risk, and deteriorating lung function.
  - Associated with neurologic complications in less than 1% of patients.
  - 20% risk of having subsequent vertebral compression fractures.
  - The mortality rate of patients with vertebral fractures exceeds that of patients with hip fractures.
  - Compression fractures can lead to early satiety (which can result in decrease intake of vitamin D, further exacerbating osteoporosis) and decreased pulmonary function.
- **Management:**
  - Early mobilization with analgesics and progressive rehabilitation (NO bed rest).
  - Cement augmentation (vertebroplasty/ kyphoplasty) can be done if the patient fails nonsurgical management. These modalities are useful only in acute fractures.
    - MRI can help distinguish between acute and chronic injuries (presence of edema in the vertebral body).
  - Kyphosis from a vertebral osteoporotic compression fracture can lead to progressive kyphosis due to load transfer to the superior adjacent vertebra. Kyphoplasty can help prevent this progression.

Gunshot injuries:

- Gunshot injuries that traverse the canal but do not affect the stability of the spine (intact pedicles) and no external leak of CSF: No need to explore the wound, instrument the spine nor repair the dura.
- Antibiotic administration:
  - Oral antibiotic if no abdominal injury or if there is solid organ injury.
  - If the bullet traversed hollow organ: IV antibiotics.
- Removal of the bullet: if in the canal with deteriorating neurological status.

Spinal Infections:

- **Discitis/osteomyelitis (see pediatric chapter, same principles):**
  - Pathology: starts in vertebral end plates (close the disc) and then moves to the disc through vascular channels.
  - Clinical presentation:
    - Pain: The most common initial presentation of a patient with lumbar pyogenic infection is low back pain.
    - Neurological deficits: can occur with progressive infection/ epidural abscesses.
  - Lab:
    - Increased ESR and CRP.
    - WBC is usually within normal.
    - Blood culture: may show the causative organism.
  - XR: narrowing of the disc space, may take few weeks to manifest.
  - MRI changes: best imaging modality for the diagnosis. *(Scenario: 67 years old, had epidural injection one week ago, now having increased pain with weakness, next step? (MRI)).*
  - MRI picture of discitis:
    - Increased signal (bright) in T2 within the disc space (free water) (inflammation).
    - T1: loss of the distinction between disc and vertebral body (both appear dark).
    - Advanced degenerative disc has a similar fluid signal within the disc space, however, in degenerative disc there is no surrounding edema or obliteration of the distinct margins of the disc.
    - T1-fat suppressed with gadolinium: will show the abscess as dark area with a surrounding rim of enhancement.
  - Management:
    - Initial management should be directed to obtain cultures (either blood cultures or needle aspiration).
      - CT guided biopsy to obtain culture is usually needed (if bacteria cannot be identified in the blood culture).
      - Treatment is usually medical: antiobiotics (long term, according to cultures). *(Scenario: 45 years, back pain for 6 months, no fever, increased ESR, CRP, MRI discitis, no abscess, blood culture positive, next step? (medical treatment according to blood culture results and brace). (Same previous scenario but with negative blood cultures, treatment? (tissue biopsy to identify the organism (CT guided) followed by intravenous antibiotics))*
    - Brace for comfort
    - Indication of surgery (aggressive debridement): Refractory infection despite medical treatment, development of deformity, abscess (epidural abscess) formation, worsening neurological affection, failure of medical treatment, instability.

- o Epidural abscess: can sometimes be managed non-surgical (however, this is debatable):
  - Absolute indication for surgery: presence of neurologic deficits (urgent decompression, with or without fusion).
  - Relative indication of surgical treatment of epidural abscess (risk factors for failure on medical treatment): CRP > 115, WBC > 12.5, history of IV drug abuse, diabetes, age older than 65, MRSA infection.
  - Relative indication of medical treatment: MSSA, age younger than 65 years, the absence of neurologic deficit, and lumbar abscess location.
  - Immunosuppression and abscess size are not risk factors for failure of medical treatment.
  - The approach depends on the location of epidural abscess (most cases need anterior approach). If debridement causes instability of the spinal segment, instrumented fixation (usually posterior instrumentation) can be added to stabilize the spine. *(Scenario: 55 years diabetic, severe back pain for 7 days, progressive weakness of the lower extremity, CRP and ESR elevated, MRI extensive discitis with abscess, treatment? (Anterior debridement with possible need for posterior instrumentation))*
  - Prognosis after epidural infection: factors associated with worse prognosis (increased incidence of neurological complication): DM, elderly, RA, HIV, cervical lesion.
- **Tuberculosis of the spine:**
  - o Pathology:
    - Relative sparing the disc until later in the disease process (unlike pyogenic infection).
    - Can track anterior and posterior to the vertebral body sparing the posterior elements of the spine.
    - Can spread to adjacent vertebrae.
    - Common in the anterior aspect of the lower thoracic and upper lumbar vertebrae. (*Scenario:12 years old, kyphos deformity, loss of weight, coughing, XR destruction of the vertebrae, diagnosis?)*
  - o Clinical presentation:
    - Insidious onset and chronic course of back pain with associated with kyphos deformity; general manifestation of TB infection.
  - o Treatment
    - Multi-drug regimen (anti-TB medications).
    - Surgery is indicated for deformity correction or failure of medical treatment.
- **Post-operative spinal infections:**
  - o Most common presenting symptom is pain at the side of surgery.
  - o Early spinal infection should be treated aggressively by surgical debridement.
  - o Instrumentation can be left in most cases of early post-operative infection (however, bone graft has to be removed in most cases).

- o The spinal surgical procedure associated with the highest rate of surgical site infection is fusion of neuromuscular scoliosis. *(Scenario: 16 years old quadriplegic cerebral palsy, had spinal fusion for neuromuscular scoliosis, developed discharge and redness, treatment? (irrigation, debridement, IV antibiotics, excision of the graft and retention of instrumentation).*
- o Epidural morphine and steroid paste after spinal surgery is associated with an 11% rate of postoperative surgical site complications and about 8 folds increase in postoperative surgical wound debridement

Spondylolisthesis (see pediatric chapter)

- **Degenerative Spondylolisthesis:**
  - o Most common location is L4-5 affecting **L5 nerve root** (manifested by EHL weakness).
  - o Degenerative spondylolisthesis with back pain and claudication (who fail non operative treatment) should be treated by decompression (laminectomy) with fusion (see lumbar stenosis)
- **Isthmic spondylolisthesis:**
  - o Most common is between L5-S1, this will affect **L5 root** due foraminal stenosis from fibrocartilagneous reparative process.
  - o Should be treated by posterior foraminal decompression and fusion at L5-S1 or L4-S1 (depending of the degree of slippage) with instrumentation and bone graft.
  - o Surgical treatment of high grade spondylolisthesis is by 360 (circumferential) fusion.

Adult deformity/ Adult scoliosis:

- Assessment of deformity by radiographs: AP and lateral long-cassette are needed for proper assessment of the deformity (Cobb angles for coronal deformity, C7 plumb line for sagittal imbalance, and a center sacral vertical for coronal malalignment).
- In cases of deformity surgery: extending the fusion to the ilium and the sacrum (rather that the sacrum alone), increase the rate of fusion of the lumbo-sacral junction.
- In osteoporotic patient with long fixation, the advantage of extending distal fixation to ilium (rather than sacrum alone) is to decrease the incidence of sacral fractures.
- The most predictive factor of disability and pain (pre and post operative) in adult scoliosis is the sagittal plane imbalance.
  - o Restoration of the sagittal balance results in relief of low back pain and neurological claudication.

- Kyphosis at the lumbosacral junction can lead to sagittal imbalance problems. The surgeon should try to restore lumbo-sacral lordosis and L5-S1 disc height (e.g. by insertion of interbody strut) to prevent sagittal imbalance (see below).
- **Pelvic incidence (PI):**
  - Definition: the angle between a line perpendicular to the sacral plate at its midpoint and a line connecting this point to the femoral head axis (the midpoint of a line connection the center of the two femoral heads (Fig 4).
  - PI = pelvic tilt + sacral slope.
  - Pelvic tilt should be less than 20°, it is affected by pelvis version.
  - PI should be equal to lumbar lordosis (with upright posture).
  - PI is not affected by pelvic rotation (unlike both pelvic tilt and sacral slope)
  - Patients with increased PI will require increased lumbar lordosis to restore sagittal balance.
    - If lumbar lordosis is not restored (PI 10° more than lumbar lordosis), there will be positive sagittal imbalance and increased risk of proximal junctional kyphosis.
  - PI correlates with the incidence and severity of spondylolisthesis.
- **The sagittal vertical axis (SVA):**
  - Definition: The distance between the C7 plumb line and the posterosuperior corner of S1 in the sagittal plane.
  - Positive balance: the axis is more than 5 cm anterior to the S1
- Patient with sagittal imbalance:
  - Will try to bend the knee to keep their upright posture.
  - If after posterior spinal fusion, the patient still has positive sagittal imbalance (failure to restore lumbar lordosis), the patient will have increased risk of proximal junction kyphosis.
- **Kyphos deformity:**
  - Operative treatment is by posterior extension osteotomies, fusion with internal fixation (see later for type of osteotomies).

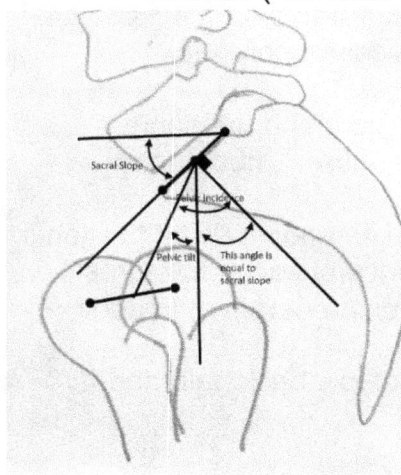

Fig 4: Pelvic incidence is the angle between a line perpendicular to the slope of upper sacrum and line from the middle for the upper sacrum to the point between the 2 centers of the femoral heads.

Lumbar Disc Herniation (Herniated Nucleus Pulposus) (HNP):

- TNF-alph is the main inflammatory/ pain mediator in cases of HNP.
- Clinical presentation/exam:
  - Back pain radiating to the leg (distal to the knee).
  - Straight leg raising (SLR): the increased tension generally occurs between 30°to 60°.
  - Contra-lateral SLR (raising the non-affected side causes pain in the affected side): more specific than SLR, occurs more with axillary HNP.
  - Waddell's signs:
    - Tenderness to light touch, over-exaggeration, pain in non-anatomic distribution (not following dermatomal distribution).
    - Presence of three of five positive Waddell signs indicates nonorganic disease (non-radicular pain) (do **not** do surgery).
- Recurrent lumbar disc herniation: MRI with gadolinium is the imaging modality of choice.
- Sequestered disc herniation: Separation of a herniated fragment from the disc.
- Spontaneous resorption of herniated discs can occur (possibly mediated by macrophages and neovascularization) and it can frequently be detected by MRI.
- Treatment:
  - Initial treatment is non operative: activity modification (short time bed rest); anti-inflammatory medications, and judicious use of pain medications
  (Scenario: 40 years old, 6 months of leg pain and weakness, no improvement with medical treatment or therapy, MRI shows postero-lateral disc herniation, treatment?).
  - Epidural steroids injection (ESI):
    - ESI can be trans-laminar or trans-foraminal. Trans-foraminal ESI is more effective (especially for lateral lumber HNP) and last for longer time.
    - ESI should not be given more than 4 times per year. If the initial response to ESI was only transient, further injections are not indicated.
    - ESI can give long term pain relief (75% of patient had pain relief at 3 years follow up).
  - Operative Vs conservative:
    - Indication for operative treatment: absolute indications are cauda equina syndrome and a **progressive** neurologic deficit; relative indication is failure of non-operative treatment (persistence of pain, persistence of weakness).
    - With failure of non-operative treatment: surgical treatment is fenestration and discectomy/ micro-discectomy (laminectomy is not indicated in simple lumbar HNP).
    - The prognosis of herniated lumbar discs is generally good for both operative and non-operative treatment. Patients who had surgery improved quicker than patients who were treated non-operatively; however, at 5 years point, the outcomes are equal to each other.

- Both groups will have similar results with medium term follow up (4-5 years). However, early follow up (one year) shows better results for operative group.
        - Nerve root injury, recurrent disc herniation, and discitis are complications of surgical treatment.
        - At 5 years after surgery for lumbar disc herniation: about 70% of the patients will report improvement of their symptoms and 20% will have had another surgical procedure in first 5 years.
    o Micro-discectomy (limited discectomy): removal of the herniated disc material with no laminectomy.
        - If there is recurrent disc herniation: the procedure can be repeated.
        - No difference in functional clinical outcomes, complications, or rate of revision surgery between tubular micro-discectomy and open conventional microsurgical lumbar discectomy.
        - Minimal invasive techniques have been associated with an increased rate of dural tear.
    o Complete (subtotal) discectomy: can reduce the recurrence of disc herniation, however, can lead to more post-operative back pain.
    o Post-operative protocol for primary micro-discectomy: patients can resume activity (up to high intensity exercises) as early as 4-6 weeks post-operative. This was found to decrease disability and pain.
    o Far lateral disc herniation can be approached by far lateral approach (paramedian approach between the paraspinal muscles (multifidus and longissimus) then release the intertransverse membrane).
    o The workman's compensation patients undergoing lumbar discectomy for HNP and radiculopathy shows significantly greater likelihood of continuing to receive disability benefits.

Thoracic Disc Herniation:

- Symptomatic cases of thoracic disc herniation are rare compared to lumbar and cervical disc herniation:
    o Most of the thoracic disc herniation seen in MRI are asymptomatic.
    o Most common levels for thoracic herniation are the lower thoracic spine.
- Clinical presentation:
    o Radicular pain (posterolateral herniation): radiating pain along the chest to the anterior wall.
    o Upper motor neurological signs (clonus, positive Babinski (down going response)) in the lower extremity: due to compression on the cord by a central disc.
- Treatment (after failure of medical treatment):
    o Posterolateral (transpedicular, transfacetal, or costotransversectomy) or an anterior approach.

- Avoid posterior decompression (laminectomy and discectomy) as it can cause neurologic injury by manipulating the cord to reach the disc anteriorly.
  - Calcified discs have higher risk of adhesions between disc and dura and higher incidence of dural tears.

Facet Disease:

- Pathology: arthritis and degeneration of the facet joint, can be a source of back pain.
- Nerve supply to the facet: *medial branch of dorsal primary rami* (after it exits the neuroforamen above and at the level of the facet) and sinuvertebral nerve.
- Facet joint disease can cause **synovial cyst** and development of lumbar canal stenosis.
  - Synovial lumbar cyst: fluid filled cyst in the lumbar spine (mostly at L4-5) related to facet joint disease (and possibly attributed to instability).
  - MRI: High signal cyst in T2 weighted images.
  - Treatment is initially non operative. If there is failure of non-operative treatment: surgery is indicated (laminectomy (decompression), synovial cyst excision, possible fusion (for instability).

Cauda Equina Syndrome:

- Due to central compression (eg disc herniation, retro pulsed fragment in fractures) at the level of L2 or lower.
- **Prognosis**: expected to have improvement in pain and weakness symptoms with less predictable recovery of the urinary and bowl function.
  - For patients presenting more than 48 hours, less than 40% will recover their bowl and bladder function.
- Clinical presentation (table 1 comparing cauda equine to conus medullaris):
  - Generalized lower extremity weakness and hyporeflexia, back pain, saddle paresthesia (perianal sensory deficit), difficult urination (urinary retention and/or urinary incontinence), and loss of rectal tone.
  - Urgent MRI is needed.
  - The condition is considered surgical emergency (to try to maximize the chances of recovery of urinary and bowl function).
  - Timing of surgery (the earlier the better) is closely related to the outcomes following the surgical treatment of cauda equina syndrome.
  - Surgery: Decompression (discectomy or removal of the compressing bone). *(Scenario: A 52-year, L2 burst fracture 3 weeks ago. He was neurologically intact and treated with conservative management, now complains of an inability to void and weak anal sphincter tone. Treatment?)*

Conus Medullaris Syndrome:

- Injury to the lower part of the cord at the at T12-L1 (eg burst fracture or herniated disc) which will have mixed spinal cord and nerve roots injury (mixed upper and lower motor neuron injury). The cord usually ends at L1-2 disc or lower part of L1 vertebra.
- Clinical presentation:
    - Loss of control of bowl and bladder with possible lower extremity weakness (hypertonic).
- Treatment is emergent surgical decompression. *(Scenario: L1 burst fracture, weak ankle dorsiflexion, loss of rectal tone, what is the type of injury?)*

	Cauda Equina	Conus Medullaris
Pathology	At the level of the roots causing lower motor neuron (usually bilateral)	At the level of the conus resulting in combination of upper and lower motor neuron (usually unilateral)
Pain	More back pain, usually sudden onset	More radicular pain, usually gradual onset
Deep reflexes	More affection of ankle reflexed	Affection of both reflexes
Sensory	Mainly over the perineal area, bilateral, symmetrical	Mainly over the saddle area, can be unliateral, asymmetrical
Bowl and bladder	Early affection	Can be early or late

Discogenic Low Back Pain:

- Pathology: degeneration of the intervertebral discs.
- The best initial study for the diagnostic back pain evaluation is plain radiographs.
- Discography involves injection of dye into an intervertebral disc space. It works by pressurizing the disc with a non-noxious fluid to stimulate nerve endings in degenrated discs.
    - The dye injected into the disc and the patient's response to the injection is noted.
    - A positive study: provocation of pain that is similar to the patient's existing back or neck pain (concordant pain) (suggests that the disc might the source of the pain).
    - Lumbar back pain with "non concordant" results at discograpms (pain not similar to the patient pre-existing pain) are better treated non operatively (by cognitive intervention and exercises).
- Patients with low back pain who are poor surgical candidate (smokers, diffuse pain, depression), with no root compression in MRI, management should be non-operative (cognitive intervention, exercise, and smoking cessation). No need to perform discogram.

- MRI: decrease signal intensity of the disc in T2 images.
- Beware of lower back pain that it due to other reasons (eg stress fracture of hip or hip arthritis). *(Scenario: 70 years old, left hip pain with lower back pain, MRI: lumbar stenosis and left hip stress fracture, treatment? (management of stress fracture)). (Scenario: patient has low back pain with hip and knee pain, MRI: degenerated disc, surgery done for discogenic lumbar pain, 2 weeks after surgery patient is having pain in the hip and knee with gait with limping, reason? (preexisting missed Hip OA))*
- Back pain with red flag for tumor or infection (pain at rest, pain at night, fever, weight loss) and negative radiograph, next step is lab work (CBC, ESR, PSA, urinalysis) and MRI.
- Highest intra-discal pressure: sitting bending forward position (with weight in the hand), and lowest is supine position (see biomechanics in the beginning of the chapter).
- Pain modulators in discogenic pain: TNF-α, IL-1, MMP (matrix metalloproteinase).
- Treatment:
    - Non operative treatment is the mainstay treatment (more than 90% will improve with non-surgical approach).
    - Operative treatment: outcome is very unpredictable. Worker's compensation state is the most important predictor of negative outcome.
    - Fusion is the main treatment for discogenic lumbar pain. Lumbar artificial disc replacement is an option (variable outcome in different studies)
- The sacroiliac joint accounts for 15% of lower back pain. Physical examination tests are poor predictors of sacroiliac joint pathology.

Muscular (Mechanical) Axial Low Back Pain:

- Clinical presentation: Short-term history of activity-related, low back pain without radiculopathy or focal neurologic findings or systemic symptoms.
- Up to 85% of people will experience low back pain at some point in their lifetime.
- Management should include reassurance, limited analgesia and range-of-motion exercises (**Nonsurgical**).
    - No need for radiographs of the lumbar spine in the early stage. *(Scenario: mechanical back pain, no bowel or bladder difficulties and no constitutional signs. No focal neurologic deficits or pathologic reflexes are noted. Management?)*
    - Spinal manipulation:
        - Controlled passive motion that moves the joint past physiologic motion, causing joint cavitation, can help with the short-term acute pain relief (not indicated or effective in treatment of radiculopathy or myelopathy).

Lumbar Canal Stenosis:

- Imaging: defined as an AP canal diameter of less than 10 mm or a cross-sectional area of less than 100 mm² (as measured on CT).
- **Clinical presentation:**

- o Back pain, radicular symptoms (leg pain is usually more than back pain).
- o **Pain with walking** that is relieved with sitting or with rest and bending forward (neurological claudication).
  - Pain gets better with forward bending (going uphill or bending on shopping cart).
- o Mild weakness (usually in the L4 or L5 distribution)
- **Imaging:**
  - o XR: may show the spondylolithesis.
  - o Flex/ ext views to assess instability.
  - o MRI will show the stenosis and possible lithesis.
- **Management:**
  - o Initial treatment is non operative: most patients will have some pain relief. Delay in surgical treatment does not adversely affect the final prognosis.
  - o Operative: Treatment according to the stability (as judged by XR):
    - **Stable spine**: no spondylolisthesis and no motion with flexion/extension:
      - Decompression (laminectomy for central canal stenosis and/or lateral recess decompression (medial facetectomy) for lateral canal stenosis). *(Scenario: 55 years old, radicular symptoms, pain with walking, relieved by bending, XR no spondylolisthesis and no instability, MRI shows stenosis (central and lateral), treatment?)*
      - The most common reason for persistent lower extremity pain following lumbar laminectomy for stenosis is residual foraminal stenosis.
      - With complete removal of one facet joint or more than 50% of bilateral facet joint, or iatrogenic pars fracture: fusion should be added to avoid instability.
      - Interspinous process decompression (X-stop) can be used in selected cases (the device block extension of the spine which help to reduce pain).
    - **Unstable spine**: spondylolisthesis or motion of L4 on L5 with flexion extension or degenerative scoliosis:
      - Decompression with fusion and instrumentation. *(Scenario: 60 years old, neurological claudication, XR spondylolisthesis, treatment?)*
      - Patients with lumbar stenosis associated with degenerative spondylolisthesis and leg pain will have better results with surgical management compared to non-surgical management.
  - o If suspecting vascular claudication (pain improve by stopping to walk with no need to sit): start with non-invasive test (ankle brachial index). *(Scenario: 65 years, smoker, right leg pain with walking, standing stops pain. Forward bending and sitting does not provide improvement of the symptoms. Leg pain is worse at night and relieved by hanging the leg over the side of the bed. Next step?)*

- o If lumbar stenosis is associated with upper extremity symptoms, it may due to associated cervical stenosis. _(Scenario: clinical picture of lumbar stenosis with numbness of both upper extremity, next step? (MRI for possible cervical stenosis))._

Ankylosing Spinal Disorders:

- Includes ankylosing spondylitis (AS) and Diffuse Idiopathic Skeletal Hyperostosis (DISH).
- Will result in rigid non-flexible spine (risk of instability and neurological injury even with minor trauma).
  - o Delay of diagnosis of instability after trauma is common.
  - o Extensive work up (CT and/or MRI) for minor trauma should be performed for patient with ankylosing disorders to exclude unstable fracture (Fig 5)
  - o Spinal fractures in both AK and DISH have high risk for complications and death.
    - ▪ AS has higher risk than DISH.
  - o Posterior multilevel spinal instrumentation is usually required to obtain adequate spinal stabilization in these patients.
- **DISH:**
  - o Middle-aged to older patients.
  - o Three diagnostic features in XR:
    - ▪ Ossification along the anterolateral border of at least four contiguous spinal segments (**non marginal osteophytes**) (Fig 6).
    - ▪ Preservation of disc height in the involved segment.
    - ▪ Absence of sclerosis or anklyosing of facets or sacroiliac joint.
- **AS**
  - o XR:
    - ▪ The anterior osteophytes are smaller than in DISH (5).
    - ▪ Marginal thin syndesmophytes. _(Scenario: 70-year-old male with ankylosing spondylitis sustains a minor trip and fall, increased mid back pain, XR and CT are normal, next step? (MRI spine))._ Diffuse syndesmophytic ankylosis can give a "bamboo spine" appearance.

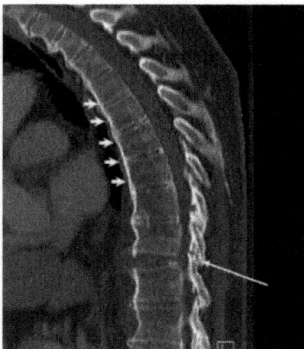

Fig 5: 70 years old male with long history of AS. Patient had a minor fall followed by news onset mid back pain. XR could not show obvious fracture. Sagittal CR shows the fracture in the posterior vertebra and the extension deformity with distraction of the anterior vertegra (arrow). The upper thoracic vertebrae show the "Marginal thin syndesmophytes" (arrow heads) characteristic of the AS. The syndesmophyes extends from the margin of the vertebra and less dense the DISH.

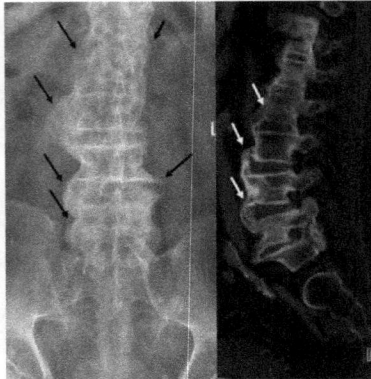

Fig 6: 65 years old male with DISH. Notice the large non-marginal syndesmophytes that can be seen in the AP XR (black arrow) and sagittal CT (white arrow). These syndesmophytes span the whole lumbar spine with preservation of the disc height.

Spinal Surgeries/ Procedures/ Post-Operative Complications:

- The most common sentinel event related to spine surgery is wrong level Surgery.
- Post-operative epidural hematoma: Can cause compression of the cord or the nerve root. If causing neurological manifestation, will require ixmmediate surgical exploration and hematoma drainage. *(Scenario: 65 years old, fusion L4-5, post-operative day 2 developing lower extremity weakness and saddle paresthesia, MRI shows hematoma, treatment?).*
- Pedicle screws spinal fixation has the highest bone-implant interface pullout strength.
- **Disc replacement surgery/ artificial disc:**
  - Mal-positioned disc replacement or those who show early migration can be safely (relatively) revised within the first 2-weeks.
  - Serum ion levels in patients with metal-on-metal lumbar disc arthroplasty are similar to values measured in patients with metal-on-metal total hip arthroplasty.
- **Spinal osteotomy:**
  - pedicle subtraction osteotomy:
    - Pedicle subtraction: removal of the body through the pedicles, wedge shaped excision.
    - 3-column osteotomies: posterior column (lamina, facets, pedicles), middle column (posterior vertebral), anterior column (part of the anterior body)
    - For localized curve (eg ankylosis spondylolitis).
    - Corrects about 30° per level
  - A Smith-Petersen osteotomy:
    - Single- posterior column osteotomy.
    - Relatively easy technique, less blood loss than other osteotomies.
    - Correct about 10° per level.
      - Can be used on 3-4 contiguous levels in large curve to give the correction needed. (*scenario: 21 years old, Scheurman, 90° thoracic curve, which type of osteotomy?)*
  - Vertebral column resection:

- Can correct large curves.
- Technically demanding procedure, require extensive monitoring.
- Massive amount of blood loss.
- **Spinal fusion:**
  - Lumbar fusion results in increased stresses on the adjacent levels. The rate of symptomatic degeneration at an adjacent segment after lumbar vertebrae fusion requiring surgical intervention for the adjacent segment is about is about 3%/ year (about 15% at 5 years and 35% at 10 years). *(Scenario: 45 years old, L4-5 fusion 5 years ago, now has low back pain radiating to the legs, most likely cause of the new onset low back pain?)*
  - For anterior cervical fusion with plate: if the upper end of the plate is close to the disc proximal to the fusion level, this may lead to osteophyte formation around the proximal disc.
  - Interbody fusion:
    - Obtaining spinal fusion by removing the intervertebral disc then inserting a bone graft between the two vertebral bodies. A "cage" is sometimes used to restore disc height.
    - According to the approach: interbody fusion can be: posterior interbody fusion (PLIF); lateral interbody fusion (LIBF); anterior interbody fusion; trans-foraminal interbody fusion (TLIF).
    - Direct lateral interbody fusion: the fusion devise is inserted through a lateral window in the psoas muscle.
      - The lumbo-sacral plexus lies within the psoas muscle.
      - The femoral nerve and the lateral femoral cutaneous nerve exit from the lateral border of the muscle, the genitofemoral nerve exits directly anterior to the muscle, the obturator nerve and lumbosacral trunk exit from the medial border of the muscle.
      - The plexus is more ventral in the distal part of the lumbar spine.
      - Lateral interbody fusion has highest risk of injury to lumbo-sacral plexus at the L4-L5 fusion (plexus becomes more ventral close to dilators and retractors).
  - Posterolateral fusion:
    - Obtaining spinal fusion by decorticating the posterior and posterolateral elements (lamina, spinous processes, the transverse process) and application of bone graft over these structures.
  - Interbody fusion is associated with more blood loss compared to posterolateral fusion.
    - Main advantage of interbody fusion compared to posterolateral fusion is the restoration of disc height and restoration of neuroforaminal height (which help relief the pain associated with foraminal stenosis).
  - Nonunion (pseud-arthrosis) after spinal fusion:
    - Risk factors: NSAIDs, positive sagittal balance > 5 cm, kyphosis > 20° degrees, age > 55 years, smoking, the use of allograft (Vs allograft),

extension of fixation to S1. See below for details on effect of smoking and medication of healing.

- o Effect of medication on spinal fusion:
    - Alendronate inhibits spinal fusion if given in the early post-operative period.
    - NSAIDs inhibit spinal fusion.
    - The main advantage of Use of rhBMP in spinal fusion surgeries is that it eliminates the need for autograft harvest.
- o Effect of smoking on spinal fusion:
    - Smoking is the most significant risk factor for nonunion after spinal fusion and should be strictly avoided.
    - Significant improvement in the rate of lumbar fusion is seen in patients who cease smoking for six months **postoperatively**.
    - The proposed mechanism of cigarette smoking inhibition of spinal fusion is diminished revascularization of the bone graft
- o Smoking is associated with lower functional outcome scores after spinal procedures, decrease fusion rate, increased risks for pseudarthrosis, postoperative wound infection, and reoperation rates.
- o Cervical fixation:
    - C1, C3-6: lateral mass screws:
        - C3-6 the direction of the screws in 20° lateral and 30° cranial and the start point is midpoint of the lateral mass and screw length of 13 mm).
        - C1: has the advantage (over the trans-articular screws) that it is not affected by the presence of anomalous vertebral artery; the trajectory for lateral mass screw is 10 degrees medial and 22 degrees cephalad.
    - C2 and C7: pedicle screws
- **Spinal monitoring:**
    - o **Somatosensory-evoked potentials (SSEP)**
    - o **Transcranial motor monitoring** is considered the most effective method of monitoring for identifying motor tract injury during cervical and thoracic spine surgery.
    - o **EMG triggering of the screws:**
        - Thresholds > 15 mA indicate a well-placed pedicle screw.
        - Thresholds < 6 mA indicate a screw that is in contact with a neural structure (dura/root).
        - Thresholds from 10-6: breach of pedicle by the screw, but most probably not in contact with neural structure (can be left in place)
    - o **Significant change** (indicative of a possible significant intra-operative neurologic complication):
        - Complete loss of potential.
        - Sustained decreased SSEP amplitudes of greater than 50%.

- Decreased transcranial Motor-Evoked Potentials (tceMEP) amplitudes of greater than 75%.
    - o Inhaled halogenated anesthetic agents (eg isoflurane) can affect the signal from spinal monitoring. Intravenous anesthetic agents (e.g. propofol) does not cause same effect.
    - o Monitoring changes during spinal procedure (especially deformity correction): The following step can be taken:
        - Assess that the lead position is correct.
        - Assess patient position.
        - Assess with the anesthiologist that hemodynamics/anaesthesia is not the cause.
            - Keep mean arterial blood pressure above 80 mmHg.
        - Reverse the correction and consider wake up test.
        - Possible steroid mega dose (not well established, controversial).
- In general, minimal invasive spinal surgeries (as compared to open conventional surgeries), will lead to similar outcome, however, MIS have the advantages of shorted hospital stay and less bleeding.
- **Iatrogenic Dural tear:**
    - o Can be closed with water tight repair with no adverse effect on long term results.
- **Iatrogenic spondylolithesis:**
    - o If remove of pars or 100% of one joint or 50% of bilateral facet: should instrument the spine otherwise will cause instability.
- Post laminectomy back pain with no signs of infection or instability is treated non operative.

Tumors of the spine (See Oncology chapter)
- Common spine tumors:
    - o Secondaries; osteoid osteoma; aneurysmal bone cysts; hemangiomas; eosinophilic granuloma; and giant cell tumors
    - o Tumors affecting mainly the vertebral body: secondaries, osteosarcoma; hemagioma.
    - o Tumors affecting mainly posterior element: osteoid osteoma, osteoblastoma, osteochondroma and aneurismal bone cyst.
    - o Osteoblastic lesion in the thoracic spine: mostly prostate metastasis. Order prostate-specific antigen (PSA) level to start the work up.
- **Osteoid osteoma in the spine:**
    - o Clinical presentation for osteoid osteoma of the spine:
        - Back pain (at night), with curvature (the tumor is in the concavity of the curve).
        - Pain is relieved by NSAIDs

- o Management:
    - ▪ osteoid osteoma close to spinal cord (in the posterior part of the vertebral body) can be treated surgically by en block excision. Radiofrequency Ablation can affect the cord (by thermal injury). *(Scenario, 10 years old girl, back pain for 6 months, XR 15 lower thoracic curve, CT shows lesion in the lamina of T10, treatment?)*
- **Hemangioma of the spine:**
    - o Characteristic finding in the CT is vertical striations (draw).
    - o MRI: thickened bone trabeculae will appear as low signal in both T1 and T2. The Tumor itself with have high intensity signal in T1 (due to high fat component of the tumor), and high intensity signal in T2 (due to high water content (blood)).
- **Chordoma (see oncology chapter):**
- **Metastatic spinal tumors (see oncology chapter):**

Tips:
- Both L4-L5 degenerative spondylolithesis and L5-S1 isthmic spodylolithesis will affect L5 root
- Most common lytic lesion in the spine: chordoma (sacrum), metastasis and ABC.
- Osteoid osteoma: pain and curve.
- DISH: non-marginal syndesmophytes; Ankylosing spondylitis: marginal syndesmophyts. Sport Medicine/ General Aspects

Chapter 13:   Sport Medicine/ General

General Aspects of Training:

- Knee Articular cartilage adapts to exercise by increasing the glycosaminoglycan content, which can improve cartilage condition.
- Anaerobic weight training in **pre-pubescent male athlete:**
  - Has been shown to be safe and do not damage the growth plates or joints.
  - Can increase efficiency of muscle action; however, there is insufficient testosterone to allow for muscle hypertrophy.
- Immobilization of a skeletal muscle will result in disuse atrophy and increased fatigability.

Delayed Onset (Post-Exercise) Muscle Soreness (DOMS):

- DOMS is a muscle ache and pain that peaks at 24 to 72 hours after intense exercise; most commonly affecting type IIB fibers (See muscle tissue in basic science chapter), and is associated primarily with **eccentric** exercise.
- Best characterized as inflammation of the muscles.

Endurance Training:

- Consists of decreased tension and increased repetitions.
- Induce hypertrophy of slow twitch fibers (type I).
- Will result in **increases capillary density** (most import adaptation as it will improves blood and nutrient delivery and elimination of metabolic waste), increased mitochondria, and oxidative capacity (increase in the enzymes activity of the Krebs cycle which increases the capacity for aerobic ATP re-synthesis during exercise), increased storage and utilization of intramuscular lipids.
  - The greater use of lipid reduces the contribution of carbohydrate to ATP re-synthesis and preserves muscle glycogen. It also increases resistance to fatigue during endurance exercise (decrease in the rate of glycogen depletion which has been linked to fatigue).
- It improves blood lipid profiles.
- Endurance training blunts the catecholamine response and contributes to the reduction in heart rate observed for the same exercise intensity following training.
  - Well-conditioned athletes have decreased resting heart rate (due to increase stoke volume (amount of blood ejected per heart beat) and increase para symptathetic tone)
  - Cardiac output equals stroke volume by heart rate.
  - When compared with static exercises, dynamic exercises have the advantage of improving the athlete's cardiac output by increasing the stroke volume.

- Endurance training will cause a net increase in type I collagen in tendons (increase turnover, synthesis and degradation).
- **Carbohydrate loading:** The practice of decreasing training and increasing carbohydrate intake (to maximize glycogen stores and delay fatigue) the week before an endurance event (e.g. Marathon running).
  - Side effects of this practice: possible weight gain and water retention.
- Best action to enhances performance in mid level endurance activity (e.g. 10K race) is adequate hydration prior to the race.

Strength/Resistance Training:

- **Hypertrophy** of type II muscle
- Resistance exercise above 60% of 1-repetition maximum (1RM) induces the most myofibrillar muscle protein synthesis (MPS)
- With resistance training, initial gain in strength is mainly by an increase in the number of motor units recruited to perform certain movement. After 4-6 weeks, individual myofibers begin to hypertrophy.

Sport injuries:
Head Injuries and Concussion:

- **"No return to play on the same day of an injury."** This is according to The Consensus Statement on Concussion in Sport and The National Collegiate Athletic Association's (NCAA) 2011 guidelines regarding concussion management.
- A graduated return to play for future games is recommended after the patient is completely asymptomatic. Patient has to remain asymptomatic in each step of the graduated return *(Scenario: 14 years old, football player, tackling, head injury, mild confusion for 3 minutes, now completely normal and symptoms free, next step? (Never return to game in the same day)).*
- With any symptoms (headache, confusion), the athlete is not permitted to return to play. The athlete's neurological examination (cognitive, cranial nerve, and balance testing, neurological assessment tests) must return to baseline before resuming exercise.
- Concussion grading scales (and its recommendation for return to play) are rarely used nowadays to guide return to play. Symptom-based, individual approach now guides return to play.
- No longer are athletes allowed to return to game the same day if their Standardized Assessment of Concussion (SAC) instruments are similar to his baseline scores obtained during the preseason (see before).
- Concussions can occur with or without LOC (loss of consciousness). The vast majority of concussions (more than 95%) do not result in LOC.

- o Brief (less than 1 minute) LOC does not reflect injury severity or predict time to recovery. Prolonged LOC (greater than 1 minute) was associated with delayed return to play.
  - o Amnesia is not predictive of severity of concussion.
- Young athletes take longer time to recover (compared to adult athletes). Post concussive symptoms may be prolonged in young patients.
- Brain MRI has no role in evaluating athletes for return to play.
  - o Mild traumatic brain injury: Most imaging studies will be normal.
  - o Neuropsychologic testing is the most sensitive test in assessing mild deficits after mild TBI.
- **Second impact syndrome (SIS):**
  - o It occurs when return to activities is allowed prior to complete resolution of the symptoms of the first head injury.
  - o A second, minor, head injury (after the athlete is allowed to return back to sport) can lead to a devastating rapidly progressive series of events that can result in sudden death (affection of the brain stem).
  - o This is preventable complication of head injury.
- **Chronic traumatic encephalopathy (CTE):**
  - o Neurodegenerative disease that occurs long time after repeated head trauma.
  - o Early behavioral manifestations include apathy, irritability, and suicidal ideation and poor memory.
  - o Onset most often occurs in midlife after athletes have completed their sports careers.
- "**Lucid interval**" is a temporary improvement in a patient's condition after a traumatic brain injury, after which the condition deteriorates.
  - o A lucid interval is mainly associated with epidural hematoma, 20-50% of patients with epidural hematoma experience a lucid interval.

Maxillofacial Trauma:

- The most serious, acute complication that can occur with multiple mandibular fractures or combined maxillary, mandibular, and nasal fracture is **airway obstruction** that can result in early death.
- **Crown fracture**: An incomplete loss or fracture of the tooth enamel without loss of the toot root.
  - o The most common maxillofacial/dental injury in ice hockey.
- **Acute tooth displacement** (luxation, tooth avulsion):
  - o Loss of the tooth together with the root.
  - o Management is immediate repositioning or replantation of the tooth. Transfer the patient to the closest dentist urgently.

- o The tooth should be transported in saline solution, milk, or saliva on gauze. The tooth should be handled gently by the crown and not by the root.
- o To clean the tooth, pour or rinse in water or saline. No brushing should be done.

Traumatic Optic Neuropathy:
- Occurs after trauma to the eye (eg boxing), resulting in reduced visual acuity and color vision, and a visual field defects.
- May be associated with hyphema.
- Urgent CT is needed to assess the presence of orbital or optic canal fracture, optic nerve sheath hemorrhage, or associated brain injuries.

Equestrian Injuries (Horseback Riding):
- Helmets provide the greatest reduction of the incidence of equestrian injuries.
- Head and spine injuries are more common in recreational and non-helmeted riders (more serious injuries).
- Extremity injuries are more common in professional and helmeted riders.
- Long term effect of horseback riding: spondylosis of the cervical spine and lumbar spine.

Hyponatremia:
- Occurs in athletes who are sweating profusely and drinking large amounts of water (replenishing the lost water, but not salt).
- Athlete will suddenly collapse with violent muscle contractions from hyponatermia.
- Treatment by oral rehydration by salty solution (avoid too rapid correction).

Dehydration:
- Due to excessive sweating.
- Cessation of sweating (at the extremes of dehydration) can lead to a fatal increase in core body temperature.

Frost bite: (See hand chapter)
- Treatment is by warming the extremity in water bath, delay the surgical debridement till the gangrenous part becomes fully demarcated.

Heat-related conditions
- **Heat cramps**: muscle cramps.
- **Heat exhaustion**: cramps associated with headache and weakness, and the skin is pale and **moist** (the temperature is less than 40)

- **Heat stroke:**
  - Hyperthermia (>40), central nervous system dysfunction (confusion, bizarre behaviors, seizures) and cessation of sweating with hot, **dry** skin, due to failure loss of thermoregulatory function.
  - It is a medical emergency (transfer to emergency department) with high death rate and requires rapid reduction in body core temperature.
    - Immediate initiation of rapid and effective cooling of the core temperature is important to save the patient. If possible, cooling should be initiated while the patient is awaiting transport.
    - Cooling methods generally are categorized as external or internal. External methods include evaporative and immersion cooling, with evaporative methods being most commonly used in the field. In evaporative cooling, a mist of cool water is sprayed on the patient's skin.

Tension Pneumothorax:

- Life threatening emergency.
- Patient will complain of dyspnea, tachypnea, tachycardia. Examination will show decrease air entry to affected side and shift of the mediastinum towards the other side.
- Urgent treatment is insertion of wide bore needle into the second intercostal space in the mid clavicular space, then transfer to hospital for chest tube insertion.

Abdominal Injuries:

- Blunt trauma can cause abdominal bleeding. The Patient will present with abdominal pain followed by vomiting and nausea.
- The spleen is the most common organ injured (with blunt abdominal injury) and is the most common cause of death after an abdominal injury (due to bleed).

Hypertrophic Cardiomyopathy

- Obtaining adequate history from athletes (history of chest pain, syncope, or family history of early cardiac death) is the most cost-effective method of screening for idiopathic hypertrophic cardiomyopathy. The diagnosis is confirmed by Echocardiography.
  - History and Physical exam is the most important part of sport-pre participation physical.
- The condition is absolute contraindication to vigorous exercise
  - Most common cause of cardiac death in athlete is hypertrophic cardiomhyopathy.

Commotio Cordis:

- Lethal arrhythmia that occurs as a result of a direct blow to the area directly over the heart.
- The athlete will collapse, becomes apneic and unresponsive, with absent radial pulse.
- Extreme emergency: the treatment is immediate protection of the airway, starting CPR, and early cardioversion (cardiac defibrillation) *(Scenario: Hockey player was hit be a bat over the left chest area, he is apneic with no radial pulse. Treatment?)*

Practice Related Issues:

- The team physician must advise his/her athletes and the school as to the best course of action to keep the students safe. In case of an athlete with a medical condition that the team physician feels it poses a significant physical risk if the athlete continues to participates in sports, the team physician should ban the college student from participating in sports (even if the student is on sport scholarship).
- Team physician is obligated to inform the players and the team organization (college administration) of all athletically relevant medical issues. This is different than if a player sees an orthopedic surgeon (who is not the team physician) in his/her office.

Arm Weakness Due to Sport Injury:

- **Stinger (Burner) syndrome:**
  - Due to injury to the brachial plexus.
    - The most commonly involved level for brachial plexus traction injuries in young athletes is the **upper trunk (C5-6).**
    - Caused by forced stretching of the neck to the contra lateral side resulting in stretch of the upper truck (Erb's point).
  - Clinical presentation:
    - Immediate severe burning pain and paresthesia radiating from the neck and extending to the arm and fingers.
    - **Unilateral** weakness of the shoulder abductor (deltoid), elbow flexor; decreased sensation over the lateral aspect of the left shoulder and radial aspect of the forearm.
    - Non-tender range of motion of the cervical spine.
  - Lasts for about 15 minutes then resolves spontaneously with no residual symptoms.
    - Most cases last less than few minutes, however some cases continue to have shoulder weakness for few hours or days.
  - Return to Play:

- After motor and sensory examination findings and reflexes have normalized, the athlete can return to play.
- **Cervical spinal stenosis (see also spine chapter):**
    - Presents with repeated attacks of arm tingling and weakness (**usually bilateral**) with sports, after which the exam is normal.
    - Diagnosis is confirmed by MRI or CT (MRI will show the possible compression on the root and/or the cord). A cervical canal of less than 13 mm diameter is considered relative stenotic whereas a diameter of less than 10 mm is considered absolute stenosis. Cross area of less than 100mm^3 is also considered stenotic
    - Management:
        - In the acute attack: remove the mask and keep the helmet.
    - If there is evidence of stenosis: athlete cannot return to games.
        - **Cervical spinal stenosis is a contraindication to participation in contact sports.** (*Scenario: 17 years old football player, complained of tingling in arms after tackling, neurological exam normal, CT shows stenosis (10mm), what is the next step?*).

Female Athletic Triad:

- Occurs in high level female athletes.
- Clinical presentations: amenorrhea, eating disorders and osteopenia/ osteoporosis.
- Can sustain stress fractures (excess training and osteoporosis).
- Workup should include obtaining a **menstrual history**, obtaining a nutritional consultation, and obtaining a bone density. (*Scenario: collegiate female athlete, had stress fracture of the 5th MT, what is important aspect of the history? (obtain menstrual history)) (Scenario: High level runner, has stress fracture of neck femur and h/o foot stress fracture; in addition to fixation, you should you obtain what history?*)
- Athletes with amenorrhea are at higher risk of developing stress fractures.
    - History of amenorrhea for one year prior to participation in intense exercise programs (e.g. new military recruits) is a risk factor for a hip stress fracture.
    - The cause of amenorrhea in these female athletes is insufficient caloric intake (due to poor diet or eating disorders).
    - Secondary amenorrhea is defined as absence of menstrual bleeding for 6 months or the absence of three to six consecutive menstrual cycles after normal menses has begun and in the absence of pregnancy.
    - The prevalence of amenorrhea among female athletes is about 15% in women who exercise vigorously and about half of elite runners and professional ballet dancers.

- Anorexia athelitca: athletes who reduce their body weight and maintain an abnormally low weight, relying on compulsive participation in excessive exercise to achieve their goals.
  - Anorexia athletica requires the absence of any affective disorder (e.g. depression).

Infection in Sport Medicine:
- **Prevention:**
  - Proper hygiene: (frequent showering using sandals (not barefooted), hand washing, wearing breathable clothing, and no sharing of towels or equipment).
  - Daily skin surveillance by athletes and trainers for early detection.
  - Frequent disinfecting of shared equipment.
  - Covering open lesions with occlusive dressing during practice.
  - Preventing athletes with infected lesion from participating.
- **Infectious mononucleosis (IMN):**
  - Viral (Epstein-Barr virus) infection that mainly affects adolescents.
  - Diagnosed with monospot test.
  - About half of the cases can be associated with splenomegaly.
    - The risk for spontaneous splenic rupture is highest in the first 3 weeks after the onset of disease, so avoid contact sports for 4 weeks from the onset of symptoms provided that the spleen has returned to normal size.
- **Herpes simplex in athletes:**
  - Contact sports athletes (e.g. wrestling) should not be allowed to participate in sports if they have active skin herpes lesion.
  - Return to sport: when they are free from systemic symptoms and all the lesions are crusted and dry and **there are no new lesions for at least 72 hours.** At least **5 days of anti-viral therapy** should have been started.
- **Warts:**
  - Cover lesion before participation.
- **Community-Acquired Methicillin-Resistant Staphylococcus Aureus (CA-MRSA):**
  - Most common mode of transmission between athletes is through disruption of the skin integrity (abrasions) and close physical contact between athletes.
  - If an athlete presents with cellulitis that does not improve on regular antibiotic, physician should have a high index of suspicion that it is due MRSA infection, and should treat accordingly (no need for culture, start with oral antibiotics for 10-14 days, see below)

- o Lesion is usually described by athletes as **"spider bite"**.
    - The cytotoxin Panton-Valentine leukocidin (produced by CA-MRSA) is responsible for tissue necrosis, and rapid development of an abscess simulating the appearance of a spider bite (see basic science chapter).
- o **Return to play**: at least **48 hours with no new lesions**, and **on treatment for more than 72 hours.**
- o **Treatment:**
    - Cellulitis: antibiotics effective against MRSA (eg oral trimethoprim-sulfamethoxazole, doxycycline or clindamycin for 10-14 days).
    - Abscess: Incision and drainage followed by antibiotic treatment. *(Scenario: athlete, ankle pain of 4 days with redness, swelling, fever, vomiting, area of skin induration, treatment?) (15 years old, soft tissue abscess over the tibia shin, treatment by cefazolin, no improvement, next step?)*
- **Septic knee bursitis**: is initially treated with antibiotics. Surgical drainage is required if the infection does not respond to antibiotics alone.

Performance Enhancing Agents:

- **Anabolic steroids:**
    - o Lead to increased muscle mass through increased production of messenger RNA.
    - o Adverse effects of anabolic steroid include: gynecomastia, acne, testicular atrophy, alopecia, electrolyte disturbance, hypertension, left ventricular hypertrophy, hypercoagulability, thrombosis, hostility and aggression, psychosis, depression, growth retardation/cessation and manic behavior.
    - o The **irreversible** adverse effects of anabolic steroids include alopecia and growth retardation (due premature closure of the growth plate).
    - o Personality effects and acne are reversible after stopping the medication.
    - o Most common behavioral effect of anabolic steroid use in athletes is increased aggression
    - o Concerns during anesthesia in patient on anabolic steroids
        - Less sensitive to anesthetic agents due to induction of the hepatic enzymes.
        - Salt and water retention due to mineralocorticoid effects.
        - Most anabolic steroid users use also diuretics to mask of water retention. Steroids and diuretics will both cause fluid and electrolyte imbalances.
        - High ventilatory requirements caused by increased oxygen consumption and carbon dioxide due to large muscle mass and high calorie intake.

- o Causes a decrease in high-density lipoprotein (has no effect on low-density lipoprotein levels). *(Scenario: Athlete, blood work shows marked decrease in HDL, possible reason?).*
- o Effect on muscle contusion (basic science study on an animal model):
  - **Anabolic steroids** can promote the speed recovery of muscle strength after muscle contusion in the long term.
  - **Corticosteroid** can cause irreversible damage to healing muscle in the long term (disordered fiber structure and a marked diminution in force-generating capacity).
- **Creatine:**
  - o An oral supplement that increases muscle mass and improves sprint times (short-term), and may allow for increased anaerobic resistance performance.
  - o Most common complication associated with creatine is muscle cramps/dehydration

Tips
- Not every "athlete" question is a sport question. It can be other pathology (e.g. Osteosarcoma).

Chapter 14:   Sport Medicine/ Lower Extremity

Hip Injuries:

- Avulsion fractures of the pelvis are generally treated with rest and symptomatic treatment (see pediatric trauma chapter).
- Hamstring injury: can be avulsion of the ischial tuberosity or proximal tear.
    - Injury of the hamstrings occurs with hip flexion and knee extension injury (position of maximum tension of the muscle) (eg water skiing).
    - Indication for surgical repair of proximal hamstring tear: three tendons tear or more than 2 cm displacement.
    - The most likely site of hamstring injury during endurance exercises: musculotendinous junction.
- Avulsion injury of ASIS (contractions of the sartorius and tensor fascia lata):
    - Occurs with hip extended and the knee flexed
    - Treated with rest and protected weight bearing with crutches until pain subsides.
- Avulsion fracture of the ischial tuberosity:
    - Due to hamstring pull.
    - Avulsion fracture of the ischial tuberosity is the fracture most prone to nonunion among pelvis avulsion fractures. Most patients have few symptoms but some have trouble sitting and returning to sports. Excision of the avulsed fragment is indicated for painful nonunions of the ischial tuberosity. _(Scenario: avulsion fracture of the ischial tuberosity 6 months ago, now still in pain with resisted hip extension, treatment?)_
- Labral tears lead to increased instability of the hip joint and increased movement of the femoral head relative to the acetabulum. Labral tears repair (in comparison to shaving) result in better sealing effect of the joint.
- Pulled groin:
    - Injury to the adductor muscle group, caused by forceful external rotation of an abducted leg resulting in avulsion injury of the adductor muscle from the pubic ramus.
    - Patient will have groin and medial thigh pain, examination will show tenderness and ecchymosis. MRI will show edema, avulsion injury and hemorrhage.
    - Treatment is mainly rest, ice, and rehabilitation.
- Adductor-related groin pain in a competitive athlete with **normal findings on MRI** can be treated with steroid injection into the pubic cleft with expected long time relief of the pain
- Osteitis pubis:
    - Supra pubic pain with tenderness over the symphysis pubis and pain with resisted rectus abdominus contraction.
    - XR and CT will show degenerative changes within the Pubic Symphysis.
    - Initial treatment is by rest, nonsteroidal anti-inflammatory drugs. _(Scenario: 21 athletes had suprapubic pain for the few months. A radiograph and CT scans shows degenerative changes in the symphysis, diagnosis?)_

Snapping Hip (Coxa Saltans):

- External-type (lateral)
  - o Snapping sensation around the lateral side of the hip.
  - o Caused by snapping of the ilio tibial band (most commonly) over the greater trochanter causing inflammation of the bursa. It can be reproduced by hip flexion.
  - o Positive Ober test (patient in lateral position with the tested side up, assessment of hip adduction with the knee extended comparing this to when knee is flexed and to the contralateral side): decrease hip adduction with the knee extended indicates tight ilio-tibial band.
  - o Management is mainly non operative (stretching of ilio-tibial band and NSAIDs, steroid injection).
    - ▪ If non operative fails: Z-lengthening of the ilio-tibial band (complete release from the Gerdy's tubercle is not recommended).
- Internal type (anteromedial):
  - o Caused by the iliopsoas tendon gliding over the iliopectineal eminence and produced by hip extension from a flexed position or flexion with external rotation and abduction.
  - o Common in ballet dancers.
  - o Ultrasonography will confirm the snapping structure. XR may show calcifications near the lesser trochanter at the insertion of iliopsoas tendon.

Sports Hernia (Athletic Pubalgia)

- The exact pathology is not well understood.
- Presents with lower abdominal pain after muscular exertion (possible radiation of pain into the testicles and/or adductor region).
- On examination: pain with resisted hip adduction. No palpable inguinal hernia with a Valsalva's maneuver.
- Imaging studies (CT, MRI) to exclude hernias or other pathologies.
- Treatment (after failure of non-operative treatment) is surgical intervention to strengthen the anterior pelvic musculature (laparoscopic hernia repair).

Impingement: See Hip Chapter

Femoral Neck Stress Fracture:

- Usually occur with recent increase in exercise activity (e.g. new recruits).
- Clinical presentation: progressive deep groin pain which is worse with weight bearing activities.
- MRI will show the lesion and edema around it.
- Treatment:

o On tension side (superior neck): internal fixation is needed (cannulated screws or sliding hip screw).
o On the compression side (inferior neck) and more than 50% of the width of the neck: internal fixation.
o On the compression side and less than 50% of the width of the neck: initial treatment is crutches with protected weight bearing with close follow up for assessment of healing.

Hip Arthroscopy:
- Complications are mainly related to traction.
- See the anatomy chapter for portal of entries.

Knee:

Meniscus Pathology/ Injury/ Repair:
- With medial meniscal tears, McMurray sign will be positive with the leg in valgus external rotation (and vice versa with lateral tears)
- Flipped bucket handle tear in the notch:
  o Patient presents with locked knee (inability to fully extend the knee).
  o MRI: double PCL sign (Fig 1).
  o Treatment is arthroscopic meniscectomy or repair. The tear is usually in the red-red zone and amenable to repair.
- Meniscectomy (partial or complete):
  o The meniscus works to distribute force through its compartment by increasing the contact area between the distal femur and proximal tibia.
    - Partial or complete meniscectomy increases peak loads in the affected compartment.
  o Posterior horn of the medial meniscus is an important secondary stabilizer to anterior tibial translation.
    - Stresses in the reconstructed ACL are increased with the excision of posterior horn of the medial meniscus.
  o Meniscal cysts: usually associated with middle third **lateral** meniscal horizontal tears.

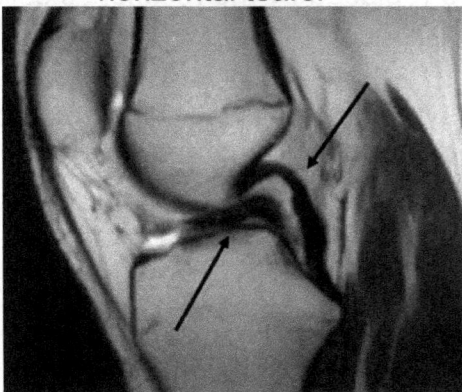

Fig 1: Sagittal MRI of the knee showing "double PCL" sign (indicating bucket handle meniscal tear).

- Meniscal repair:
  - Mainly for red-red (peripheral) tears in young adults.
    - During healing of meniscal tears in the peripheral vascular zone: Inflammatory cells infiltrate the injured area.
  - The gold standard treatment: inside out vertical mattress.
  - Post-operative weight bearing is restricted for about 3 months (in contrast to partial meniscectomy).
- Discoid lateral meniscus
  - Lateral discoid menisci are more common than medial.
    - Discoid lateral meniscus will cover almost the entire lateral tibial plateau.
  - Sagittal MRI will show contiguous meniscus or "bow tie" sign on three consecutive images.
  - For asymptomatic discoid lateral meniscus discovered accidentally (e.g. in an MRI study or during knee arthroscopy performed for other reason): No surgical intervention is needed for the discoid meniscus.
- Meniscus allograft transplantation:
  - **Indications/prerequisites:** prior total meniscectomy, clinical symptoms of meniscal deficiency (recurrent effusions, pain in the involved tibiofemoral compartment), age younger than 50 years (relative), BMI less than 30, 2 mm or more of tibiofemoral joint space (on a 45-degree weight-bearing AP radiograph), ligamentous stability, normal alignment (high tibial osteotomy can be added to correct deformity if needed), and no radiographic evidence of advanced arthrosis (eg flattening of the femoral condyles).
    - Mechanical alignment should be corrected prior to or concomitant with the transplant.
    - Meniscus transplant can be performed with concomitant correction of limb malalignment or concomitant ACL reconstruction.
    - For medial meniscus transplant: better results achieved if the alignment is within two degrees of valgus limb alignment.
    - Use of fresh-frozen irradiated meniscal allografts gives better results.
    - Most important factor to the success is accurate graft sizing. Donor cell viability is not mandatory as they are replaced by the recipient's cells within several weeks.
- Pediatric (adolescent) meniscal tear:
  - Peripheral meniscus tears without locking symptoms can be initially treated nonsurgically. Operative treatment can be performed if non operative treatment fails.

Persistent Knee Pain in Athletic Patients:

- Beware of missed tumor or infection (see tips of general sport chapter).

- If there is persistent symptom despite rest and therapy, or if there is night pain, proceed with further diagnostic studies (do not recommend additional treatment (eg therapy or steroid injection) before further investigating the cause of the pain.
  - The image of choice is usually MRI. Bone scan may be useful, however, it may miss a soft-tissue mass. *(Scenario: 40 years old male, twisting injury few months ago, NSAIDs and rest, still in pain, O/E posterior tenderness, negative meniscus signs, next step?)*

ACL Injuries and Reconstruction (See anatomy section):

- Anatomy: see anatomy chapter.
- **Mechanism of injury:**
  - Can be noncontact or contact injuries. Both will lead to anterior translation and **internal rotation of tibia** causing the injury (valgus **external rotation of the femur on a fixed tibia**).
    - Noncontact injuries occur with the knee in slight flexion, valgus, and internal rotation (valgus component causes lateral compartment bone bruising which can be detected in MRI)
    - Contact injuries: lateral-side impact producing a valgus force to the knee.
    - In the ACL-deficient knee, posterior horn of the medial meniscus provides secondary restraint to anterior tibial translation.
- **Clinical presentation:**
  - History of knee trauma followed by popping, immediate swelling, pain, and inability to walk is highly suggestive of ACL injury (around 70% sensitive).
  - Physical exam: positive Lackman's test, anterior drawer and pivot shift.
    - The AM bundle controls translation, especially during flexion (90°), whereas the PL bundle controls rotation (detected by Pivot shift, see later) and translation in early flexion (30°).
  - Quads avoidance gait:
    - Abnormal kinematics in ACL-deficient knee: absence of the normal femoral internal rotation and decreased anterior translation of the tibia during late swing (due to adaptive decrease in quadriceps contraction and increase in hamstring contraction).
  - Positive Pivot shift:
    - Technique: a valgus force to the fully extended and internally rotated knee. As the knee is brought into flexion, a clunk occurs around 30° of flexion.
    - Detect the rotational stability function of the ACL which is mainly by the PL bundle.
    - Explanation: With an ACL-deficient knee the lateral tibial plateau subluxates anteriorly with full knee extension and internal rotation. With

knee flexion, the lateral tibial plateau slides posteriorly into a reduced position, producing the clunk. The ilio-tibial band with flexion moment helps reduce the tibia in the pivot shift test.
- Pivot shift can detect failure to construct the PL bundle (leading to rotation instability).
- The pivot shift test is significantly associated with patient satisfaction, activity limitation, and sports participation.
- XR: Segond fracture (avulsion of the **anterolateral** capsule attachment of the proximal tibia).
- MRI picture (Fig 2):
  - Will show the ACL injury.
  - **Posterolateral** tibia and **lateral** femoral condyle bone brusing.
- Associated meniscal injury:
  - Acute ACL injury: most commonly associated injury is concomitant **lateral** meniscal tear.
  - Chronic ACL injury: can lead to bucket handle **medial** meniscal tear most likely secondary to its role as a secondary restraint.

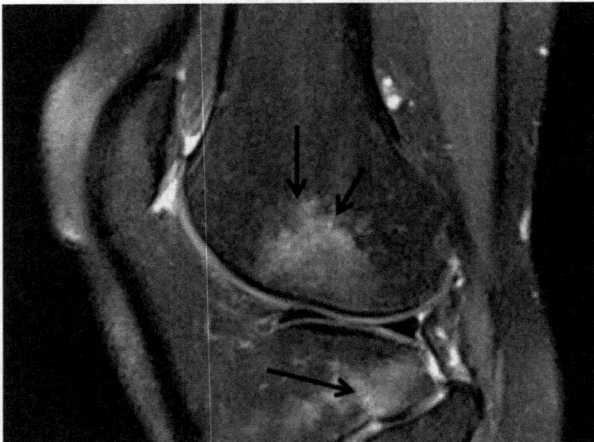

Fig 2: Bony lesion in ACL injury. Notice the edema (bony contusion) in the lateral femoral condyle and and postero-lateral tibial condyles (arrow).

- **Management:**
  - Initial acute management of ACL injury is physical therapy for regaining the range of motion and strength.
    - Immediate ACL reconstruction carries an increased risk for postsurgical stiffness. Delaying the surgery after regaining the range of motion of the knee is preferred by most surgeons.
  - Hamstring strengthening support the ACL ligament by resisting anterior translation of the tibia.
  - **Definitive Treatment:**
    - If the patient wants to go back to sport activity: delayed ligament reconstruction.

- For pediatric patient: bracing can be tried, however, bracing and continued activity can lead to meniscal and chondral lesion.
- **Double bundle reconstruction:**
  - Biomechanical studies have shown that double-bundle reconstruction more closely duplicate normal knee kinematics (compared to single bundle); however clinical outcomes, were found to be the same between both techniques
- **Tunnel position**
  - Vertically oriented graft (femoral tunnel at 12 position) will fail to reconstruct the PL bundle leading to decreased rotational stability and instability with cutting movements. It will also impinge against the PCL. *(Scenario: ACL reconstruction at 12 o'clock position, physical exam will show? (positive pivot shift)).*
  - The most common cause of failure of primary ACL reconstruction is **surgical technical error.**
    - **Most common surgical error is tunnel malposition.** *(Scenario: ACL reconstruction, 8 months' later failure, most common cause?)*
  - Most common tunnel mal position is **anterior position of femoral tunnel** (anterior to the intercondylar ridge).
    - Most common technical error.
    - Will cause the graft to be **tight in flexion (loss of flexion)** and lax in extension
    - Associated with adverse effect on clinical outcomes and can result in stretching and failure of the graft. *(Scenario: ACL reconstruction, patient had limited flexion, and then had failure of fixation, what is the possible cause?)*
  - Tibial tunnel:
    - Should be placed posterior to a line extending from Blumenstat's line when the knee is in full extension.
    - Center of tibia tunnel placement should be along the posterior aspect of the anterior horn of the lateral meniscus
    - A tibial tunnel drilled too anteriorly will limit full extension (due to notch impingement of the graft) and causes tightness in flexion.
  - Trans-tibial drilling:
    - The tibial tunnel will influence femoral tunnel placement.
    - Tibia tunnel placed too anteriorly can lead to a vertical graft orientation (rotational instability and PCL impingement, see before).
    - The surgeon should assess the position of femoral tunnel after the tibial tunnel is drilled, and if it will lie in a vertical position (1, 12 or 11), a separate portal for femoral drilling (antero-medial) with the knee hyper flexed should be done.
  - Impingement of the graft on the femoral notch is caused by anterior placement of the tibial tunnel or inadequate notchplasty.
  - Graft-screw divergence (angle between bone plug of BTB and interference screw) > 15-30° may lead to failure of fixation due to loss of pull-out strength leading to early ACL failure. Efforts should be done to decrease this angle to less than 15°.
- **Post-operatively rehabilitation:**

- o Lowest strain exercises are isometric hamstring contractions at 60 degrees of knee flexion.
- o Isometric quadriceps contraction with knee extended (e.g. straight leg raises or quads set) places little stress on an ACL graft.
  - Isokinetic and isotonic quadriceps strengthening are generally not recommended in the first 6 weeks.
- o Open chain leg extension exercises (e.g. seated leg extension exercises or non-weight bearing terminal knee extension) place the greatest amount of anterior shear stress on the anterior cruciate ligament.
  - This shear is greatest between 0-30° of extension. *(Question: what exercise to avoid after ACL reconstruction?) (Question: what degrees in seated leg extension cause most shear stress on the ACL graft?) (Question: what exercise causes significant anterior tibial translation?)*
- o Early accelerated vs non-accelerated rehabilitation has no significant difference in long term results regarding number of graft failures, laxity or knee scores.
- **Graft in ACL surgery:**
  - o Graft incorporation
    - The first phase: inflammatory response with donor cell degeneration. The graft will act as a scaffold for host cell migration (first 3 weeks).
    - The second phase: revascularization with host cell fibroblast migration into the graft structure (up to 6 months).
    - The final phase: remodeling of the graft into a more organized pattern of collagen structure.
  - o Initial graft tension will decrease shortly after the graft is applied (stress relaxation)
    - Preconditioning an ACL graft can reduce the amount of stress relaxation by up to 50%
    - Stretching of the graft occurs over time as the graft is loaded (Creep).
  - o Quadruple semitendinosus and gracilis tendons graft has the highest biomechanical maximum load to failure (more than native ACL).
  - o Bone-patella tendon-bone (BTB) autograft harvesting can be complicated by patellar fracture or patellar tendon rupture. *(Scenario: ACL with BTB bone graft, 2 weeks follow up, unable to extend the knee, XR patella alta; diagnosis?)*
  - o Horizontal incision for BTB graft harvesting is associated with less injury to the intra patellar branches of the saphenous nerve and better cosmetic scar, however it is technically more difficult.
  - o BTB (compared to hamstrings graft):
    - Has the advantage of faster incorporation into the bone tunnels.
    - Is associated with higher incidence of anterior knee pain.
    - Has higher rate of second surgery for manipulation of the knee with or without lysis of adhesions.
    - Other less significant differences: BTB has better stability on KT-1000, and lower incidence of graft failure. The hamstring graft has higher incidence of hardware removal.
  - o **ACL Allograft (see also general chapter):**

- The incidence of pre-implantation positive cultures of allografts used for anterior cruciate ligament reconstruction is about 10%.
  - The treatment of low- virulence organisms (eg coagulase negative staph) is unnecessary if there is no evidence of clinical infection.
  - The routine culture of allograft tissue is not recommended.
- Antigenicity in allograft is mainly related to bone component more than soft tissue component.
  - BTB allograft has more immunogenicity than hamstring allograft.
- Compared to similar autograft, allografts showed a prolonged inflammatory response, slower rate of biological incorporation and remodeling, and a higher proportion of larger-diameter collagen fibrils.
- The intra-articular portion of an allograft undergoes an initial phase of necrosis followed by invasion by host synovial cells forming an acellular collagen scaffold.
- Cryopreservation uses chemicals to remove cellular water to prevent ice crystal formation. Allograft is stored in a cryoprotectant solution of dimethyl sulfoxide or glycerol to displace the cellular water
- **Sterilization:**
  - Low dose gamma irradiation (less than 3 megarads) with antibiotic soaks is the most commonly used method for sterilization.
  - Sterilization by gamma irradiation at or higher than 3 megarads significantly decreases the structural and mechanical properties of an allograft.
  - Elimination of HIV with gamma irradiation requires doses greater than 3.5 megarads which can alter the mechanical properties of the allograft.
  - Ethylene oxide sterilization can be complicated by post implantation chronic inflammatory process.
- **Female Patients with ACL injury:**
  - Female athletes have higher rate of ACL injury than male athletes (5-8 times more):
    - Most import factor for higher rate of ACL injuries is neuromuscular factor (muscular imbalance and relative weakness of the hamstrings**).**
    - Techniques which focus on increasing patient neuromuscular control during playing are effective at preventing female ACL injuries (however, there are some controversies around this topic).
    - Females have greater total valgus knee loading during landing and greater maximum valgus knee angle than males (the more valgus moment, the more prone to ACL injury).
    - Other reasons: smaller notch size, generalized ligamentous laxity.
- **Post-operative complications of ACL surgery:**
  - **Acute Infection after ACL:**

- Will present with increased pain, swelling and discharge few days after surgery.
- Initial management is aspiration and culture.
- When diagnosis if confirmed: urgent irrigation and debridement.
- Preservation of the graft is possible in cases of early infection.
  - o Infrapatellar contracture syndrome after ACL surgery:
    - A complication of ACL surgery characterized by: patella baja, decreased active knee extension, decrease range of knee flexion (active and passive).
  - o Disease transmission:
    - The incidence of HIV disease transmission by allograft is about 1 in 1.6 million in adequately screened specimens (see general chapter).
  - o Postoperative hemoarthrosis:
    - Clinical presentation: knee pain and swelling in the first week after ACL reconstruction with inability to perform a straight leg raise or activation of quadriceps. Limited ROM. No signs of infection (clean incision).
    - Treatment: knee aspiration.

PCL Injury and Reconstruction:

- Bundles: see anatomy chapter. Anterolateral bundle PCL is at maximum tension with the knee in 90 flexion (the posteromedial bundle tensions both in extension and in high flexion).
- Classic mechanism for injury is anterior blow to the flexed tibia with plantar flexion of the ankle. *(Scenario: skate board injury with laceration on the anterior surface of the tibia and ankle, what injury is suspected?)*
- Complete rupture of the PCL leads to increased contact pressures in the patellofemoral and medial compartments of the knee.
  - o Late cartilage injury can occur in the medial femoral condyle and patella in cases of untreated PCL.
- On exam: posterior drawer test and quadriceps active tests.
  - o Quadriceps active test: patient lies supine with hip and knee flexed. In PCL deficient knee, the tibial will be sagging and when patient tries to activate his quadriceps to extend the knee, its first action will be pulling the tibia anterior to its normal place.
- **Treatment:**
  - o Isolated PCL injury: non operative treatment is sufficient in most cases.
  - o The PCL can be reconstructed using either single bundle or double bundle technique.
    - Single bundle PCL reconstruction: should be tightened at 90 flexion.
    - Double-bundled PCL reconstruction: the anterolateral bundle is tensioned with the knee in a position of mid flexion and the posteromedial bundle is tensioned in extension (tensioning of the posteromedial bundle in extension to protect against hyperextension).

o Advantage of the tibial inlay fixation (compared to transtibial tunnel technique) is the elimination of the 90-degree "killer" turn at the tibial aperture of the tunnel.

o For PCL deficient knee, therapy will be in the form of quads strengthening to prevent posterior translation of the tibia in relation to the femur.

Postero-Lateral Corner (PLC)

- **Dial test:**
  - o Increased external rotation of the tibia at 30: injury to PLC.
  - o Increased external rotation of the tibia at 30 and 90: combined PLC and PCL
- If PLC injury is associated with a varus knee alignment, treatment should include a valgus-producing HTO. *(Scenario: 26-year-old, positive dial test, had reconstruction 2 years ago, now has recurrence, XR shows 7 degrees of mechanical varus, treatment?).*
  - o Varus knee alignment is the most predictive factor of failure following PLC reconstruction
- Late failure of ACL or PCL reconstructions: most commonly due to missed PLC injury.

Medial collateral ligament (MCL) injury:

- Valgus stress test:
  - o If positive at 30° knee flexion: MCL injury.
  - o If positive at 0° knee flexion: MCL plus ACL injury
- **Treatment:**
  - o Nonsurgical management (functional rehabilitation and early motion) is preferred for MCL tears
  - o Tibial sided tear has the higher risk of failure to heal with non-operative treatment.
  - o Femoral sided (proximal) tears heal fast with non-operative management. These proximal injuries are more prone to calcification which is characterized clinically with temporarily increased pain and stiffness.

Prophylactic Knee Brace:

- Can decrease the incidence of medial collateral ligament injuries.
- Not effective for prevention of ACL, PCL or meniscal injuries.
- Can increase the incidence of ankle injuries.

Ganglion cyst of the cruciate ligaments:

- Clinical presentation: knee pain with limitation of both knee flexion and extension.
- MRI scans will show a fluid-filled lesion with an increased signal on T1- and T2-weighted images (in contrast to lipoma which would be bright on the T1-weighted image only).

Proximal Tibio Fibular Ganglion Cyst:

- Treatment is by proximal tibio-fibular joint fusion (especially after recurrence).

Knee Arthroscopy (See Anatomy Chapter):

- For loose body in the posterolateral compartment of the knee, the arthroscope can be placed between the ACL and the lateral femoral condyle for better visualization.

Cartilage Injuries and Repair:

- Before cartilage repair procedures, the surgeon should make sure that the lower limb is in proper alignment. Osteotomy to correct the alignment (if needed) can be done either before or at the same time of the cartilage repair procedure.
- **Micro-fracture:**
  - Activation of marrow mesenchymal cells by subchondral drilling of the osteochondral defect
  - The defect will be replaced mainly with fibro-cartilage (Type I and some type III collagen).
  - Used mainly for contained defects less than 2cm^2.
  - Good outcome with micro-fractures are associated with:
    - Low body mass index, high fill-rate on follow-up MRI of the defect, short duration of preoperative symptoms.
    - Patellar micro-fracture results are generally not good.
- **Osteochondral Autografts (Mosaicplasty, Osteochondral Autograft Transfer System (OATS)):**
  - The resulting healing will be predominantly type II collagen.
  - The transplanted chondrocytes remain viable and articular cartilage heals with surrounding cartilage.
  - Graft fixation strength initially decreases during the early healing phase, then increases with healing of the subchondral bone to the surrounding bone.
  - The post-operative regimen should avoid full weight bearing for the first 12 weeks to allow for integration of the bone plug.
  - Indication: distal femoral condyle articular cartilage small defects less than 3 cm in diameter, symptomatic, with intact menisci and absence of arthritis and proper mechanical alignment.
    - Larger diameter (equal or >3 cm in diameter) defect can be treated by OATS but my lead to donor side morbidity (not preferred). These lesions are better treated with osteochondral allograft or autologous chondrocyte implantation (ACI). *(Scenario: young male with 2 cm cartilage defect in the femoral condyle, had failure of micro-fracture, treatment? (OATS)), (same scenario with 3.5 cm (allograft)).*
  - The donor site for OATS: distal/medial surface of the trochlea (proximal to sulcus terminal) (lowest contact pressure) or the superolateral intercondylar notch.
- **Autologous Chondrocyte Implantation (ACI):**
  - It provides predominantly type II collagen in the repair tissue.

o Chondrocytes are obtained from cartilage harvested from non-weight-bearing areas of the knee then the harvested cells are tissue cultured to obtain 20 to 50 times the original number of cells to transplant.

o Osteochondral lesions of up to 8 mm depth may be treated with ACI alone; larger depth lesions need bone grafting.

o After about 14 weeks, the transplanted cells will integrate with the surrounding normal margins, and become part of the repaired tissue.

o Indications: grade 3 or 4 defects on the patella or trochlea.

o Contraindication: Cartilage loss with diffuse arthritis (relies on full-thickness cartilage margins to maintain transfer tissue to fill the defect). (_Question: what is contraindication for ACI (diffuse joint narrowing indicating diffuse arthritis))._

Patellofemoral Joint:

- For knee flexion of less than 30°, there is minimal articulation between the patella and the trochlea. At 30°, the patella starts to engage in the trochlea.

- **Exam and radiographs:**
  o J sign: a shift of the patella laterally in the trochlear groove and is most pronounced during 30 to 90° of the flexion arc.
  o XR: Lateral patellofemoral angle provide the best radiologic indication for lateral retinacular release (see fig 3).

- Lateral retinacular release is mainly indicated in the treatment of lateral facet compression syndrome.

- **Patellar dislocation:**
  o History of previous patellar dislocation is the most important predictive factor for recurrent instability (another future dislocation).
  o The patella will dislocate laterally, causing possible osteochondral lesion which usually occurs in the medial patellar facet and/or lateral femoral condyle. Small medial patellar ship fractures can occur due to avulsion of the MPFL.
  o Treatment:
    ▪ Immobilization in extension is recommended for first-time acute patellar dislocations.
    ▪ Surgical treatment for a first-time patellar dislocation is recommended if there is an associated displaced osteochondral fragment.
    ▪ MPFL reconstruction is the main current treatment for recurrent instability.
    ▪ MPFL femoral foot print: between medial epicondyle and adductor tubercle.
    ▪ MPFL has the highest tension at about 30° of knee flexion (position of tightening the graft in MPFL reconstruction).
    ▪ **Anteromedial (Fulkerson) tibial tubercle osteotomy:**
      ▪ Advantage/indications: reduce lateral patellar subluxation/dislocation; unload areas of arthrosis on the **distal and lateral** aspects of the patella.

- Contra indications: **medial or proximal patellar** articular cartilage, medial condylar femoral lesions.

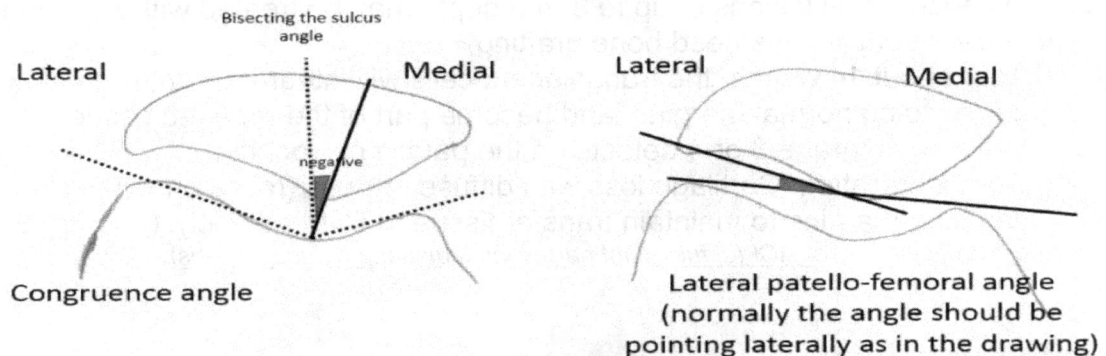

Fig 3: Two measures for patellar position using Mechant views. The Congruence angle is done by first identifing the highest point of the medial and lateral condyles and the lowest point of the intercondylar sulcus (the sulcus angle) then bisecting that angle; then the angle is drawn between the bisector of the sulcus angle and another line from the median ridge of the patella to the lowest point of the intercondylar sulcus. If the line from the notch to the lowest point in the patella is medial to the bisector of the salcus angle (as in the example) it will be considered negative. Normal angle is −16°. The lateral patello-femoral angle is the angle between a line from the highest point of the condyles and one along the lateral condyle. The normal angle should be open lateral (as in the example).

Valgus Producing High Tibial Osteotomy (HTO) (See Knee Chapter):

- If instability (ACL deficiency or PLC deficiency) is associated with varus deformity, correction of the instability should be combined with HTO (simultaneous). _(Scenario: 30 years old soccer player with ACL injury few months ago, on exam there is obvious lateral thrust with gait and XR shows 8° of varus deformity, treatment?)._
- Changing the tibial slope during HTO can help with instability. Decreasing the tibial slope can help with anterior instability after ACL injuries. For patients in which ACL reconstruction is not preferred (e.g. with arthritic changes affecting the knee joint), HTO with decreasing the tibial slope can be an alternative approach. _(Scenario: 45 years old, ACL injury 5 years ago, having medial joint pain and instability, XR medial joint arthritis changes, 7° varus deformity, treatment?)_

Patellar Tendinopathy (Patellar Tendinitis) (Jumper's Knee):

- Patellar tendinitis is common in jumping sports such as basketball. The pain is localized to the inferior border of the patella and is exacerbated by active extension of the knee.
- Treatment is rehabilitation through eccentric training:
  - Indication for surgical treatment (debridement and repair of the patellar tendon): If there is failure of non-surgical treatment or if there is associated disruption of the extensor mechanism (MRI finding or start of a new complaint (e.g. inability to jump)).
  - Cortisone injection is contraindicated.

Iliotibial Band Friction Syndrome
- Due to friction between the iliotibial band and the lateral femoral condyle
- Common in runners.
- Clinical presentation: localized tenderness over the lateral knee at 30° of knee flexion, positive Ober's test.
- Treatment:
  - Initial treatment is ice, NSAIDs and iliotibial band stretching.
  - Corticosteroid injection to the iliotibial bursa if the above fails.
  - Surgery for resistant cases: Z-lengthening, or iliotibial band bursectomy.
  - Iliotibial band excision is not recommended.

Ruptured Patellar Tendon:
- Pathology: avulsion of the patellar tendon from the lower end of the patella.
- On exam: inability to actively extend the knee or keep it extended against gravity.
- XR (lateral): proximal migration of the patella (patella alta) (Fig 4).
- Treatment is by open repair of the patellar tendon to the inferior patellar pole (anchor suture or bone tunnel).

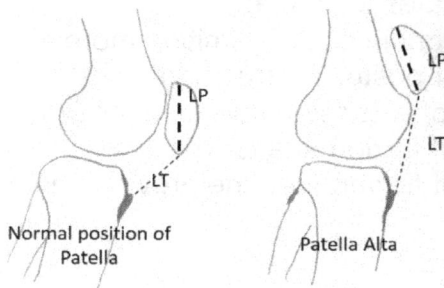

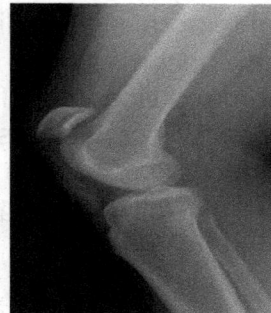

Fig 4: Patella alta. The Insall-Salvati ratio (length of patellar tendon (LT)/ length of Patella (LP)) should be around 1. If the ratio > 1.2, it indicates patella alta. XR shows patella alta in patient with patellar ligament rutpture.

Rupture Quadriceps Tendon:
- History of non-contact sport injury followed by pain and swelling.
- On exam: extension lag, defect above the superior pole of the patella.
- XR: no patella alta (in contrast to patellar tendon rupture)
- Treatment: surgical repair of the rupture tendon to the superior pole of the patella.

Chronic Exertional Compartment Syndrome (CECS):
- Intra-compartmental pressure thresholds diagnostic for CECS are 30 mmHg at one minute post exercise pressure and 20 mmHg at 5 minutes post-exercise pressure.

Stress Related Injuries of The Tibia:
- Will result in tibial pain following recent increase of physical activity.
- **Shin Splint:**
  - Inflammation of the muscles, tendons, and bone tissue around the tibia.

- o Pain typically occurs along the medial border of the tibia.
- **Stress fracture:**
  - o Localized failure of the bone structure with very localized point tenderness along the tibia.
- A bone scan can differentiate between shin splint and stress fracture:
  - o Increased uptake in the tibial cortex in a diffuse, longitudinal orientation is consistent with shin splints compared to a more discreet, localized uptake which is seen with a stress fracture.

Foot and Ankle: See Foot and Ankle Chapter.

Tips:
- Adductor related hip pain: can be treated by cortisone injection; lower abdmonimal hip pain (athletic pubalgia): needs referral for general surgery.
- Both Achilles insertional tendinopathy and patellar tendinopathy are treated with eccentric rehabilitation program.
- ACL rehab: hamstring strengthening, PCL Rehab: quads strengthening.
- Knee XR: Segond avulsion (lateral capsule from tibial side) indicates possible ACL tear; Pellegrini Stieda (on medial femoral side) indicates MCL tear.
- In the knee joint, anterior structure becomes more tight in flexion (limiting more flexion) and less tight in extension and vice versa for posterior structures.
- ACL repair: tibial tunnel too anterior will cause loss of extension due to notch impingement while posterior tunnel will cause loss of flexion due to PCL impingement. Anterior femoral tunnel will cause tight flexion (see the previous point). Vertical ACL will cause less rotational control.

Chapter 15:   Trauma/ General

Biomechanics of Plates:

- locked screw plate construct:
    - Act as fixed angle construct.
    - The screw locks in the plate, does not bring the bone to the plate.
    - Cannot be used as a template for reduction.
    - Mode of failure: simultaneous failure of the screws (catastrophic failure).
    - Indication for locked plating:
        - Osteoporotic bone and metaphyseal fracture. Locked plate system is best used in comminuted metaphyseal fractures especially in osteoporotic bone.
        - Bridging of fracture: bridge plating can be done with both locked and non locked constructs (if the patient has osteoporosis, locked plate is preferred).
        - Locking plate is also indicated in periprosthetic fractures. This will allow the use of locked uni-cortical screws in combination with circlage cables as there is no room for bicortical screws due to the stem in the medulla.
- Non locked plate construct:
    - Act by friction between the plate and bone (plate-to-bone compression).
    - The screw pulls the bone towards the plate.
    - Can help in obtaining reduction (act as a reduction tool).
    - Mode of failure: sequential failure of the screws.
- When using hybrid locked/ non locked plate fixation, the combination of non-locked and locked screws will allow lagging fracture fragments first then locked screws provide fixed angle support.
    - Start first with non locking screw (to reduce the plate to the bone) then use locking screws ("lag" then "lock") (general rule). Starting with locking screws may prevent reduction.
- A non-locking end screw can decrease the peri-prosthetic fracture risk caused by locked plating in the osteoporotic diaphysis (decrease the stress concentration). It also increases the bending strength by 40% (compared to locking end screw).
- Locking screws have more resistant to axial loading (compared to non locking screws).
    - Uni-cortical locking fixation has more axial fixation strength than non-locking fixation.
- Torsional load:
    - When plates are loaded in torsion, the unicortical locked screw constructs is inferior to bicortical locked screw constructs.
    - Unicoritcal locking screws have less rotational strength than bicortical screws.

- o The rigidity under torsional load is determined by the number of screws (not its position in the plate).
- **Mechanism of action of plates (Bio-mechanics of the plates):**
  - o **Compression**: compression applied by peripheral position of screws.
    - ▪ To obtain compression of both cortices (near and far), compression plate should be pre bent concavity towards bone), (Fig 1).
    - ▪ Screws must be placed eccentrically in the hole (away from the fracture)
  - o **Neutralization**: the fracture is fixed with lag screw (providing compression), then the plate is applied to provide neutralization for shear, bending and rotational forces (see Fig 2).
  - o **Buttress**: The plate is used to support the partial articular segment; it will resist shear force at the joint surface.
    - ▪ For buttress fixation (lateral condyle split depressed fracture, medial femoral condyle fracture, volar Barton fracture): must use non-locking screws to push the plate to the bone (locking screws will not push the plate to bone, see before) (See Fig 3).
  - o **Tension band**: the plate is applied to the tension side of the fracture to convert the tension force to compression force across the fracture.
    - ▪ If a plate applied on the tension side of the bone, it will act as a tension band and when the bone is loaded, the axial and bending loads are transmitted through the bone as a compression force minimizing the bending stresses on the plate (provided there is bone contact on the opposite side of the bone).
  - o **Bridging plate**: The plate is used to fix the proximal and distal fragments spanning the injury zone with indirect reduction of the fracture (alignment, length and rotation). The biology helping fracture healing (fracture hematoma) is left intact (hence called biological fixation).
    - ▪ Locked plate in bridging mode act biomechanically like external fixator without compression.
    - ▪ Bridge plating is mainly used in cases of comminution to avoid stripping of the fragments.

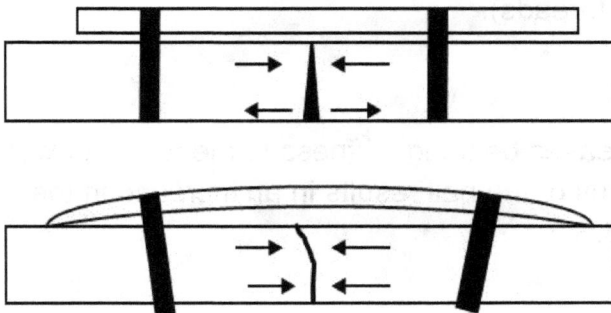

Fig 1 showing distraction of the far cortex with plate compression. To obtain compression on both far and near cortices, the plate should be "pre bent" so the concavity is towards the bone

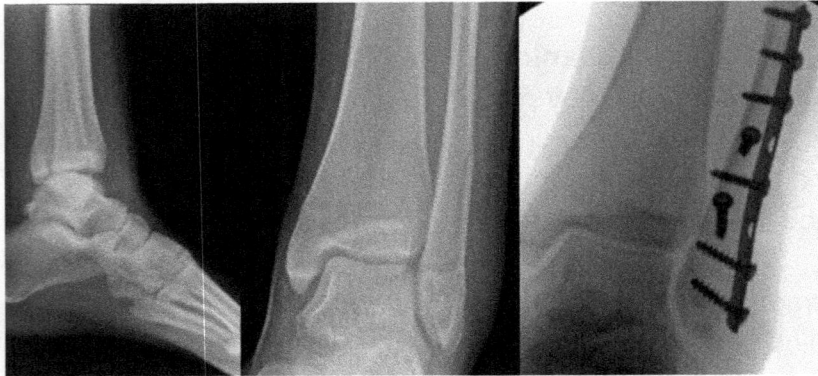

Fig 2: Supination external rotation ankle fracture. After reduction, the fracture was first fixed with 2 compression lag screws then a neutrization plate was added to the contruct.

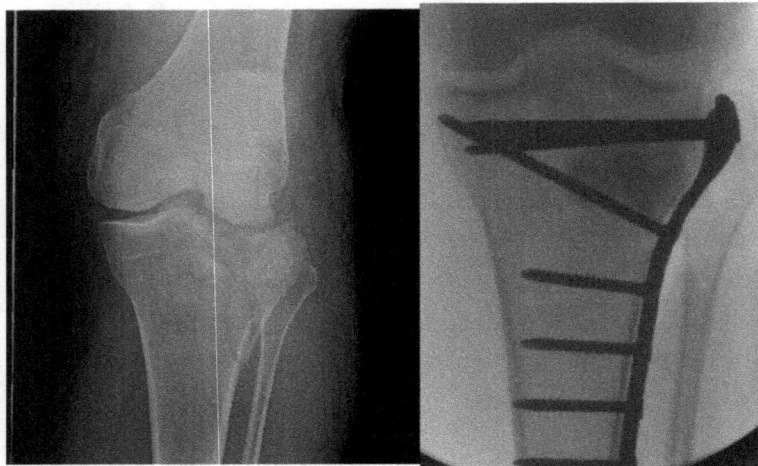

Fig 3: XR of left knee showing Schatzker type II (split depressed) tibial plateau fracture. The fracture was reduced, and plate was used in the "buttress" mode to support the laterally displaced articular fragment. Notice that all distal screws are "non-locking" screws to be able to push the plate to the bone.

Biomechanics of Screws:

- Inner diameter of the screw is the same as the diameter of the drill bit for the threaded hole.
- Screw factors associated with higher pullout strength (bone quality is the most important factor related to pullout strength):
  - Smaller inner diameter.
  - Larger outer diameter.
  - Fine pitch (distance between two threads).

Biomechanics of Nails:

- Increasing the diameter of solid nail increases bending stiffness to the fourth power.
  - This means that doubling the radius of the nail results in an increase in the bending stiffness by a factor of 16.

- Both torsion and bending rigidity of nail is proportional to the 4th power of the diameter.
- The longer the working length (distance between the fracture and the locking screws), the less rigid is the nail (the more motion at fracture side).
  - The shorter the effective working length of the nail fixation, the stiffer the device.
- Causes of less rigid nail: titanium nails, less thickness (less diameter), longer working length of the nail.
- Dynamic locking screw: placed **away** from fracture in the oblong hole (to allow dynamizaiton).

Biomechanics of External Fixation:

- Methods to increase the rigidity of an external fixator:
  - Pins: increasing pin diameter, increase pin number, increased pin spread within each segment.
  - Rods: increasing the number of connecting rods (stacking), decrease the bone-rod distance, multi planar rods.
    - The single most important factor is the pin diameter because it has an exponential effect
- Methods to increase the rigidity of a ring fixator:
  - Increasing the number of wires, tensioning the wires, lower ring size (closer to body), wires closer to fracture, using two rings (stack) on each side, increasing the number of connecting rods (between the rings on opposite sides of fracture.

Biomechanics of Fractures/ Injuries/ Fixation/ Repair (See Also Biomechanics Chapter):

- **Stability**
  - Relative stability:
    - Examples: bridge plating, IM fixation, casting.
  - Absolute stability:
    - Examples: compression plating (with anatomic reduction).
    - Articular fractures usually require absolute stability.
- **Fracture Gap Strain:**
  - The relative change in fracture gap divided by the fracture gap (fracture gap strain = $\Delta L/L$)
    - No unit is used for strain (length divided by length)

- Anatomically reduced fracture with compression across the fracture has low fracture strain (small change in fracture gap).
- A comminuted fracture has a low fracture strain (large gap).
- Incompletely reduced fracture fixed with compression plating has high fracture strain (large change in fracture gap)

- **Stress:**
  - Force divided by the area over which that force is distributed. Increasing the area will result in decreasing the stress.
- **Working length of the plate**
  - The distance from the fracture to the nearest screw is the working length of the plate.
    - The smaller the working length, the stiffer the construct (bending stiffness).
    - Bridge plating with empty screws in the plate (at the fracture level) has flexible construct which allows the plate to avoid "Stress concentration" (see below).
- **Stress distribution and stress concentration**
  - If central screws (the ones closest to the fracture ends) are **close** together, this will result in concentrating the stress on a small area (**stress concentration**).
    - This can result in failure of the implant under less amount of force or under less number of fatigue cycles.
  - If central screws are further **away** from each other, this will result in distributing the stress on a wider area (**stress distribution**).
    - If suspecting motion at the fracture site (bridging technique), it is advised to leave empty holes in the plate construct to apply the concept of stress distribution.
- **Stiffness:**
  - Use of multiple locking screws and use of screws close to the fracture increase the construct stiffness.
- **Biology of fracture healing**: see basic science chapter.
- **Mechanism of fracture and fracture pattern:**
  - Torsion: spiral fracture (eg skiing injury).
    - When bone is subjected to a torsional force, the maximum tensile load is generated in a plane 45° to the long axis of the bone.
  - Bending:
    - Uneven bending: oblique fracture.
    - Even pending: transverse fracture.

- Bending and compression: oblique/ transverse fracture with butterfly fragment. The fracture will start as failure in tension in the opposite side of the force, then progress to the other side as failure in compression with butterfly segment (e.g. If the force is hitting the bone form lateral to medial, the fracture will start on the medial side failing in tension, then will progress laterally failing in compression with butterfly segment).
  - Bone is stronger in compression than in tension, so in cases of bending stress, the fracture will start first on the side subjected to tension (convex) then travel to the side subjected to compression (concave)
    - Four-point bending: segmental fracture (e.g. hit by car bumper).
  - High-speed torsion or crush mechanism: comminuted. *(Scenario: 40 years old, presenting with fracture femur, XR transverse fracture, what was the mechanism of injury?)*
  - **Stress fracture**: due normal bone subjected to abnormal stress (repeated prolonged stress), more common in females, caused by bone resorption due to continued loading without having time for healing.
  - Pathological fracture (insufficiency fracture) abnormal weak bone subjected to normal stress.
- **Maximize pullout strength of screws:**
  - Large outer diameter.
  - Small inner diameter.
  - Fine pitch.
    - Bone quality is the prime determinant of screw holding power in osteoporotic bone (same applies for pedicular screws).
- Implants should not be removed before 12 months from the fixation as it will increase the possibility of re-fracture
- Gunshot injuries:
  - Gunshot bullet velocity below 3,000 ft/sec is considered low velocity.
- Airbag reduce severity (not incidence) of brain injuries and facial fractures after motor vehicle collisions.
- Post-traumatic stress disorder should be suspected if the patient thinks that the emotional component of the trauma is more difficult the physical part.

Bone Biomechanics (See Also Biomechanics Chapter):

- Cortical bone is anisotropic, (mechanical properties are different in different directions) (strongest in compression, weakest in torsion) (see material chapter).
- Stresses on bone are highest at the periosteal surface.

Open Fractures:

- In open fractures, the hematoma that forms around the fracture ends (contains growth factors and cytokines from the platelets) is lost from the open wound and from the irrigation process.
    - o This will result in losing the factors that initiate the inflammatory phase of fracture healing leading to delayed bone healing. Infection may also result in delayed healing.
- Timing of antibiotic administration and adequacy of debridement of devitalized and necrotic tissues are the most important factor in determining development of infection in open fracture.
    - o Acute culture of the wound (at the time of the first debridement of the open fracture) is not indicative for later development of infection or the causative organism (if infection occurs).
- Farm injuries are automatically considered a grade III open fracture regardless of size, energy, or additional soft-tissue injury due to the likelihood of substantial contamination.
    - o Antibiotic recommendations for farm injuries include a first- or second-generation cephalosporin and an aminoglycoside with added penicillin for anaerobes from farm contamination.
- **Irrigation of open fracture:**
    - o Bulb irrigation with saline provides the most sustained reduction of bacterial count in the wounds.
    - o Bulb irrigation and low pressure irrigation have lower rate of rebound wound contamination (compared to high pressure irrigation).
    - o Compared to bacitracin, castile soap has lower primary wound healing problems.

Soft Tissue Coverage:

- Negative pressure wound therapy (NPWT) (e.g. Vacuum Assisted Closure (VAC) device):
    - o Advantages/ indications:
        - ▪ Can be used as temporizing dressing (prevents external contamination, reduces edema around the wound, increases oxygen tension in the wound, and promotes the formation of granulation tissue).
        - ▪ Remove excess interstitial fluid (improve tissue edema), which promotes increased local **vascularity and perfusion** and, promotes/accelerates granulation tissue formation (compared to conventional wet-to-dry dressing changes).

- Can be used over exposed bone. However, in most patients (except young patients with very high healing potential) it will not be able to form granulation tissue over an exposed bone or implant.
- Occasionally (especially in children) granulation tissue may form over bone or tendons. In these cases, closure can be achieved by split graft, avoiding a more complex coverage procedure by a flap. *(Scenario: 8 years old, open tibial fracture, debridement done, defect of 5cm by 5cm with bone and tendon exposed, next step?)*.
- Separate the wound from the external environment which thus decreasing the risk for wound infection (however, it does not remove bacteria from the wound).
- Helps to prevent contracture of the wound (increasing the chance of delayed primary closure).
- In cases of split thickness skin graft, it promotes skin graft incorporation (non-adherent dressing should be applied between the sponge and the graft).
  - o Complications/ disadvantages/contraindications:
    - Most common complication: skin rash (due to contact with a suction sponge).
    - Most serious complication: hemorrhage. Risk factor is using the sponge over major vessel that has been ligated (NPWT should not be used directly over exposed major vessels). Specialized sponges can be used to decrease adherence to vessels, exposed nerves, or exposed bone. If major bleeding occurs, the surgeon has to take the patient to the operating room to explore the wound.
    - Should not be used with exposed tumor tissue.
  - o Incisional NPWT:
    - Can be used for wound with persistent serous discharge (seal the wound and lower the risk of infection) (achieve better result than regular compressive dressing).
    - Can decrease wound complication for "high-risk wound" (e.g. calcaneus ORIF, pilon ORIF).

Shock:
- **Definition of shock:** tissue under-perfusion (inadequate tissue perfusion).
- Bleeding in trauma patients will lead to hypovolemic shock which will result in: decreased cardiac output, decreased pulmonary capillary wedge pressure, decreased central venous pressure, and decreased mixed venous oxygen saturation and increased systemic vascular resistance (catecholamine response).

- o **Compensated shock:** normal vital signs but with **hypoperfusion** of organs due to selective perfusion of the heart, brain and kidney (detected by serum lactate or base deficit, see below for resuscitation).
  - This leads to systemic inflammatory response and increased risk for a primed immune system due to the ongoing stimulation of the immune system. This primed immune response can lead to exaggerated response to a second stimulus (e.g. surgery or infection).
  - 48-96 hours after injury: increased inflammatory response (increased circulating cytokines) (try to avoid major intervention).
  - IL-6 has been closely associated with the magnitude of the systemic inflammatory response to trauma and with the development of multiple organ dysfunction syndrome (MODS). Persistent elevated levels of IL-6 (> 800 pg/mL) indicate an exaggerated systemic inflammatory response to trauma and have been associated with the development of MODS.
  - IL-6 has been identified as a marker that correlates with orthopedic injuries and surgical interventions of these injuries (eg repair of femur fracture).

- **Stages of hemorrhagic shock**

Stage	Blood loss	Response	Treatment
I	< 15% (750 ml)	Minimal increased heart rate (90-100), normal blood pressure (**with widened pulse pressure**), normal mentality.	Minimal support.
II	15-30% (750- 1500 ml)	Increased heart rate (100-120), normal (or mild drop) in blood pressure, decrease pulse pressure, anxiety, decrease UOP	Crystalloid
III	30-40% (1500-2000 ml)	Marked increased heart rate (120- 140), low blood pressure (with decrease pulse pressure), marked decrease UOP (5-15 ml/h), confusion	Colloid and blood transfusion
IV	>40% (>2000 ml)	Marked increased heart rate (>140), marked drop in blood pressure (with very narrow pulse pressure), decreased Ph (acidosis), UOP <5 ml/h (negligible), lethargy.	Colloid and blood transfusion

Pulse pressure (difference between systolic and diastolic blood pressure); UPO (urine output).

Resuscitation:

- Signs that a polytrauma patient is **not** fully resuscitated (borderline trauma patient) (vital signs may return to normal values):
  - Base deficit more than 2 mmol/L, urine output less than 0.5 ml/kg, elevated serum lactate (normal < 2.5 mmol/L), and lowered core temperature.
- When polytrauma patients had been adequately resuscitated:
  - Base deficit becomes less than 2 mmol/L, urine output > 0.5 ml/kg.
  - Can have their definitive internal fixation.
  - Presence of lung injury that had been treated (eg. hemothorax treated with chest tubes) is not contra-indication for Intra medullary fixation. *(Scenario: poly trauma patients with bilateral femur, hemothorax, chest tube inserted, resuscitated, next step in management? (bilateral IM nail)).*
  - The most accurate method to assess resuscitation is by assessing tissue oxygenation **(base deficit and lactate level)**.
    - Patients with compensated shock (see definition above) should have their resuscitation monitored using parameters other than vital signs (blood pressure, heart rate, and urine output).
    - Resuscitation of a patient with hypovolemic shock is complete when aerobic metabolism has been restored in all tissues. *(Question: poly trauma patient, best method to assess resuscitation?) (Scenario: poly trauma patient, BP, Pulse and urine output all are normal, what is his resuscitation stage? (cannot be determined)) (Question: what is the marker that indicates that the injured patient had been resuscitated and he will have minimal perioperative complications following definitive stabilization of long bone fractures? ((Serum lactate <2.5 mmol/L or base deficit less than 2))*
    - Base deficit can be used as a predictor of mortality and a measure of resuscitation.
- For massive blood resuscitation in hemorrhagic shock (especially with patients who are still actively bleeding): the transfusion of packed red blood cells (PRBC), fresh-frozen plasma and platelets should be administered in a 1:1:1 transfusions ratio from the beginning of resuscitation
- **Neurogenic shock and spinal shock: see spine**

Damage Control Orthopedics VS Early Total Care:

- **Damage control:**
  - The patient condition is stabilized by temporary measures (this will be followed later on by internal fixation when the condition of the patient improves). This will help avoid "second hit" (impact of surgery after impact of trauma).

- o Indications (debatable): multiple injuries with severe pelvic/abdominal trauma and hemorrhagic shock, Injury Severity Score (ISS) > 40, ISS >20 with thoracic trauma, severe pulmonary contusion, severe head injury, hypothermia < 35°C.
- o Damage control includes external fixator for the pelvis and lower extremity fracture, I&D of open fractures, splinting of upper extremity fractures and reduction of dislocated joint. *(Scenario: MVC, femur fracture, open tibia fracture, humerus fracture, base deficit 8 mmol/L, urine output 0.3 ml/kg, what is the next step?) (Note: for femur fracture: external fixator is better than skeletal traction)). (Scenario: poly trauma patient, serum lactate 5 mmol/L, next step for femur fracture?) (Scenario: poly trauma, pelvic injury, femur fracture, exploratory laparotomy done, now patient pulse 110, BP 100/50, temperature 35, management of femur fracture?) (Scenario: young female, fall from a height, AP III pelvis, femur fracture, open tibia fracture, both bones forearm fracture, blood transfusion, BP 90/60, base deficit -8, treatment now?) (Scenario: middle aged female, ATV accident, intra cranial bleed, bilateral hemothorax, humerus fracture, open tibia fracture, distal femur fracture, hip dislocation, initial management?)*
    - ▪ For femur fracture: if the external fixator is left less than two weeks, there is minimal risk of infection (similar infection rate of IM nail of the femur in cases of DCO and ETC if the subsequent nailing was performed within two weeks from external fixation).
    - ▪ Contamination rates in external fixator pin sites increase when left in place for more than 2 weeks
- Early total care: early stabilization of fractures in patients can lead to earlier mobilization and rehabilitation leading to diminished pulmonary complications. *(Scenario: young patient with femur fracture, AP III pelvis. Adequately resuscitated, initial management: IM nail of the femur and ex fix of the pelvis).*
- Patients with a closed head injury and a lower extremity long bone fracture: the fracture can be acutely treated by intramedullary nails (early total care) so long intraoperative hypotension is avoided (early IM nail was found not to compromise the outcome related to the head injury so long hypotension is avoided).
    - o **Hypotension** and hypoxemia are major determinants of morbidity and mortality in patients with severe head injuries (GCS <9). *(Scenario: severe head injury, ipsilateral femur and tibia fracture, while doing surgery: what to avoid?)*
- Both DCO and ETC has equal union rates.

Polytrauma:
- Patients with poly trauma and upper extremity fractures that can usually be managed conservative (minimally displaced ulnar fracture, metacarpal fracture), are better treated with ORIF for these upper extremity fractures to allow early mobility.
- Mortality in trauma patients who sustain head, chest, and abdominal injury that requires surgical intervention exceeds 90%. *(Scenario: poly trauma patient with subdural*

bleeding (required decompression), hemothorax (required chest tube insertion) and splenic injury (required splenectomy), what is the mortality rate?)

- **Cervical spine clearance:**
  - o Trauma patients who are non responsive should be evaluated by CT of the cervical-thoracic area before clearing their cervical spine.
- **Metabolic response to major trauma:**
  - o Increased catabolism.
  - o Carbohydrate: increased glycogenolysis (glycogen change to glucose) and hepatic gluconeogenesis (formation of glucose from non carbohydrate materials).
  - o Increased insulin resistance of tissues and hyperglycemia.
  - o Lipid: increased lipolysis. Free fatty acids will be used as energy substrate by tissues.
  - o Protein: Skeletal muscle breakdown.
    - Amino acids converted to glucose in the liver and used as substrate for acute-phase protein production.
    - Negative nitrogen balance.

Pregnancy:

- Pregnant female with trauma and hypotension should be placed in left lateral position to relief pressure on the IVC by the uterus and allow more blood return to the general circulation.
- Pregnancy is not contra indication for fixation of pelvic and/or acetabular fractures.
- Factors associated with increased fetal mortality in pregnant trauma patients: increase ISS, high energy injuries and maternal hemorrhage.
  - o Surgical approach, fracture classification, fetal position, and the trimester of pregnancy have not been shown to be associated with increased fetal mortality.

Scoring System for Trauma:

- **ISS (Injury Severity Score):**
  - o Anatomic system based on the six body regions (head, face, chest, abdomen, extremities (including pelvis), and external (skin and muscle)).
  - o Calculated as the sum of the **squares** of the **three** highest Abbreviated Injury Scale (AIS) scores in each of the six body regions.
    - Abbreviated Injury Scale is a score from 1 (minor) to 5 (critical)
  - o Used for triage and as a predictor of length of hospital stay and mortality.

- o ISS does not consider multiple injuries within each anatomic region (bilateral femur fractures will have the same score as unilateral femur fracture)
    - NISS (New Injury Severity Score), the calculation of the sum of the squares of the three highest AIS scores, regardless of whether they are in the same body region or not (the NISS will be the same or higher than the ISS in any example). *(Scenario: Poly trauma: Bilateral femur fracture (AIS 3); kidney contusion (AIS 2); Pulmonary injury (AIS 4), what is the ISS and NISS? (ISS = 9+16+4= 29. NISS = 9+9+16= 34))*

Abuse:

- Domestic (intimate partner) violence: can be suspected with repeated visits to the physician's office or the emergency department. It is not mandatory to report.
- Elderly abuse: mandatory reporting.
- Child abuse (non accidental trauma (NAT)): see pediatric orthopedic chapter.

Nonunion:

- The nonunion can be septic or aseptic
    - o Aseptic nonunion can be biological or mechanical (or combined).
        - Hypertrophic nonunion is an indication of mechanical instability.
        - Atrophic nonunion is an indication of biological failure.
    - o According to morphology: nonunion can be atrophic (or oligotrophic) or hypertrophic
- For any nonunion: infection has to be excluded first.
    - o Fever or wound discharge does not have to be present in cases of infected nonunion. (*Scenario: humerus fracture 6 months ago, wound healed, patient started in the last weeks to complain of newly onset pain, XR: nonunion with broken hardware. next step? (Blood work to exclude infection)).*
    - o Intra-operative cultures should be taken from nonunion site in every case of nonunion.
- Before surgical treatment of nonunion of fractures that commonly heal without surgery (eg humeral shaft fracture), the patient should be evaluated for metabolic or endocrine abnormality that may had contributed to the nonunion (e.g. Vit D deficiency)
- Broken hardware is a sign of nonunion.
    - o For biological failure: If the fracture is fixed with a plate, the failure of fixation construct will be through plate breakage (rather that pulling out of the screws). (*Scenario: clavicle fracture, 6 months while push up patient developed pain, XR shows nonunion with broken plate, reason for failure? (Biological (e.g. infection))).*
- In general: aseptic nonunion is treated by bone grafting (to improve biology) and compression across the fracture (to improve mechanics).

- The best bone graft option for treatment of nonunion is autogenous bone graft (eg iliac crest bone graft or reamer irrigation aspiration (RIA)).
- Treatment of hypertrophic nonunion is usually by increasing mechanical stability.
- **Nonunion of tibia and femur:**
    - Aseptic nonunion after IM nail cases: treatment can be by exchange nailing (success from 60-80%).
        - If exchange nailing fails, treatment is bone grafting and compression plating.

Infection after internal fixation:

- Early infection (first two weeks): can be treated with irrigation and debridement without implant removal.
- For late infection (more than 6 weeks): should be treated with irrigation and debridement. The implant should be removed especially in cases of infection with high virulence organism (staph aureus). *(Scenario: ORIF of tibia by plate 8 weeks ago, discharge from wound, culture staph aureus, treatment?)*

Compartment Syndrome:

- Pathology: increased pressure within a closed osteofascial compartment.
- Clinical presentation:
    - Severe uncontrolled pain, swollen non compressible compartments, pain with passive movements of the toes or the fingers.
    - Tingling, numbness, paresthesia.
    - Pulses can be normal or mild decrease.
    - 4 Ps (pulseness, palor, paralysis and Poikilothermia (coldness)) are late signs and may never occur. Pain on passive stretch is an early sign.
- Absolute pressure will be > 30 mm Hg, or the difference (delta Δ) between diastolic pressure and compartment pressure is less than 30 mm Hg (e.g. diastolic pressure 45 and compartment pressure 28, so delta is 17).
    - If assessing the compartment pressure while patient is under anesthesia, remember that diastolic blood pressure is usually lower than normal (by about 20 mmHg). This difference (if not accounted for) may result in false positive results.
    - If the patient is intubated and the leg/forearm is swollen, pain cannot be assessed; so diagnosis will depend on compartment measurement.
        - If difference between diastolic and compartment pressure is more than 30 mm Hg, follow up serial measurement (or continuous compartment monitor) should be done.

- o Compartment pressure is best assessed by less than 30mm difference between diastolic and measured compartment pressure
- If a patient in a cast started to develop symptoms of compartment syndrome (tingling, numbness, increased pain), the first thing to do is to split, bivalve and spread the cast. All dressing should be removed to avoid any external compression, and then re assess. If this fails to control symptoms: urgent fasciotomy. *(Scenario: tibial fracture treated in cast, with increased pain, and numbness; what is the first thing to do?)*
- Lower leg compartments:
  - o Anterior leg competent: deep peroneal nerve, anterior tibial vessels, TA, EHL, ED, peroneus tertius.
    - ▪ Weakness of the extensor hallucis longus is seen in cases of anterior leg compartment syndrome.
  - o Lateral leg compartment: superficial peroneal nerve, peroneus longus and brevis.
    - ▪ Superficial peroneal nerve is at risk of injury when releasing the lateral compartment of the lower leg.
  - o Superficial posterior leg compartment: Soleus and Gastrocnemius (NO neurovascular structures).
  - o Deep leg compartment: tibia nerve, posterior tibial vessels, peroneal vessels, TP, FHL, FDL.
    - ▪ Deep posterior compartment syndrome causes pain with dorsiflexion of the toes (toe extension), anterior compartment syndrome causes pain with toe flexion.
  - o Treatment of leg compartment syndrome:
    - ▪ Two incisions. anterolateral (for anterior and lateral compartments) and medial (for superficial and deep posterior compartments).
    - ▪ Soleus muscle must be released to reach the deep posterior group from the medial incision.
- Foot compartment syndrome:
  - o Nine compartments in the foot.
  - o Treatment: three incisions
    - ▪ Two on the dorsal foot and one medially. *(Scenario: 30 years old, a 400 stone fall on the foot, took 10 minutes to remove it, severe pain, swelling, XR multiple fractures of the metatarsus and phalanges, treatment?)*

Chapter 16:   Trauma/ Upper Extremity

Sterno-Clavicular (SC) Joint

- **Anterior SC Dislocation:**
  - The preferred treatment is observation.

- **Posterior SC dislocation:**
  - Treatment is closed reduction with a towel clip. Open reduction with reconstruction of the joint if closed reduction fails.
    - A thoracic surgeon should be available prior to beginning these procedures.
    - Main stabilizer for the SC joint: posterior capsule (see anatomy chapter).
  - For patients less than 20 years old, the injury usually occurs as a physeal Salter Harris injury of the medial clavicle (which is still not ossified). MRI can confirm the diagnosis. Management is observation (remodeling is expected).

Acromioclavicular (AC) Joint Separation:

- To be able to visualize AC joint, Zanca view should be used (10° cephalad with dose of 50% of the standard shoulder penetration)
- Classification of AC separation:
  - Type I: sprain (both AC joint and CC ligament are intact).
  - Type II: Subluxation (disrupted AC joint, CC ligament is intact), widening of the AC joint with near normal CC distance.
  - Type III: dislocation of the AC joint (disrupted AC joint and CC ligament), widening of the AC joint and increase in the **CC distance** (25%-100% increase compared to the other side).
  - Type IV: posterior displacement of the AC joint (through the trapezius).
  - Type V: disruption of the AC, CC ligament, detachment of the deltoid fascia (**CC distance** increase on the affected side by more than 100% compared to the other side).
  - Type VI: inferior (exceedingly rare).
- Treatment:
  - Type I, II: non-operative.
  - Type IV and type V: surgical treatment.
  - Type III: controversial, most cases can be managed non-operative.
    - Operative and non-operative treatment for type III AC joint separation lead to similar outcomes, however, operative treatment has higher complication rate.
  - Pinning across the AC joint (compared to coracoclavicluar screws) has more complications related to hardware migration.

- Coracoclavicular screws usually break, so routine removal after 6 weeks is recommended to prevent screw breakage. Other common mode of failure of fixation is loss of thread purchase in the coracoid.
- Closest neurological structure at risk during insertion of coracoclavicular screw is the musculocutaneous nerve.

Scapula-Thoracic Dissociation:

- Internal degloving of the upper extremity, usually associated with injury to the neurovascular bundle (nerve, artery or both).
- Imaging/diagnosis: The distance between the spinous process and the shoulder is increased on the affected side.
- Neurological affection/status is the most important determinant for outcome.
- The condition has high mortality and morbidity (about 50% flail arm, 25% early amputation, and 10% mortality).
- Management:
  - Assessment of the pulses in the affected extremity. (May need more invasive vascular study if there is decrease of pulse).
  - Neurological assessment (if the patient is not intubated). *(Scenario: 45 years old, fall from a tree, clavicle fracture, glenoid fracture, hypotension, no pelvic injury, next step? (assessment of the pulse)).*

Scapula/Glenoid Fracture:

- **Glenoid fracture:**
  - Displaced intra articular fracture (glenoid fossa) (more 4mm) should be treated with open reduction (or arthroscopic assisted reduction) and internal fixation.
  - Glenoid rim:
    - Indications for operative fixation include: displaced fractures > 10 mm, involvement of > 25% of joint surface or associated subluxation or instability of humeral head.
    - Shoulder dislocation with bony Bunkart: internal fixation of the fragment if possible (large enough for fixation); otherwise if the fragment is small, it should be captured with the its capsular attachment (see shoulder chapter).
- **Scapular neck fracture**
  - Scapular neck fracture with angulation > 40° or > 2 cm of medial translation should be treated by ORIF.
- **Scapular body fracture**

- o The most commonly associated injury with body fracture is chest injury.
- o The vast majority can be treated non-operative (sling for comfort).
- **Acromion and scapular spine**
  - o Displaced scapular spine fracture resulting in shoulder weakness may be treated by internal fixation (to restore deltoid function and avoid subacromial impingement due downward tilt of the distal fragment).

Fracture Clavicle:

- For shaft fracture: the lateral segment is displaced inferiorly by gravity (weight of the upper extremity) which is transmitted to the distal piece through the CC (coraco-clavicular) ligament.
- Open fracture clavicles are associated with high incidence of pulmonary and closed head injuries.
- Indication for surgery: Z-fracture pattern (see Fig 1), more than 2 cm shortening, polytrauma (multiple bones fractures), open fractures, fractures tenting the skin (pending open fractures).
- Complications/outcome of **non-operative treatment**:
  - o Malunion: nearly all patients treated non-operatively will have some degree of malunion. Symptomatic malunion occurs in about 9% of patients.
  - o Nonunion: about 15% of patients.
    - Risk factors of non-union with non-operative management of clavicle fracture: advancing age, **female** gender, **significant displacement,** significant comminution and severity of trauma (which affect the comminution and displacement).
    - Symptomatic nonunion of the clavicle is treated with open reduction and internal fixation (by plating) and bone grafting.
  - o Non-operative treatment of the mid shaft clavicle fracture with ≥ 2 cm shortening (malunion) will result in weakness of shoulder muscle and deficits of shoulder endurance and strength. **ROM will be maintained.**
  - o Comminuted mid shaft clavicle fractures treated non-operatively have higher rate of nonunion and lower patient satisfaction.
  - o Clavicle fractures with greater than 100% displacement: surgical treatment has higher union rates are higher and better functional outcomes when compared with nonsurgical management.
  - o Figure of eight and simple arm sling give the same results regarding union rates and alignment (with higher degree of discomfort related to the use figure of eight band and better satisfaction with slings).
- Plate fixation of the clavicle can be either anterior-inferior or superior (similar union rates).

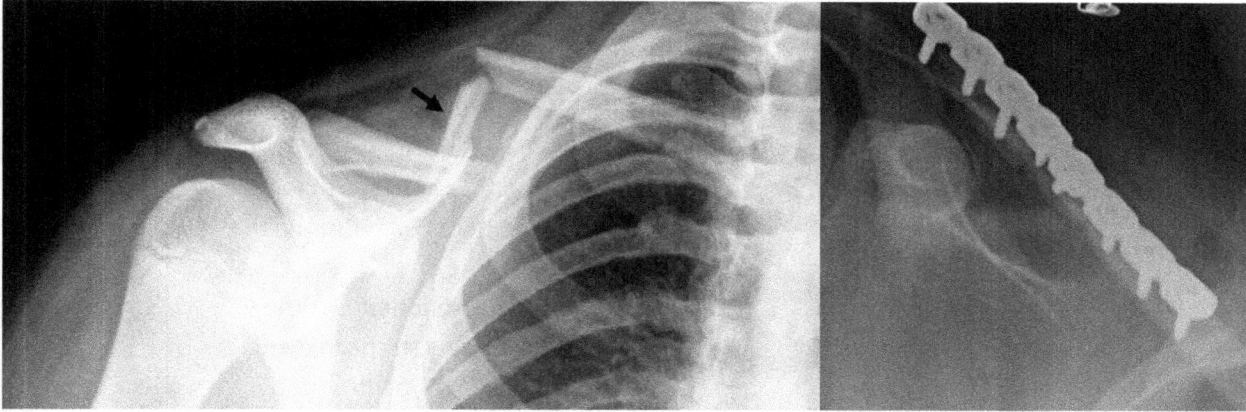

Fig 1: XR right clavicle showing segmental clavicle fracture with the middle part of the bone (arrow) lying vertically between the medical and lateral ends (Z-pattern). The fracture was fixed using pre-contoured plate.

- o Superior plating: technically easier, biomechanically stronger, does not need detachment of the deltoid origin.
    - o Anterior-inferior plating: **reduced implant prominence (only proved significant difference)**, possible longer screws (clavicle wider front to back than top to bottom), and a potential for decreased risk to the subclavian structures.
- Implant removal (due to irritation/ prominent implant or infection) is the most common reason for revision surgery.
- Nonunion after operative treatment is uncommon (fewer than 2% of cases).
- **Lateral clavicle fracture:**
    - o Classification (Fig 2):
        - ▪ Type I: occur lateral to coracoclavicular ligaments (trapezoid (lateral), conoid (medial)) or interligamentous (between the conoid and the trapezoid parts), usually minimally displaced and stable (intact CC ligament). Treatment is non-operative (sling).
        - ▪ Type II A: Fracture occurs medial to intact conoid and trapezoid ligament (usually displaced and needs surgery).
        - ▪ Type II B: Fracture occurs between ruptured conoid and intact trapezoid (usually displaced and needs surgery).
    - o Displaced distal clavicle fracture in a professional athlete: treatment is open reduction and internal fixation to provide the best chance to heal and retain shoulder function.

Trapezoid ligament

Conoid ligament

Type I

Type IIA

Type IIIA

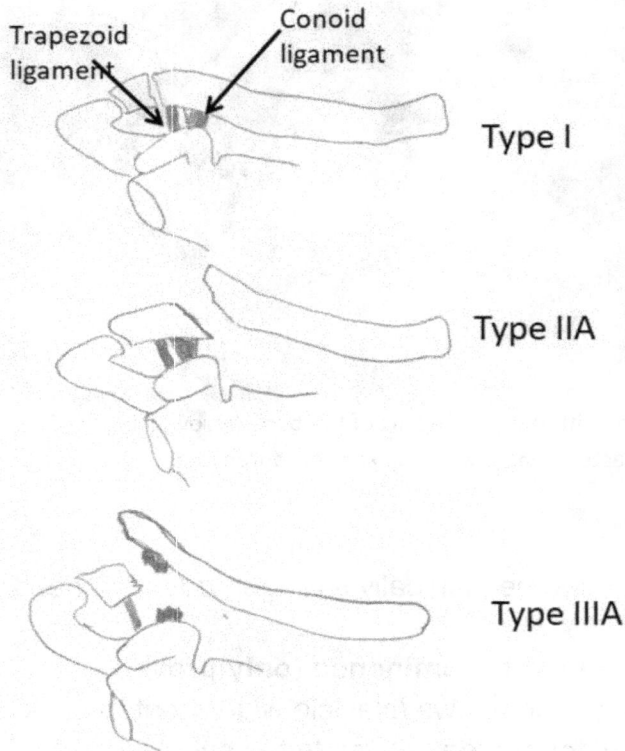

Fig 2: Classification of lateral clavicle fracture. Type I: minimal displacement due to fracture line lateral to CC ligament. Type IIA: the fracture line is medial to the two components of the CC ligmanets (trapezoid and conoid). Type IIA: the fracture line is in between the two component of the CC ligament; however the part medial to the fracture (conoid) has also been ruptured.

Proximal Humeral Fracture:

- Assessment: XR shoulder trauma series (AP, scapular Y and axillary view (or Velpeau axillary view)) should be obtained to assess the position of the humeral head in relation to the glenoid (see posterior shoulder dislocation in Shoulder chapter). *(Scenario: 65 years old, fall, shoulder pain, AP view shows no fracture or mildly displaced fracture, next step?) (Complete the XR series))*
- Osteonecrosis of the humerus head after proximal humerus fracture:
  - Risk factors: 4-parts fractures, angular displacement of the head (greater than 45°), shoulder dislocation, head-split, length of the metaphyseal head extension (calcar segments) less than 8 mm, loss of the integrity of the medial hinge.
  - Highest risk for osteonecrosis: four-part fractures with associated dislocation.
- **Treatment:**
  - Minimally displaced proximal humerus fracture is best treated non-surgically (Sling, early range of motion).
    - Pendulum exercises with elbow range of motion within 1 to 2 weeks of the fracture. Proximal humerus have a good outcome if range of motion exercises are initiated within 2 weeks of the injury.

- Early ROM and age of patient are the most important factors in determining outcome in cases of non-surgically treated proximal humeral fractures. *(Question: most important factor determining the outcome after minimal displaced proximal humeral fracture?)*
- Acute physical therapy and activity as tolerated shortly after fracture cannot be initiated because of the resulting pain.
- No further imaging studies (e.g. CT or MRI) are needed for this type of fracture (other than the complete trauma XR series).

o Displaced fracture in young patient: ORIF
- Restoration of the medial support (medial calcar) is the most important factor to avoid failure of fixation. Other techniques to prevent failure: incorporation of the rotator cuff into the construct, fibular strut allograft, adequate length of the screws to reach subchondral bone.
- When performing percutaneous pin fixation, using a pin fixation through the anterior cortex can place the biceps tendon at risk.
- Most common complication of ORIF in elderly patient is **screw cut out and penetration of the joint.**
- External rotation places the greatest stress on lesser tuberosity fixation (see the shoulder chapter).
- After ORIF of proximal humerus, decrease ROM of the shoulder is commonly due to post-operative scarring.

o Elderly patient with head split or displaced 4-parts fracture in active elderly: arthroplasty (hemi or reverse shoulder arthroplasty (RSA)) is the preferred treatment.
- Hemiarthroplasty: possible complication is nonunion of the tuberosity fragments (predictor for a poor outcome). Using RSA avoids this complication (see shoulder chapter).

o Greater tuberosity fracture more than 5mm (3 mm for athletes) should be treated by internal fixation to avoid later impingement.
- Mal-union will lead to impingement, mechanical block, and altered shoulder mechanics.

o Fracture-dislocation of the shoulder (fracture of the greater trochanter with anterior shoulder dislocation): treatment is closed reduction of the shoulder then assessment of the amount of greater tuberosity displacement. If greater than 5mm after shoulder reduction: ORIF of the greater trochanteric fracture.

Humerus Shaft Fracture:

- Most humeral shaft fractures can be treated non-operatively (starting with coaptation splinting then later conversion to a fracture brace). *(Scenario: 40 years old, mid shaft short oblique humerus fracture, closed, isolated injury, treatment?) (Scenario 50 years old, spiral fracture in the lower 1/3 of the humerus shaft, radial nerve palsy, treatment? (Functional brace)).*

- o Hanging cast: less commonly used now as a treatment option. To assess the success of the hanging cast to reduce the fracture, the follow up radiographs should be obtained in the sitting/ standing position (not supine).
- o Nonunion of shaft humerus after non-operative: treatment is open reduction and compression plating with autograft.
- Indication for operative treatment:
  - o Failure to obtain and maintain adequate closed reduction (shortening > 3cm, rotation > 30°, angulation > 20°).
  - o Pathological fractures.
  - o Open fractures and those due to high velocity gunshot injuries.
  - o Associated injuries: vascular injuries, **brachial plexus injuries**, ipsilateral elbow, shoulder or forearm fracture (floating elbow), bilateral humerus fracture, lower extremity injuries requiring upper extremity weight bearing.
  - o Segmental fractures (higher risk of nonunion at one or both fracture site).
  - o Patients-related factors: polytrauma, major chest injury, poor compliance/ tolerance with the brace, big breasts.
    - ▪ Floating injuries: ORIF of both arm and forearm fractures.
  - o Comminuted fracture (even with radial nerve palsy (either starting pre reduction or post reduction)) are **not** by themselves an indication for surgery (see below for details).
- The surgical treatment of choice is either antegrade locked intramedullary nailing or plate osteosynthesis.
  - o Plate Vs Nail: both have similar results regarding union, however, nail has statistically significant higher incidence of **shoulder pain**. IMN has higher rates of **re-operation** compared to plating (but similar healing rate).
    - ▪ Most common complication for IM nail for humeral shaft is shoulder pain.
  - o Anterior to posterior distal locking screws are close to median nerve and brachial artery (see anatomy for muscles supplied by median nerve).`
- Humeral shaft fracture with associated radial nerve palsy:
  - o Radial nerve with closed humeral shaft fracture (post injury, post reduction and post-surgery) (including Holstein-Lewis lesions (oblique distal third fractures of the humerus with post reduction radial nerve palsy)): treatment is observation for 2-3 months (coaptation splinting for 1 to 2 weeks, followed by a humeral fracture brace with cock-up splint for the radial nerve). *(Scenario: 45 years, motor vehicle collision, transverse humeral fracture, complete radial nerve palsy, treatment?) (Scenario: 34 years old male, altercation, humerus shaft fracture, intact radial nerve, closed reduction done, post closed reduction radial nerve palsy, treatment?)*

- EMG and nerve study should be obtained for the first time around 6 – 12 weeks (earlier test will give false results).
- If there are no clinical or EMG signs of recovery at 6 months: nerve exploration is recommended. *(Scenario: Humerus fracture closed, radial nerve palsy, at 6 weeks EMG showing no signs of recovery, what next? (observe))*
  - About 90% to 95% of the radial nerve palsy will spontaneously recover.
  - Open fracture with radial nerve palsy: I&D and open reduction and internal fixation with radial nerve exploration
  - Radial nerve palsy at the level of mid arm: First muscle to recover (clinic monitor recovery): BR, last EIP (index extension) (see radial nerve in the anatomy section).
- Distal extra articular humeral shaft fracture can be treated either operative or non-operative.
  - Both have similar rates of healing.
  - Operative treatment achieves more predictable alignment and potentially quicker return of function but risks iatrogenic nerve injury, infection and possible need for reoperation.
  - Functional bracing can be associated with skin problems and varying degrees of angular deformity, but function and range of motion are usually excellent.
- Open fractures (I, II, IIIA) of the upper extremity (humerus and forearm) can be treated with debridement of the wound followed by open reduction and internal fixation in the same setting (in contrast to lower extremity). *(Scenario: open grade II of humerus and both bones forearm, patient stable, debridement done, next step? (ORIF all fractures)).*

Intra-Articular Distal Humerus Facture:

- Intra-articular distal humerus fractures are best approached through posterior approach, using olecranon chevron osteotomy to clearly visualize the reduction of the articular surface.
  - Fixation is strongest with dual column plating (90-90 (perpendicular) or parallel plating). Recent biomechanical studies indicate that **parallel medial and lateral plates provide greater rigidity than perpendicular 90-90 plating**.
  - The most common complication associated olecranon osteotomy for fixation of distal humerus fracture is symptomatic hardware (about 70%).
  - Most common post-operative complication after ORIF of distal humeral fracture is loss of ROM of the elbow (stiffness).
  - Prognosis after treatment: loss of some of the range of motion of the elbow and about 25% loss of flexion strength.
  - Triceps splitting is an alternative to olecranon osteotomy.

- Displaced, comminuted, intercondylar distal humerus fracture in patient older than age 65 years (especially in those with comorbidities affecting bone health (eg osteoporosis, rheumatoid arthritis and oral corticosteroid use)): preferred treatment is total elbow arthroplasty as it can produce better outcome compared with open reduction and internal fixation. *(Scenario: 75 years old female with distal humerus fracture. XR: osteoporosis and a severely comminuted intra-articular fracture, treatment?) (Scenario: 78 years old, male, lives alone, fill down, XR: osteopenia and distal humerus fracture with small distal piece, treatment?) (Scenario: 65 years old, rheumatoid arthritis, on chronic steroid medication, have comminuted distal humerus fracture, treatment?)*
- For any elbow fracture: early ROM is the goal.
  - In the early post-operative period after elbow fracture ORIF: if the patient is presenting with stiffness and XR shows no malunion, the treatment is formal physical therapy and static progressive splinting

Capitellar Fracture:

- Classification: Type I: the broken capitellum is composed of bone and cartilage (small part of trochlea can be part of the fracture); Type II: small fleck of cartilage with minimal subchondral bone; Type III: comminuted; Type IV: the fracture extend medially to include most of the trochlea.
- XR will show "double-bubble" sign in the lateral view (See Fig 3).

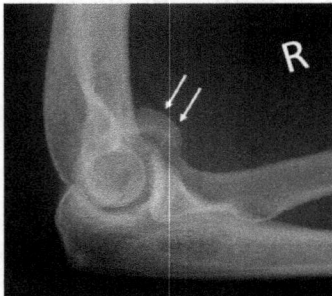

Fig 3: Right elbow lateral XR of 35 years old with elbow pain and swelling after trauma. Note the capitellum fracture which is displaced anteriorly (arrows). The fracture cannot be seen obviously in the AP view.

- Treatment is open reduction and internal fixation.
  - If fixation cannot be done (as in some cases of type II and III): excision of the fragment.
  - Approach: direct lateral approach. *(Scenario: 45 years old, fell down, elbow pain, XR appears normal in the AP view, lateral view (Fig 3) (the fracture capitellum can be seen anterior to tear drop), treatment?) (Scenario: 45 years fell down, CT shows partial articular fracture of the lateral distal humerus fracture (capitellar fracture) and Mason type II radial head fracture, treatment? (ORIF of both fractures)).*

Fracture Radial Head:

- Type I: non-displaced; treatment is sling followed by ROM
- Type II: fractures of a single piece with greater than 2mm displacement; treatment is assessment of stability and rotation.

- o If there is no bony block or instability, sling and early ROM.
- o If there is bony block for supination/pronation or instability: treatment is ORIF.
- Type III: comminuted, displaced fractures.
  - o ORIF for three or less pieces.
    - During a posterolateral approach for ORIF of a radial head fracture, the arm is kept in pronation position to avoid injury to the posterior interosseous nerve (see approached in anatomy chapter).
    - When applying fixation, the arm should be in neutral position (to avoid impingement in the PRUJ during rotation). The fixation should be applied in 90 arc which is outlined by the radial styloid and Lister tubercle.
  - o For more than 3 fragments: excision or prosthetic replacement.
    - If there is wrist pain (suggesting an injury to the interosseous membrane (Essex-Lopresti lesion)): excision is contraindicated.
    - If there is evidence of elbow instability (e.g. history of elbow dislocation, coronoid fracture): excision is contraindicated. *(Scenario: 35 years old, radial head fracture, displaced, 3 pieced, wrist pain, treatment? (ORIF)) (same scenario: comminuted pieces, treatment? (Prosthetic metallic replacement))*
- For type I and type II not causing block to ROM: sling and early ROM (no splinting) (see above).
  - o To assess bony block for a patient with pain from the fracture: local anesthetic (lidocaine) injection in the elbow then assessment of movement.
- Indications for radial head arthroplasty (rather than simple excision) (see above):
  - o Type III Mason fracture with interosseus membrane injury (Essex-Lopresti)
  - o Type III Mason Fracture with elbow instability (elbow dislocation, coronoid fracture). *(Scenario: elbow dislocation with radial head fracture (displaced comminuted), elbow is reduced, how to treat radial head fracture?)*
    - In the above cases, radial head excision can lead to complications including chronic wrist pain, and proximal radius migration (in cases of interosseous membrane injury) or progression of elbow instability.
- Assessment of the length of the radial head replacement:
  - o The most sensitive method is to visually assess the lateral aspect of the ulnohumeral joint with the radial head resected and then with the trial radial head to assess the appropriate length of the radial head.
  - o Intra-operative fluoroscopy can be added (assessment of the radial side of the ulnohumeral join).

Simple Elbow Dislocation:

- Elbow dislocation with no associated fracture.

- Disrupted LCL with intact MCL will show more stable the elbow with the forearm in pronation.
- Management:
  - Closed reduction and assessment of the stability of the elbow through the ROM. In simple elbow dislocation the elbow is usually stable after reduction through a full arc of ROM.
    - In posterior dislocations, the elbow is typically more unstable in extension, so immobilization should be in at least 90° of flexion.
    - If the elbow is stable, immobilization for 5 to 7 days followed by ROM to avoid stiffness.
    - If the arc of stability is not the full ROM, hinged elbow brace in the stable arc can be used.
    - If the MCL (anterior band) is disrupted, immobilize the elbow in supination (as the arc will be affected (more unstable) if tested in pronation); if the LCL is disrupted, immobilize in pronation (the arc will be affected (more unstable) in tested in supination). If the LCL and the MCL are disrupted, the forearm should be positioned in neutral to off-load the lateral-and medial-side injuries.
    - If the elbow completely unstable after reduction (no stable arc): surgical reconstruction (with possible application of the hinged external fixator) is needed. The main ligament that is responsible for recurrent dislocation and needs to be addressed by surgical reconstruction is the **lateral ulnar collateral ligament.**
    - Loss of extension is the most common complication of the treatment of simple elbow dislocations.
  - Indications for surgical repair are: irreducible dislocations, associated fractures, or dislocation which are unstable after closed reduction.

Elbow Fracture Dislocation:

- Terrible triad: elbow dislocation with: radial head fracture, coronoid fracture (the medial part), lateral ulnar collateral ligament injury (avulsion from the humeral epicondyle)
- Preferred treatment is coronoid ORIF, radial head fracture repair (if possible) or replacement (if highly commuinuted), and lateral ligamentous repair. _(Scenario: 35 years old with elbow dislocation, coronoid fracture, radial head fracture, had reduction in the ER, what to expect? (Recurrent dislocation (fixation of fractures is necessary to maintain stability))._
- Most common complication after surgery for terrible triad is elbow stiffness (similar to other elbow injuries)

Olecranon Fracture:

- Simple transverse fracture at the level of the middle of the trochlear notch: treated by tension band wiring.
  - The K-wires in tension band wiring can cause injury to AIN (if they are prominent in the ventral surface.) (detected by failure to do OK sign by thumb and index).
    - If there is post-operative AIN palsy with good length of the K wire, the treatment is observation for nerve recovery.
  - K wires that penetrate the anterior cortex of the ulna in olecranon fixation can result in decrease in forearm rotation.
- Comminuted olecranon fracture or oblique fractures: treated by dorsal plating.
- Most common complication after ORIF of olecranon is prominent implant.

Coronoid Fracture:

- Anterior medial fracture is due to varus stress of the elbow (will be associated with lateral UCL injury).
  - The XR in the AP view will show progressive narrowing of the ulno humeral joint from lateral to medial.
  - Anteromedial fracture will cause posteromedial instability if not appropriately fixed.
  - Anteromedial fracture is an indication for surgical fixation.
- The most common pattern of coronoid fracture with a terrible triad injury is a transverse fracture of 2 mm to 3 mm of the tip.

Galeazzi Fracture:

- Fracture of the radius with dislocation of the distal radio-ulnar joint (DRUJ).
  - Isolated Fracture of the lower one third of the radius (within 7.5 cm from the articular joint) has a higher chance to be associated with Galeazzi lesion.
- Treatment (in adults): ORIF of the radius fracture, with closed reduction and evaluation of the (DRUJ) in supination.
  - If stable: no more intervention needed.
  - If unstable: pining the DRUL in the reduced position.
    - If irreducible (after anatomic reduction of the radius), explore the DRUJ. Assess the possibility of extensor tendons entrapment (especially **ECU**).

Monteggia Fracture Dislocation:

- Fracture of the proximal ulna with dislocation of the radial head.

- Pathology: The annular ligament is disrupted during a Monteggia fracture dislocation of the elbow.
- Bado type II (posterior dislocation) is the most common (in adults) and it has the worst prognosis.
    - Can be associated with posterior interosseous nerve palsy (due to compression by radial head), treatment for nerve palsy is observation (most cases will improve spontaneously), if no improvement by 3 months, nerve conduction test.
- Management:
    - Fixation of the ulna fracture (using dorsal plate).
    - If after fixation of the ulna fracture, the radial head is still non reducible, assess ulnar reduction (usually the reason is mal-reduction of the ulna).s
    - If associated with radial fracture (Bado variant): radial head fixation or repair (comminuted fracture especially in elderly are better treated with radial head replacement)
- Complications: stiffness and loss of some degree of ROM is common. Other complications include nonunion and implant failure.

Both Bones Forearm Fracture:
- Goal for radius reduction and fixation:
    - Restoration of radial bow, length and alignment.
    - Non-comminuted fracture: absolute stability should be achieved.
    - Communited fracture: relative stability (bridging) can be used to avoid de-vascularization of small fragment.
- Approaches (see anatomy section)
    - Henry approach: volar approach to the radius
    - Thombson: dorsal approach to the radius
        - Used mainly for proximal fractures.
        - The arm should to be kept supinated during the deep approach (to protect the PIN).
    - Single incision for treatment of both bones of the forearm fracture is associated with higher incidence of heterotrophic ossification causing bony synostosis (compared to dual incisions).
- Open fracture of the both bones of forearm can be treated by irrigation and debridement followed by immediate ORIF (same session).
- For communited open fracture:
    - If the defect is less than 5 cm: can be managed by autogenous bone grafting.

- If the defect is larger than 5 cm (especially if associated with soft tissue and skin extensive loss): free fibular graft (with possible muscle, fascia and skin from the lateral lower leg)
- For cases of heterotopic ossification: early excision (6 months rather than 12 months) with radiation therapy and indomethacin is a viable option in treating and preventing recurrent heterotrophic ossification in the forearm.
- Plates should not be removed prior to 12 months. After implant removal, the forearm must be splinted for 6 weeks to decrease the chance of re-fracture.

Ulnar Fracture:

- Isolated minimal displaced ulnar fracture: treatment is non-operative (no difference in outcomes between surgical and nonsurgical treatment).

Chapter 17:   Trauma/ Lower Extremity

Hip Dislocation:

- In polytrauma patients, the first orthopedic injury to treat is the hip dislocation *(Scenario: 35 years, MVC, hip dislocation R, open tibia L, R humerus fracture, L both bones of forearm fracture, what is the first management?) (Scenario: 40 years, fall from height, open tibia fracture, closed L distal femur, R hip dislocation, first step?) (Scenario: 35 years old, hip dislocation with posterior wall fracture, next step? (reduction (not CT, as the CT should be obtained after reduction))).*
- After reduction of hip dislocation: CT is needed to assess loose bodies in the joint *(scenario: 45 years, dislocation of the hip, reduction, next step?).*
- If after reduction of hip dislocation, there is retained bony fragment in the joint, the patient needs to have urgent open reduction and removal of the retained bony fragment (and possible internal fixation). Traction should be applied until the surgery which can be done the following day (does not have to be emergently done immediately after the CT).
- Posterior hip dislocation can cause injury to the sciatic nerve (especially the peroneal division of the sciatic nerve).
- Posterior hip dislocation can be associated with deceleration injury. This may be lead to traumatic rupture of the thoracic aorta (excruciating chest pain, radiating to the back, hypotension, tachycardia, possible lower extremity weakness (cord ischemia)).

Pelvic Fracture:

- Unstable pelvic injuries can be associated with excess internal bleeding. The first maneuver should be controlling the bleeding by application of pelvic binder (or sheet). The binder will prevent expansion of the pelvis which will decrease the pelvis volume and prevent more bleeding into the pelvis cavity. *(Scenario: 45 years, MVC, in the trauma bay, BP 80/50, XR: APC III, next step?).*
  - In hemo-dynamically unstable trauma patient with open book pelvis injury: the best method of initial stabilization (of the fracture and general condition of the patient) is application of pelvic binder (or pelvic sheet).
  - If the injury is vertical shear, you may add a skeletal traction pin to the limb on the involved side (with the binder).
  - For unstable patient with lateral compression, the initial treatment is skeletal traction (by application of distal femoral pin) until definitive posterior fixation can be done.
  - The binder should not be left for more than 36 hours (to avoid skin complication).
  - If the patient continues to be unstable after application of the pelvid binder (but not in extremis), patient should be transferred to interventional radiology for possible controlling of internal bleeding from the internal iliac system.

- o Pelvic packing for a hemodynamically unstable patient (for patients in extremis who cannot tolerate to go to interventional radiology suite) is performed by placing a pelvic external fixator then packing the pelvis with lap sponges via a subumbilical incision.
- Predictor of mortality for patients with pelvic fracture:
  - o The most predictive parameter of mortality is the need and the amount of blood transfusions (representing the degree of shock) required in the first 24 hours after injury.
- **Classification of pelvic fracture**
  - o Anteroposterior compression (APC):
    - AP I: widening of the anterior pubic symphysis (less than 25 mm), no disruption of the SI joint. NO disruption of the sacro-spinous or sacro-tuberous ligament. **No surgery is needed.**
    - AP II: widening of the anterior symphysis (more than 25 mm) (Fig 1). Disruption of the anterior part SI joint (anterior SI ligament), disruption of the sacro-spinous and sacro-tuberous ligament. Intact posterior SI ligament. **Fixation of the anterior pelvis (e.g. symphyseal plating) is needed, no posterior fixation needed.**
    - AP III: disruption of all ligaments (sacro-spinous and sacro-tuberous, anterior and posterior SI ligaments). Needs anterior and posterior fixation. *(Scenario: motor cycle injury, XR and CT show symphyeal widening of 30mm, no widening of the posterior SI joint, treatment? (Anterior symphseal plating, no need for posterior fixation)) (Scenario: 40 years old, fall from height, CT and XR shows AP I, treatment?).*
    - If symphyseal widening is more than 25 mm: preferred definitive treatment is anterior plating (4 or 6 holes can be used, 2 holes is not recommended).
    - AP III pelvic fractures are the most common type associated with severe internal pelvic bleeding.
    - AP injury: The vessel most likely injured is the **superior gluteal artery**. For lateral compression injury (much less risk of bleeding): obturator artery or a branch of the external iliac artery.
    - In AP injury, the most common long term sequalae is pelvic pain and sexual dysfunction.
    - Fracture of the lateral sacrum in conjunction of the AP injury (can be better seen in CT) is an indication of avulsion of the sacrospinous and sacrotuberous ligaments.

  - o **Lateral compression:**

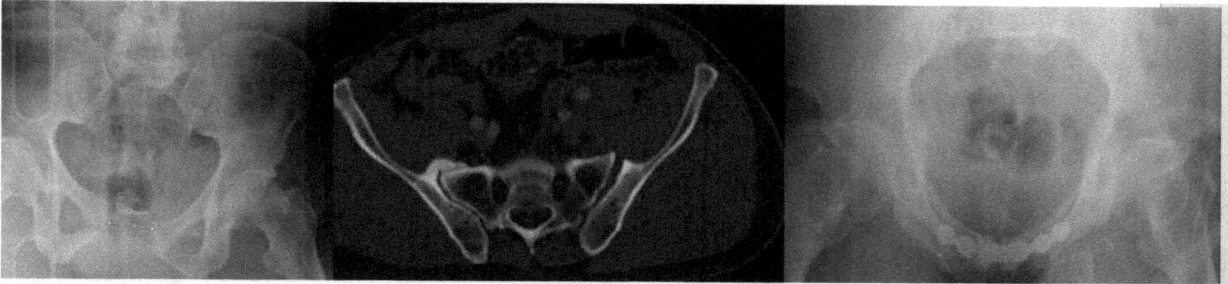

Fig 1: pelvis AP XR showing symphysial widening (47mm) and left SI widening. CT shows failure of the anterior SI ligament with intact posterior SI ligament (the joint is wide in the front and congruent in the back). This indicate AP II pelvic injury. The patient was treated with anterior fixation (symphsial plate), with no posterior fixation.

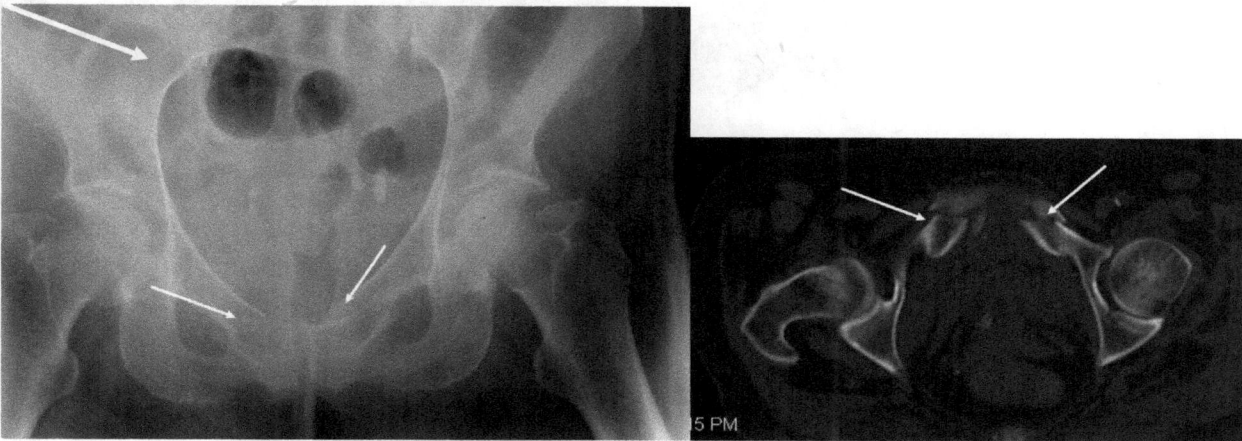

Fig 2: inlet XR on elderly patient with lateral compression injury. Notice the transverse fracture of the pubic rami in the inlet view (arrow).

- XR: will show transverse pubic fracture (seen mainly in inlet view) (Fig 2 and CT in Fig 3).
- Type one: transverse fracture of the anterior pelvis with posterior compression fracture of the sacrum.
- Type two: fracture of the anterior pelvis with posterior fracture of the ilium (crescent).
- Type three: lateral compression of one side and AP on the other side. *(Scenario: 34 years, falling, CT showing the crescent fracture, what stage?)*
- **Tilt fracture**: lateral compression fracture with displaced superior pubic ramus fracture which may cause injury to the vagina. This involves dislocation anteriorly of one pubic bone with symphyseal

disruption and anteriorly angulated ramus fractures. Careful vaginal examination is necessary to rule out open fracture (Fig 3).

- Most pelvic injuries are lateral compression injuries that can be managed by weight bearing as tolerated with no need for surgical intervention. Post ambulation radiographs are used to assess the stability of the fracture

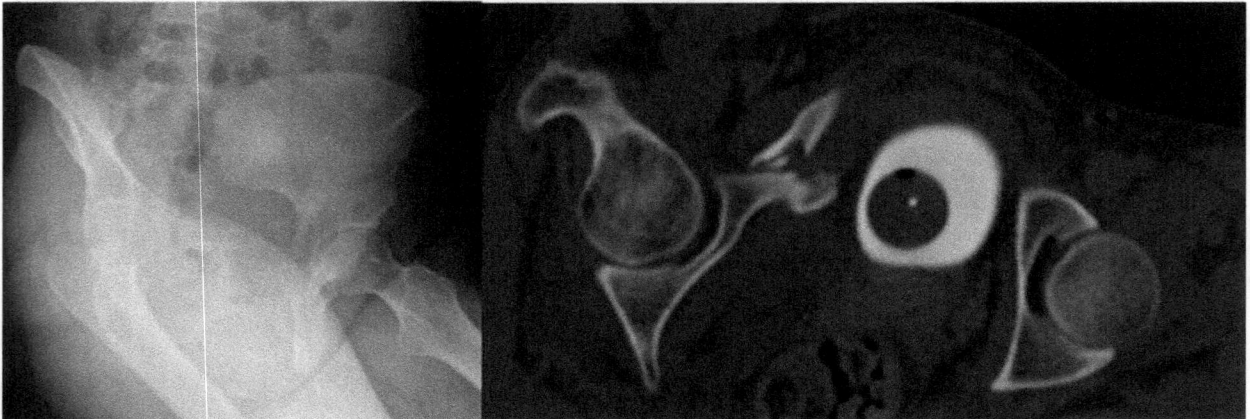

Fig 3: Pelvis AP of 26 years old female who had roll over accident by a tractor; notic the severe internal rotation of the right hemiplevis. The CT shows severe internal rotation fot the pubid fracture with posterior fragment abuting against the bladder and a transverse fracture of the pubic.

- Lateral compression pelvic fractures are associated with more head and chest injury (compared to AP injuries). Mortality often occurs from associated injuries (**head injury**). *(Question, which type is associated with higher need for blood transfusion?) (Scenario: 40 years old, MVC, XR: lateral compression, what is the most common cause of mortality? (same previous scenario: XR shows AP III, what is most common cause of mortality? (pelvic and abdominal injury))*

- **External fixator for the pelvis**:
  - Will help maintain a stable blood clot over the fracture surfaces and venous plexuses and prevent dislodgment of these clots with movement of the pelvis.
  - Two type of pins construct: iliac crest (cluster of 2-3) or anterior pins (AIIS)
    - AIIS pin for: starting point is teardrop in the **obturator outlet** view radiographs (Fig 4). The teardrop represents the column of bone from AIIS to PIIS; then iliac view should be taken to ensure that the pin is superior the sciatic notch.
    - Application of pins in the AIIS require more image guidance and longer time than iliac crest, however they are biomechanically stronger.
  - If trauma surgeon needs to perform laparotomy to address internal bleed, placement of external fixation just prior (or immediately after) to the laparotomy should be considered (if possible).

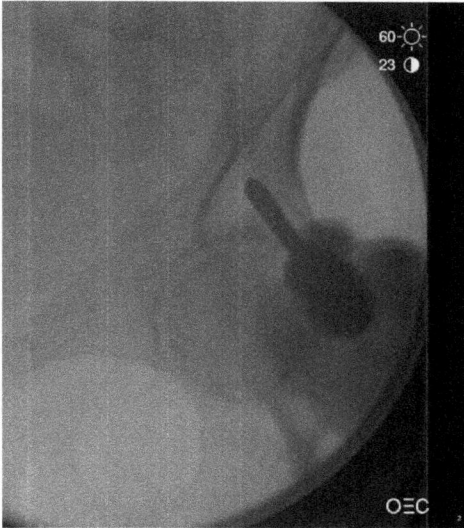

Fig 4: intra operative fluoroscopy using obturator outlet view. The "tear drop" can be seen above the acetabulum. The pins for pelvic anterior fixator are inserted in the middle of the tear drop.

- If suspecting a possible urethral injury (blood at meatus or wide separation of the symphasis (>5cm)): retrograde urethrogram is the best initial test to assess the injury of the urethra.
- The most common urologic complication in male patients who have sustained pelvic fractures with associated urethral injuries is uretheral stricture.
- Pelvic trauma in females:
    o Most common long-term sequelae are sexual dysfunction and dyspareunia.
    o Most female with history of pelvic fracture will end deliver by cesarean section (regardless of whether anterior pelvic fixation is present or not).
- **Ilios-sacral (IS) screws:**
    o Can be inserted percutaneously using image intensifier using combination of inlet view (volar/ dorsal orientation of the guide) and outlet view (proximal/ distal orientation). The lateral sacral view can also be added for confirmation of screw position (lateral view can show both volar/dorsal and proximal/distal orientation).
    o If an ilio-sacral screw pierces the anterior sacral ala (encroach over the anterior wall), it can cause injury to **L5** nerve root. *(Scenario: pelvic fracture, treated by IS screws, CT shows anterior penetration of the sacral ala, weakness of what muscle is expected? (see anatomy chapter)).*
    o To avoid injury to the L5 nerve root, the screw in the lateral view should be **posterior to the iliac cortical density (ICD)** (Fig 5), screws anterior to the ICD can be in the recessed area of the sacrum ala causing injury to L5.
    o Transiliac pelvic screw (much less frequently used now compared to the IS screws): inserted percutaneously, through both iliac wings posterior to the posterior border of the sacrum. The starting point (on lateral view) should be

at the posterior iliac crest posterior to the posterior border of the sacrum at the level of the S1 body.

- **Vertical shear:**
  - Pathology:
    - Combined anterior and posterior pelvic injury.
    - Vertically unstable injuries (posteriorly: SI joint disruption or sacral fracture; anteriorly: symphyseal disruption or superior and inferior pubic fractures).
  - Treatment: needs combination of posterior fixation (e.g IS screws/ transacral screw) plus anterior fixation (e.g. symphyseal plate).
- **Sacral Fracture:**
  - **Dennis classification:**
    - Zone 1: Lateral to the foramen, Zone 2: through the foramen, Zone 3: medial to the foramen.
  - The highest rate of associated nerve injury in sacral fractures occurs in fractures medial to the foramen (zone 3).
  - Sacral fracture with distraction and/or displacement of more than 1 cm is an unstable injury that requires posterior fixation. If there is associated anterior injury, this should also be fixed (either internal by plate or external by external fixator). **Fixation of the anterior pelvis only for combined anterior and posterior injury will not be stable pattern.**
  - **U-shaped (and H-shaped) sacral fractures:**
    - Bilateral vertical sacral fractures that connect to each other with a transverse fracture through the second or third sacral segments (Fig 5); the injury can occur without anterior pelvic injury. These patients will have spinopelvic dissociation with a high incidence of neurologic injuries.

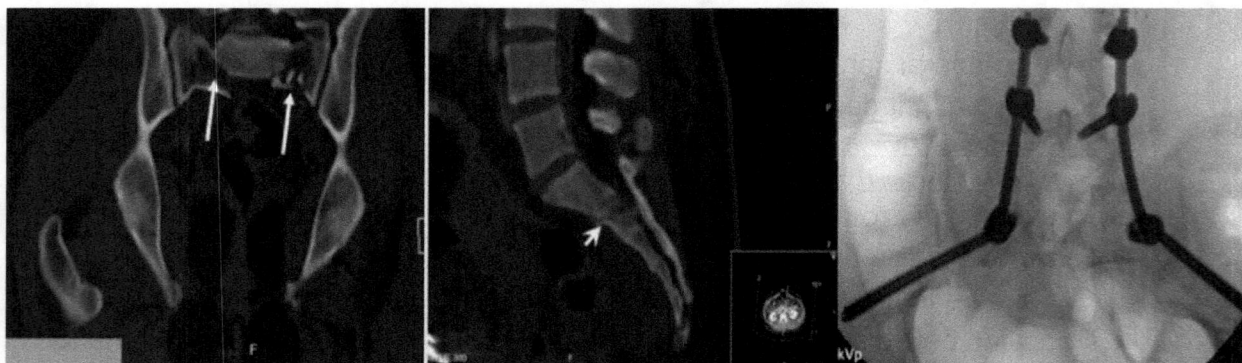

Fig 5: H-type sacral fixation. Coronal CT shows bilateral sacral fracture, sagittal reformat shows transverse fracture. The fracture was treated using spino-pelvic fixation (iliac screws connected with pedicle screws in L5 and L4.

- The lateral view (or the sagittal reformat of a CT) will show the degree of kyphotic deformity and the amount of displacement of the sacral segments. The injury can be missed if only depending on axial CT cuts, inlet and outlet views. *(Scenario: Axial CT showing bilateral sacral fracture, next step?)*
- May require decompression and possible spinopelvic fixation (fixation from L4-5 to iliac crest with/without added sacral fixation) (Fig 5).

Acetabulum:

- The most common complication following acetabular or pelvic ring injury is DVT (up to 75% without prophylaxis).
- Post traumatic arthritis will occur in about 25-33% of cases of acetabular fracture.
- Most common complication related to treatment/ reconstruction is development of HO (especially if double incisions used)
- Morel-Lavallee lesion:
  - Internal degloving the tissues around the hip/pelvis area, associated with higher infection rate.
  - Treatment: open debridement closing only the fascia and leaving the remaining wound open, or performing a percutaneous debridement with irrigation of the subcutaneous tissues.
- **XR and classification (see Fig 6):**
  - The ilioischial line (better seen in the iliac view): posterior column.
  - The iliopectineal (better seen in the obturator view): anterior column.
  - Two oblique views (obturator and iliac oblique):
    - Obturator view: will show the posterior wall and iliopectineal line (anterior column).
    - Iliac view: will show the anterior wall and ilioischial line (posterior column)
  - CT:
    - Transverse fracture runs from anterior to posterior (sagittal plane) in axial view (Fig 7).
    - Column fracture in the CT scan runs in the coronal plane (side to side).
- Acetabular surgery within two weeks of the injury is associated with better reduction and better outcomes (compared to those done after more than 2 weeks).
- Treatment:
  - Non-operative treatment:
    - Indications: non-displaced fractures, roof arc >45° (see fig 7), secondary reduction (with associate both column in which the whole

acetabulum is shifted medially; however, the relation between the acetabulum pieces and femoral head is relatively maintained).

- o Operative indication: displaced fracture (most important indication is failure to maintain the reduction of the femoral head under the acetabular dome without traction).
- o Accuracy/ quality of reduction was found to be the most important prognostic factor to predict treatment long term results and outcomes.

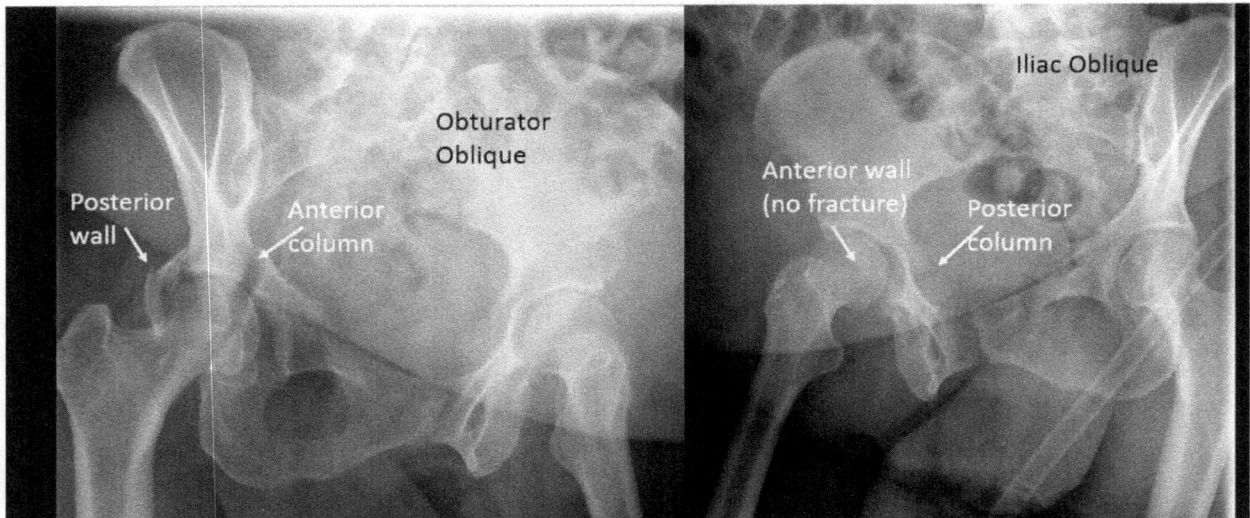

Fig 6: The two Judet views. Obturator oblique view shows the posterior wall and anterior column. Iliac oblique view shows the posterior column and anterior wall.

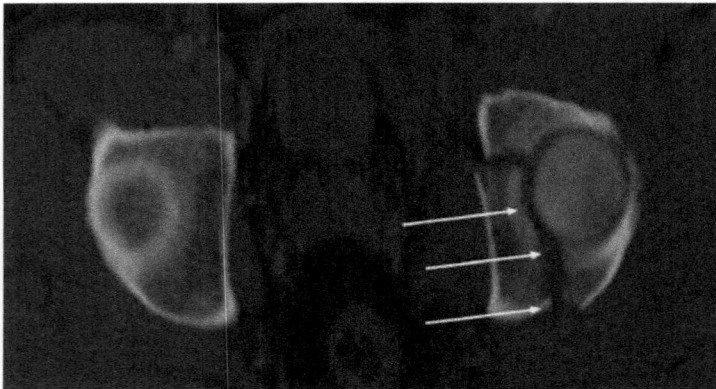

Fig 7: CT scan of tansverse acetabular fracture. Notice that the fracture line in axial CT travels from anterior to posterior.

- **Posterior wall:**
  - o If the posterior wall broken fragment is less than 20%: non-operative treatment, if it is more than 40%: surgical treatment, if it is between 20%-40% assess the stability:
    - ▪ Assessment of the stability is best performed by dynamic fluoroscopic examination under anesthesia *(Scenario: 30 years, MVC, posterior wall fracture in*

the CT about 30%, next step? (Assessment of stability)) (Scenario: 32 years, MVC, posterior hip dislocation, reduced, posterior wall fracture in the CT about 30%, next step? (Assessment of stability)).

- o Assess the marginal impaction (impaction of part of the posterior wall of the acetabulum) and loose fragment in the joint by CT scan (see Fig 8).
- o **Posterior wall fracture dislocation:** urgent reduction is needed follow by CT scan. If after reduction, there is a piece of bone that become entrapped in the joint causing incongruent reduction, management is skeletal traction (to relieve pressure on the joint and prevent articular damage) and expedient open reduction and fixation of the fracture (see hip dislocation section).
- **Associate both columns:**
  - o No connection between any part of the acetabulum and SI joint (no part of acetabulum connected to intact ilium).
  - o Spur sign in the XR (due to medialization of the femoral head in relation intact part of the ilium), can be best seen in the obturator view (Fig 9).
  - o Usually treated through anterior (ilio-inguinal) approach. *(Scenario: 40 years old, MVC, XR of acetabular fracture (obturator view showing spur sign), what type of acetabular fracture? What approach?).*
  - o Can have secondary congruency (the medialized femoral head is congruent with the displaced pieces of the acetabulum which had also migrated medially). Secondary congruency can be treated by non-operative treatment.
- Acetabular fracture in elderly patient usually involves the anterior column and medial wall (quadrilateral plate) with extensive comminution (different than regular patterns described before).
  - o Head impaction (sea gull sign) is a poor prognostic sing if fixation of fracture is attempted (relative indication of arthroplasty). These fractures can be treated with combined ORIF and THA.

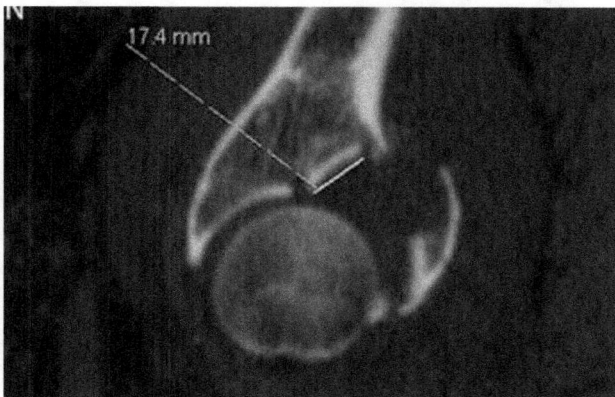

Fig 8: Sagittal CT reformat showing posterior wall fracture with impaction of part of the superior wall (measured line). Notice that the impacted part is at an angle with the rest of the articular surface.

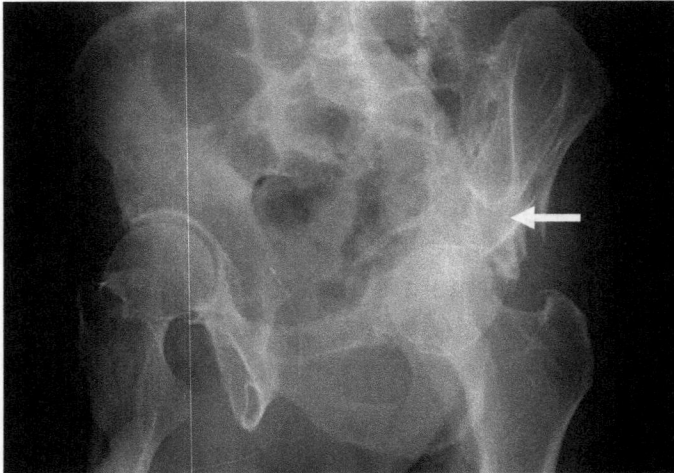

Fig 9: obturator oblique XR of the left acetabulum showing the spur sign for associated both column fracture.

- **Approaches for acetabulum ORIF:**
  - Kocher Lungenbeck:
    - Used in cases of posterior wall, posterior column, transverse with posterior wall, some cases of transverse fracture (if main displacement is posterior).
  - Anterior approaches:
    - Two common approaches: ilio-inguinal and intra pelvic (modiffied Stoppa).
    - Used for anterior wall, anterior column, anterior column posterior hemi-transverse, and most cases of associated both column fractures.
  - Combined approaches (anterior and posterior) or extended ilio-femroal:
    - Used for some cases of associated both column fracture and T type acetabular fracture.
  - For transverse fracture, the approach (anterior or posterior) depends on which side is more displaced.
  - Modified Stoppa (intrapelvic approach) exposure offers the best access to the quadrilateral surface of the acetabulum.
  - **Outlet obturator** oblique is the view needed to ensure that an anterior column screw used for acetabular fracture fixation does not penetrate the hip joint (Fig 10).

Fracture Head Femur:
- **Pipkin classification (Fig 11):**
  - Pipkin I: the fracture is inferior to the fovea (small, not in the weight bearing area). Treatment is usually by excision of the fragment.
  - Pipkin II: the fracture line starts above the fovea (large, weight bearing area); needs fixation in most cases.

o Pipkin III: I or II with associated femoral neck fracture.
o Pipkin IV: I or II with associated acetabular fracture. Treatment with usually by surgical dislocation of the hip by trochanteric osteotomy: will allow fixation of both the posterior wall of the acetabulum and the head fracture.

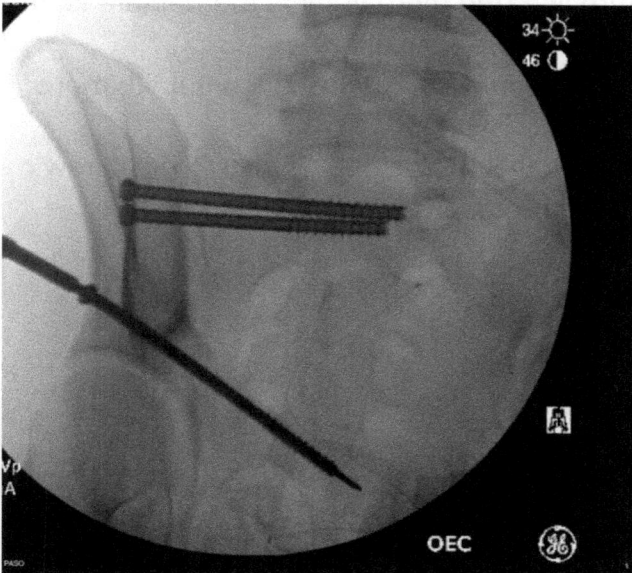

Fig 10: obturator outlet intra operative fluoroscopy used to insure that anterior column screw did not penetrate the hip joint.

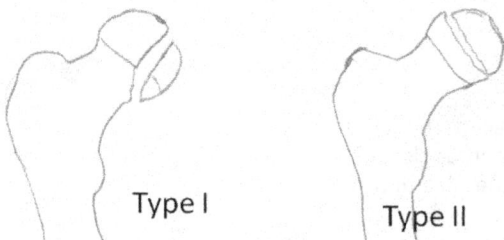

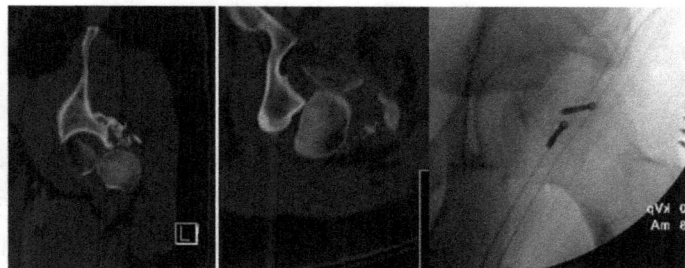

Fig 11: Pipkin classification. Type I: fracture line inferior to the fovea; Type II: fracture line superior to the fovea; Type III: associated with femoral neck fracture; Type IV: associated with acetabular fracture. CT sagittal and axial views showing type IV fracture. Intra operative fluoroscopy shows ORIF of the head of the femur by surgical dislocation and fixation of the fracture.

Fracture Neck Femur:

- **Complications:** nonunion, AVN, arthritis, failure of fixation.
  - o ANV is the most common complication in displaced fractures in young adults with displaced fracture, followed by non-union.

- o Risk factor for AVN: age (high percentage in elderly patients), displaced, female, higher energy injury.
- Delay up to 24 hours and associated femoral shaft fracture was not found to increase the incidence of AVN.
- **Powel classification:**
  - o Assess the orientation of the fracture line (the more vertical the fracture is, the more shear stress and more prone for failure of fixation).
    - ▪ I: within 30° of horizontal line, II: within 30°-50° of horizontal, III: more than 50° of horizontal.
    - ▪ Best biomechanical fixation of Powel III fractures is sliding hip screw and side plate (with possible anti-rotation screws).
- **Treatment:**

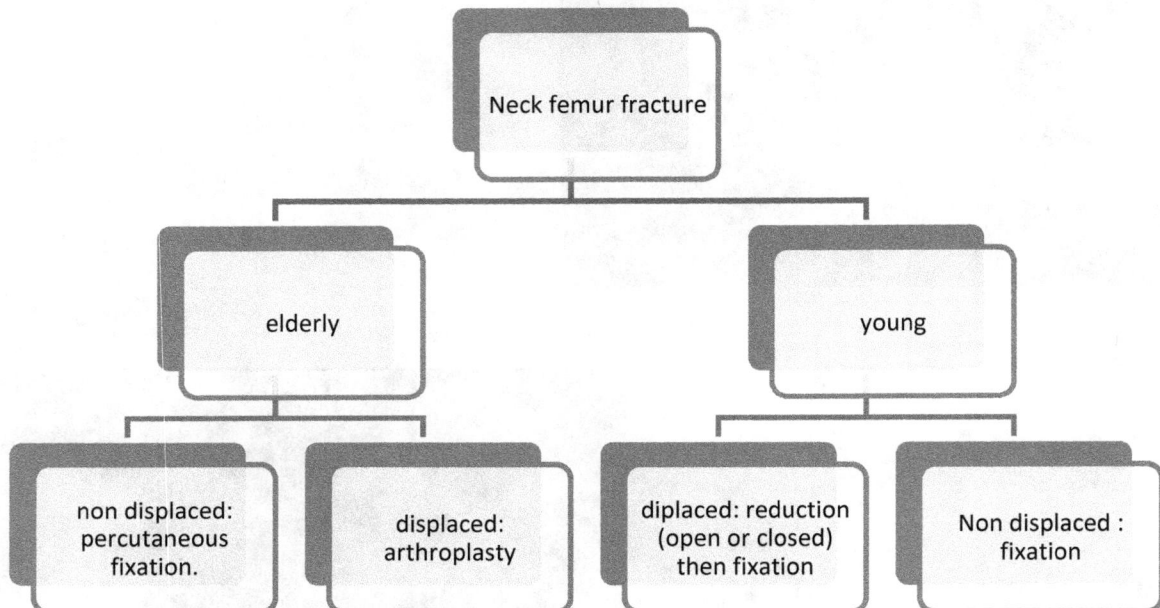

```
                    ┌─────────────────────┐
                    │  Neck femur fracture │
                    └─────────────────────┘
                    ┌──────────┴──────────┐
              ┌──────────┐          ┌──────────┐
              │ elderly  │          │  young   │
              └──────────┘          └──────────┘
              ┌────┴────┐          ┌─────┴─────┐
```

elderly		young	
non displaced: percutaneous fixation.	displaced: arthroplasty	diplaced: reduction (open or closed) then fixation	Non displaced : fixation

- o For young patients, if anatomical reduction cannot be obtained by closed method, open reduction should be done.
- o Quality of reduction and fixation are most important factors to obtain better clinical outcome.
- o Fixation of the fracture: either multiple screws or fixed angle device with side plate.
  - ▪ The construct of the 3 screws: inverted triangular. The lower screw: just above the calcar and posterior (the most important screw). The two other screws are superior.
  - ▪ 4th screw does not add biomechanical advantage.

- If using a screw construct: avoid starting below the lesser trochanter (to avoid stress riser and later subtrochateric fracture).
- Using washer provides bio mechanical advantages (more compression).

- **Nonunion of the fracture neck femur:**
  - Diagnosis: continued hip pain, varus collapse, backing out of screws.
  - Treatment: valgus intertrochanteric osteotomy *(Scenario: 40 years, femoral neck fracture, fixed by sliding screw, 3 months later still in pain, and lag screw backing out, treatment? (Implant removal and Powel's valgus osteotomy)).*

- **Femoral neck fracture in elderly (see the previous algorithm):**
  - Stable pattern (Garden 1 and 2): fixation by screws.
  - Unstable pattern (Garden 3 and 4): arthroplasty.
    - **Cemented hemiarthroplasty** used to be the gold standard, however THA and cementless femur fixation are becoming more popular.
    - Equal results with general Vs regional anesthesia.
  - Should be treated as urgent cases with surgery done once the patient condition had been "optimized", usually within 36 hours of admission if possible.
    - Surgery within 36-48 hours was found to decrease 3-month mortality.
  - If the patient presented late for any reason, screening Duplex should be obtained at admission to assess the presence of DVT.
  - It is better to have patients admitted by geriatric service (improvement in clinical outcomes within the hospital stay, a reduction in iatrogenic complications, 1-year mortality rates and readmission rate compared to the usual care given by orthopedic admission).

Trochanteric Fracture:

- If there is fracture of the lateral cortex (distal to the vastus ridge) or reversed obliquity pattern (Fig 12), treatment is by cephalomedullary nail (NOT by sliding hip screw) which will have higher failure rate. Other options (but less commonly used implant in the USA) for this type of fracture include: 95° blade plate, dynamic condylar plate or proximal locking femoral plate) *(Question: what is a significant predictor of failure following fixation of trochanteric fracture by DHS? (**lateral wall integrity**)). (Scenario: reversed obliquity fracture treated with sliding hip screw, failed, management now? (Revision to blade plate or cephalomedullary nail)).*
- Pre-injury cognitive and physical function is the most predictive factor of post-operative functional outcome after hip fracture fixation.
- Risk factor for mortality after hip fracture: chronic renal failure, obstructive lung disease, congestive heart failure.

- **Technical aspects of fixation:**
  - Tip-apex distance of greater than 25 mm (combined in both the AP and LAT views) is associated with a higher risk of screw cut-out.
  - Failure is mainly due to varus collapse.
  - Short cephalomedullary nail for fixation of intertrochanteric hip fractures are associated with increased risk of a postoperative ipsilateral femoral shaft fracture.
  - Cephalo-medullary nails (especially the old designs) for trochanteric fracture have larger diameter (less curved) than the femur diameter in elderly, this may lead to penetration of the distal tip of the nail trough the anterior cortex of the femur (mismatch between the nail diameter (larger) and femur diameter (smaller)). New nail designs have smaller radius of curvature (more bent).
  - Cases of failed fixation (cut out of the screw with varus collapse):
    - For the elderly patient: treatment is conversion to total hip arthroplasty with a calcar replacement femoral component that bypasses the hardware.
    - For young patients: revision fixation with valgus osteotomy.
  - Entry point of the cephalomedullary nails should be the tip of the greater trochanter. Entry point that is more lateral than what it is supposed to be will result in varus deformity and possible failure of fixation.

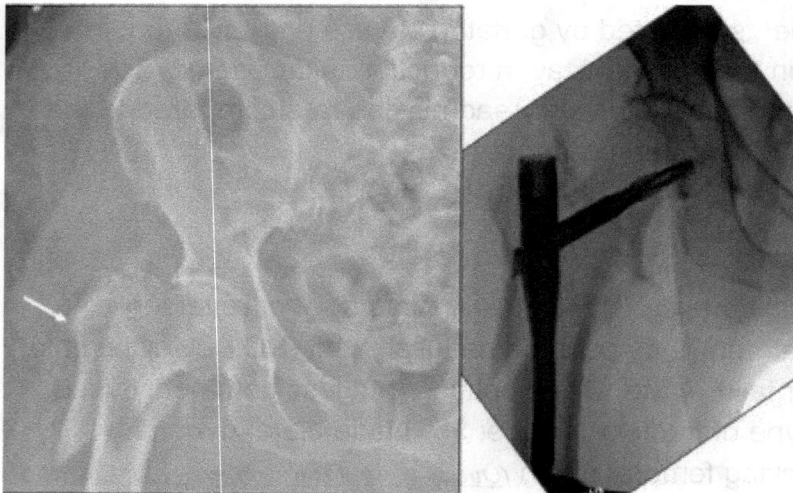

Fig 12: Unstable trochanteric fracture (reverse oblique). The arrow points to the trochanteric edge; fracture which affect the lateral cortex distal to the ridge are considered "unstable". The fracture was treated with cephalon-medullary nail.

Subtrochanteric Fracture:

- Deformity: The proximal fragment will be abducted (gluteus medius), flexed (ilio-psoas) and externally rotated (by hip external rotator).
- Treatment is by: IM nail fixation.

o Lateral positioning of the patient will allow flexing the distal fragment to align with the proximal fragment for easier reduction.

Femur Shaft Fracture:

- Ipsilateral femoral neck and shaft fractures occur with an incidence of about 5%.
    - o About 25%- 30% of these fractures are diagnosed on a delayed basis.
      (Scenario: 45 years old, fracture shaft femur, IM nail, follows up visit after 10 days complain of hip pain, next step? (Hip XR with leg internally rotated 15°))
    - o Fine-cut CT scan through the femoral neck is the best imaging study to diagnose femoral neck fractures in patients with femoral shaft fractures.
    - o The femoral neck fractures that is typically seen in association with ipsilateral femoral shaft fractures is a nondisplaced, vertical, and basicervical fracture.
    - o Treatment options: **two implants** for the two fractures (screws for fracture neck femur and retrograde nail for shaft), or a **single implant**: antegrade cephalomedullary nail/ reconstruction nail for treatment of both fractures (or less commonly long sliding plate for fixation of both fractures).
        - The use of a single implant is associated with higher mal-reduction rates of the shaft and/or neck fractures and increasing the rates of nonunion or malunion.
        - Neck femur fracture fixation takes priority and surgeon should start with it if possible.
- Bilateral femoral fractures: have higher mortality rate.
    - o Retrograde nailing is beneficial in bilateral cases (easier positioning, can be done on flat radiolucent table).
- The treatment of choice for closed comminuted diaphyseal femoral shaft fractures in adults is **reamed** (will allow placement of a larger implant) intramedullary nailing with **static** interlocking (prevent shortening or loss of reduction due to comminution).
    - o Comminution of the fracture: can lead to mal-reduction.
    - o Compared with non-reamed nailing: reamed femoral nailing has a higher rate of union.
    - o Antegrade and retrograde nail femur have similar union rate, however, there are more complications related to the knee with retrograde nailing and more complications related to the hip with antegrade nailing.
    - o External fixators: can be safely changed to IM nailing within the first two weeks after application of the external fixator with no significant increase in the incidence of deep infection.
    - o Comminuted femoral shaft fracture is better treated with 2 static distal locking screws. If only a single distal screw is used, the most likely mode of failure of

the construct is breakage of the shaft of the screw in the region that is inside the nail.
- o The entry point for antegrade femoral nail can be through the pyriformis or through the greater trochanter.
  - ▪ The proper location for starting point for nails in the lateral view is along the axis of the canal of the shaft of the femur.
  - ▪ Using a pyriformis entry nail (straight) through greater trochanter will result in varus deformity (greater trochanter entry nail must have a lateral bend to be able to accommodate the shape of the proximal femur). Using trochanteric entry nail through the pyriformis will result in valgus deformity.
- o For retrograde nailing, the proximal locking should be at or proximal to the level of lesser trochanter to avoid injury to the femoral vessels.
- o Mal-rotation is the most common deformity after IM nailing of the femur (especially comminuted fractures).
  - ▪ Assessment of the rotation post operatively is best done by bilateral lower extremity CT with cuts through the neck and through the distal femur. The angle of rotation (formed by line parallel to the posterior femoral condyles and another line along the axis of the neck) is compared between both sides (see Fig 13).
- Fracture of femoral shaft in the adolescent patients: see pediatric
- Nonunion of femoral shaft fracture:
  - o Associated with: **use of NSAID (strongest association)**, delayed weight bearing, and simple fracture patterns. Static (vs dynamic) locking do not influence the rate of union.
  - o Treatment: exchange nailing (2mm larger) (with possible bone grafting) has a high rate of success. *(Scenario: 35 years male, femur fracture, antegrade IM nail 6 months ago, persistent pain, XR nonunion with broken locking screws, treatment? (Exchange nailing) (note: dynamization is not an option as the locking screws are already broken (auto-dynamized) and the fracture still did not heal)*

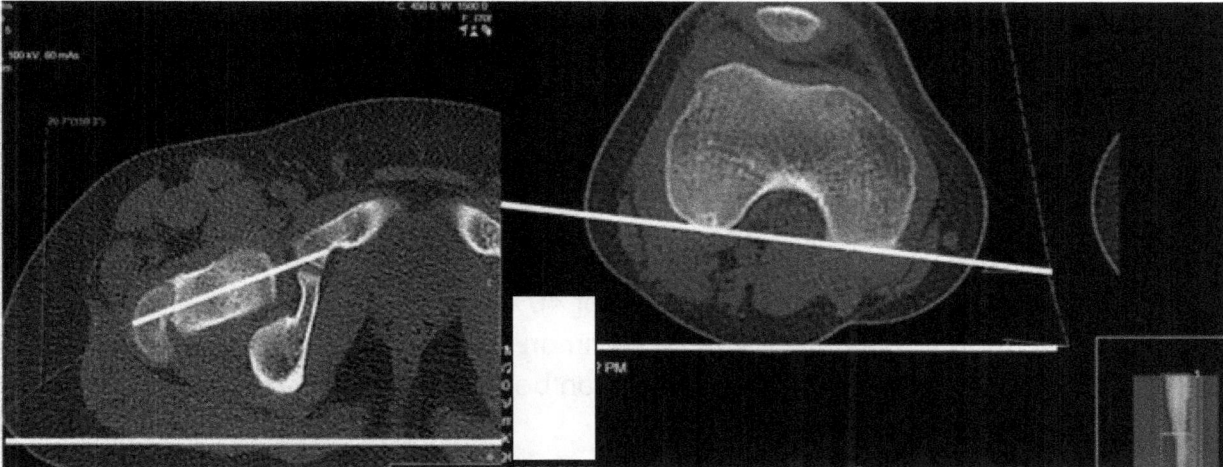

Fig 13: Assessment of version in 10 years old boy with intoeing. CT is done in which the angle between the femoral neck the transverse is calaculated. The angle between the posterior condule condyle and transverse is measured at the level of distal femur. The femoral version, is the sum of these two angles (if they are in differernt direction as in this example) of the difference between them (if they are in the same direction).

Supra Condylar Fracture of The Femur:

- Treatment: plate fixation.
- Risk factors for implant failure:
  - o **Short construct**, obesity, open fractures, smoking, diabetes and younger age.
  - o If there is osteoporosis (especially with loss of cortical contact): use a locked plate for fixation.
  - o Use a long construct is preferred (longer than 9 holes).
- Hoffa fragment: posterior condylar fracture (usually the lateral condyle); needs to be fixed, the screw will be from anterior to posterior (headless screw, counter-sunk)

Patella fracture:

- Non-displaced: assess the extensor mechanism
  - o Inject lidocaine and assess the patient ability to keep his knee extended. If intact, the treatment is non-operative (weight bearing as tolerated with knee immobilizer in extension). If not intact: fracture needs fixation.
- If displaced fracture: ORIF by tension band technique.
  - o Tension band can be done around K wires or through cannulated screws.
  - o Symptomatic implant is the most common complication.

- For small comminuted distal pole fracture: partial patellectomy can be done (with reconstruction of the patellar tendon
  - The tendon has to be attached to the **anterior** part of the distal remaining patella to avoid tilting of the patella.

Knee dislocation:

- Direction: most common types are: anterior 40% and posterior 40%.
  - Anterior dislocation is the most common type associated with arterial injury.
  - Postero-lateral rotator dislocation can be irreducible: the femur button hole in the medial capsule.
- Knee dislocations almost always involve rupture of both the anterior and posterior cruciate ligaments.
- Treatment:
  - Assessment of pulse, **emergent closed reduction**, re-assessment of the pulse and ABI and assessment of post reduction stability.
  - Admission for observation of the pulse for 48 hours.
  - Ligament repair/reconstruction/ augmentation will be needed (early Vs Late).
    - Most surgeon with go for early postero-lateral corner (PLC) repair and/or augmentation and later cruciate reconstruction.
    - Early collateral repair can be done.
  - According to pulse assessment **after the reduction**:
    - Symmetrical LE pulses and ABI ≥ 0.9: no need for invasive studies, repeat assessment for 48 hours.
    - **Absent** pulse: immediate exploration in the OR with vascular surgeon.
    - **Decrease** pulse (ABI < 0.9): arthrogram or CT angiography for assessment of intimal injury. *(Scenario: after reduction of knee dislocation, what is the next step? (Assessment of pulse)) (Scenario: patients presenting with knee dislocation and absent pulse: what is the initial management? (urgent closed reduction with re –assessment of the neurovascular condition after reduction)). (Scenario: knee dislocation on the right, reduction done, pulse is weaker on the right compared to the left, next step? (assessment of the ABI, if less than 0.8 proceed with angiogram or CT angiography)).*
    - Ankle-brachial index (ABI) can be easily performed; it is sensitive and specific. Useful for blunt lower extremity injuries and knee dislocations.
  - According to stability: patient can be maintained in knee immobilizer or will need external fixator.
    - If there is gross instability (especially if vascular repair or fasciotomy was done), spanning external fixator application across the knee should be applied to provide stability and protection of vascular repair.

Traumatic knee laceration:

- Saline load test with amount greater than 155 mL is the most sensitive method to assess if a traumatic laceration close to the knee is a traumatic arthrotomy (i.e. communicate with the knee joint).

Tibial plateau fracture:

- **Schatzker classification:**
  - Type I: split, type II: split depressed, type III: depressed.
  - Type IV (medial condyle) may represent a variant of knee dislocation and have higher incidence of compartment syndrome and the highest risk of associated vascular injury (especially those with the fracture line exiting lateral to the tibial spine).
  - Type V (bi-condylar) and VI (bicondylar with metaphysio-diaphyseal dissociation) fractures: the posterior medial condyle is usually displaced from the rest of the tibial plateau.
    - Lateral XR will show subluxation of the femur with the displaced tibial condyle. CT will show the postero-medial segment more obvious.
    - This fracture pattern will require double plating (anterolateral and posterior medial).
    - If XR or CT shows posterior subluxation of the femur with displaced posterior medial fragment, application of posterior medial buttress plate should be done to prevent subluxation of the joint.
- Peripheral meniscal tear and bony ACL avulsion are the two most common injuries associated with tibial plateau.
  - Associated meniscal injury:
    - lateral meniscus more commonly affected than medial.
    - Most common type of injury is **peripheral tear**.
    - Tear of the medial meniscus are most likely to be associated with type IV medial plateau fracture.
- Indication for fixation: more than 10-5 mm depression or **instability on stress** (detected by **physical exam**).
  - Non-displaced or minimally displaced tibial plateau fracture: most important indication for surgery is knee instability to varus/valgus stress (more than 10 degrees motion) (on physical exam). *(Scenario: 45 years old, minimally displaced tibia plateau, what will determine need for surgery?)*
  - Non-displaced or minimally displaced fracture with no instability should be treated with non-weight bearing on the affected side with ROM exercises for 6-8 weeks, followed by gradual weight bearing.

- **Operative treatment:**
  - ORIF with bone grafting of the defect (see Fig 3 in general trauma chapter).
    - For void filling: calcium phosphate is the material which has the highest compression strength (least amount of joint depression with follow up).
  - For bicondylar fracture:
    - If the medial fracture is nondisplaced with bone contact, it is possible to use one locking plate from the lateral side.
    - If the medial fracture is displaced (especially with posterior femoral subluxation): needs bilateral plating (postero medial plate and lateral plating by dual incision).
  - There is no advantage for using locking plate for split, depressed or split depressed tibial plateau fracture (type I, II, III).
    - Locking plates do not provide buttress effect when used in pure locking mode (general rule).
  - Pure medial fractures (Schatzker type IV) are best treated with medial fixation.
  - In cases of long side plates: percutaneous screws in the shaft can result in injury to the superficial peroneal nerve (same applies for tibial shaft treated with minimal invasive plating).
  - If using external fixator: wires should be at least 14 mm from articular surface specially near the posterior cortex (to avoid intra articular position).
  - For highly comminuted Schatzker type V, VI or those with associated with knee dislcaotion/subluxation with soft tissue injury, spanning external fixator can be applied initially for 10-14 days followed by internal fixation (only small portion of cases needs this approach in contrary to tibial plafond injury in which majority of cases will need staged treatment).
  - The outcome of fracture fixation is worse in elderly patients.
  - The use of small fragment fixation (3.5mm) (raft of 4 screws) is referred to maintain the joint elevation obtained by surgery (compared to thicker screws).

Tibial Shaft Fracture:

- Most cases of tibial shaft fracture are treated surgically with IM nail; however, closed reduction and casting can sometimes be used.
  - Absolute indications for treatment of the tibial fracture by internal fixation: open fracture, ipsi lateral femoral fracture, poly trauma, failure to obtain adequate closed reduction.
  - Relative indication for non-operative treatment (immobilization in a long leg cast, followed by weight bearing as tolerated in a patellar tendon bearing cast until union is achieved) (much less done nowadays compared to operative

fixation): spiral fracture pattern, low-energy mechanism, fracture of the fibula at a different level, diaphyseal fractures of the tibia with intact fibula (this pattern is more prone to varus mal-reduction).

- Acceptable reduction criteria: shortening less than 10mm, varus-valgus less than 5°, procurvatum-recurvatum less than 10°.
- Shortening is the most difficult deformity to control in cast.
- Nonsurgical treatment can lead to varus malunion is about 25% of cases.

- The best fluoroscopy view to detect the proximal level of tibial nail is lateral knee fluoroscopy.
- Most common complication after IM nail for tibial fracture is **knee pain**.
  - Removal of the nail can result in resolving the pain in about 25% and improving it in about 70%.
- Unreamed nailing:
  - Advantage: less surgical time.
  - Disadvantage: higher nonunion rates with increased hardware failure and increased time to union (reamed nailing has higher union rate).
  - The non-reamed nail (compared to reamed nailing) result in more rapid restoration of endosteal blood flow.
- SPRINT study:
  - Randomized, controlled trial
  - Reamed intramedullary (IM) nailing has less reoperation rate compared to unreamed IM nailing for closed tibial shaft fractures.
  - For open fractures: reoperation rates are similar between reamed and non-reamed (union rate and infection).
- Thermal production during reaming is mainly related to use of large diameter reamer in a small diameter isthmus. Use of tourniquet is not a major factor in generating heat during reaming (contrary to what used to be believed).
- The most statistically significant predictors nonunion: transverse fracture pattern, open fracture, and cortical contact of 50% or less.
- **Proximal tibial shaft fracture:**
  - Deformity: develop procurvatum (flexion) valgus deformity. If nailing is done, it may not correct this deformity.
    - Blocking screws can used to correct the deformity. It should be inserted in the proximal fragment in the concavity of the deformity **(lateral and posterior)** (see Fig 14).
    - Other options to control the deformity are: direct open reduction and temporary fixation by plate or reduction clamp, or using semi-extended position nailing.

- For distal tibial fracture:
    - The most common deformity after IM nailing of distal tibial fracture is rotational mal alignment.
    - Spiral distal tibia fractures can be associated with intra-articular fracture extension. CT scan of the ankle in these types of fractures is recommended to identify possible associated injury. (*Scenario: 30 years, fell, fracture distal third of tibia, next step? (ankle CT)).*
- **Stress fracture of tibia**:
    - The tibia is the most frequent bone affected by stress fracture in athletes and new military training.
    - The anterior midshaft region of the tibia is at higher risk secondary to tensile forces and relative paucity of blood supply.
    - Treated initially by rest (non-weight bearing on the affected extremity) followed by resumption of activity when symptoms resolve.
- **Late Clawing of the toes after tibia fracture:**
    - The FHL and FDL can become tethered to the fracture of the distal tibial shaft resulting in clawing deformity of the toes. The posterior tibial muscle will be normal (no varus or equines deformity and normal single heel rise).
        - Treatment: Release of the FHL and FDL from the fracture site or retromalleolar lengthening of the tendons.
    - Missed deep posterior compartment syndrome: clawing of the toes with varus and equines deformity and inability to perform single heel rise (FDP, FHL, and posterior tibial muscle are all affected).
        - Treatment is excision of the scarred muscles and tendons (FDP, FHL, and posterior tibial tendon) with Achilles tendon lengthening. *(Scenario: tibia fracture, 6 months later patient had toes clawing causing calluses on the dorsum of toes, no varus deformity, treatment?) (Same scenario with varus deformity, treatment?)*

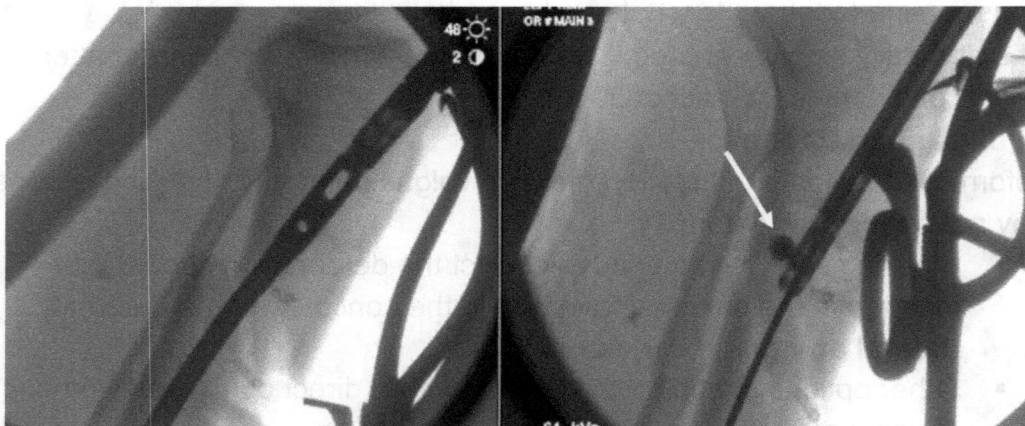

Fig 14: Usage of blocking screw (arrow) to correct flexion deformity of the proximal tibial. The screw was applied in the concavity of the deformtiy (posterior).

- **Tibia nonunion:**
  - Exchange nailing:
    - For aseptic nonunion cases.
    - Best indicated for treatment of hypertrophic nonunion and nonunion with minimal gap. *(Scenario: open tibia fracture, treated with small diameter nail, after 7 months XR shows nonunion, broken locking screws, markers of infection negative, treatment? (exchange nailing)) (Scenario: closed tibia fracture, 9 months later has nonunion, no signs of infection, next step?) (Scenario: 25 years, tibia fracture, nailing, persistent pain, fall from a height and now has severe pain, XR broken nail, treatment?)*
- **Open tibial fracture:**
  - Insensate foot in open fracture is not contra indication for reconstruction.
    - Absent plantar sensation at initial evaluation is not prognostic for long-term plantar sensory status or functional outcome.
  - Open IIIC fracture with vessel injuries amenable for repair and insensate foot should be treated with I&D, external fixator and vessel repair.
    - Nerve exploration is not indicated in the acute setting, as it will add more insult to the tissue with no clear benefit (the injury may be due to stretch of the nerve (neurapraxia) that may improve spontaneously).
  - The most important predictor of infection after an open type III tibial fracture is time to transfer to definitive trauma center, timing of antibiotic administration and quality of debridement.
  - The LEAP study showed that:
    - Loss of plantar sensation is NOT indication for early amputation.
    - The timing of wound debridement, the timing of soft-tissue coverage, and the timing of bone grafting after injury did not impact the infection or union rates and had no effect on functional outcome (however, other study (Godina, 1986) showed direct relation between risk of infection and timing of soft tissue coverage).
    - Patients who are definitively treated with external fixation had a significantly longer time to union, poorer functional outcomes, longer time to achieve full weight bearing, and more time in the hospital (these results have been challenged with the use of stronger ring fixator).
    - The most important predictors of patient satisfaction at 2 years after injury include the ability to return to work, absence of depression, faster walking speed, and decreased pain. Reconstruction versus amputation, age, education level, plantar sensation, gender, socioeconomic status did not make difference.

- The projected lifetime healthcare cost for patients treated with amputation is higher than costs for those who are treated with limb-salvage procedures (need for multiple prosthesis).
    - The negative pressure dressing (wound VAC) does not lower or raise the risk of infection in open fractures. However, the wound VAC may decrease the probability of needing free tissue coverage (can stimulate granulation tissue that will only require skin graft coverage) (see general trauma chapter).
    - Irrigation using a liquid soap additive is as effective as the use of irrigation with bacitracin with regards to the rate of postoperative infection and fracture healing, and has lower incidence of soft-tissue healing complications (see general management of open fracture in the chapter of general trauma).
- Flap coverage for soft tissue defect in cases of open fracture:
    - Upper thirds: medial gastrocnemius rotational flap.
    - Middle third: soleus rotational flap.
    - Lower third: free flap.
    - Open tibia fracture with exposed bone and tissue loss extending posteriorly cannot be treated with soleus or medial gastrocnemius rotation flap as they are part of the zone of injury. Soft-tissue coverage will require a free tissue transfer or other modalities (e.g. shortening).
- BMP: BMP 2 proved for open fractures of the tibia; BMP 7 proved for non-union.

Pilon Fracture (Tibial Plafond Fracture):
- Mechanism: Due to axial injury; most cases will be the result of high energy injuries.
- Pathology: Highly comminuted fractures. The anterolateral fragment (Chapot fragmenet) has the anterior inferior tibio-fibular ligament (See Fig 15).
- **Preferred treatment: Staged surgery:**
    - 1st stage: external fixator to maintain alignment and length and allow for soft tissue rest.
    - 2nd stage (after about 10-14 days after the first surgery): ORIF when the swelling comes down to decrease the incidence of wound complication.
    (Question: what is the difference in outcome between early and late fixation of plafond? (higher incidence of wound complication with early fixation))
- Prognosis:
    - Patients with pilon fracture continue to improve in function and pain for an about 2 years after surgery.
    - Posttraumatic degenerative arthritis is present in almost all ankles.

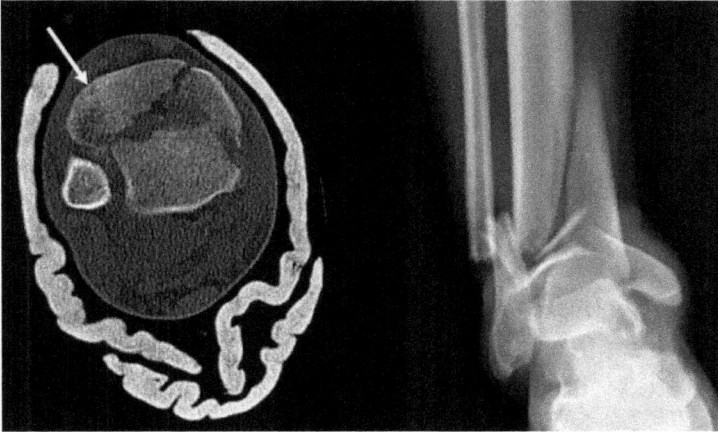

Fig 15: XR and CT of comminuted axial fracture (Pilon). Axial CT shows the anterolateral fragment of the distal tibia (arrow) that has the attachment of the ATFL. During surgery, this fragment should be reflected laterally to preserve the ligmanent attachment.

- o Patients will have limitations in recreational activities. Patients will have long-term adverse general health effects (compared to their gender and age-matched peers).
  - Studies showed that patients with pilon fracture had very low SF-36 scores their age and gender matched norms (the lower the score the worse the function).
- o Despite these adverse outcomes, small percentage of patient will need a late ankle fusion (about 13%).

Ankle Fracture (Non-Axial Injuries)

- Any lateral displacement of the talus is an indication for surgery (1mm lateral displacement of the talus leads to about 40% decrease in tibio-talar contact area) *(Question: most important factor in determining surgical indication for ankle fracture?).*
- Assessment of syndesmotic injury:
  - o Tibiofibular clear space, tibiofibular overlap and medial clear space (Fig 16).
  - o At 1 cm above the joint, the tibiofibular clear space should be ≤ 6 mm on both the AP and mortise radiographic views. Tibio-fibular clear space > 6 mm on both the AP and mortise views is the most reliable predictor of syndesmotic injury (minimal change between different ankle positions).
  - o Medial clear space (most commonly used parameter): should not be more than the superior clear space (< 5mm) (it should be measured with the ankle in 90 flexion in the mortise view).
- Talo-crural angle (between tip of malleoli and upper surface of the talus): assess lateral malleolus/ fibula length
- Anatomic reduction is the most important prognostic fracture after ankle fracture.
- **Supination external rotation ankle fracture (SER):**
  - o Occurs at the level of the syndesmosis (Weber B).

- The lateral malleolus fracture line runs from distal anterior to proximal posterior.
- **Stages:** The injury starts on the anterior talo-fibular ligament (stage I), then progress lateral malleolus fracture (stage II), then posterior syndesmosis (posterior talo fibular ligament) or posterior malleolus (rarely stays in this stage) (stage III) then goes to the medial side (deltoid or horizontal medial malleolus) (stage IV).
- **Assessment of medial side injury (differentiation between SER II and IV)**
  - The fracture stage will direct treatment. Stage II can be managed by weight bearing as tolerated with CAM boot or a cast while stage IV will require surgical fixation.
  - "Stress radiograph" is used to assess the medial side ankle injury is: external rotation stress test (or gravity stress test) is performed to assess the integrity of deltoid ligament on the medial side (by measuring medial clear space, tibio-fibular overlap and/or tibio-fibular clear space) (Fig 17).

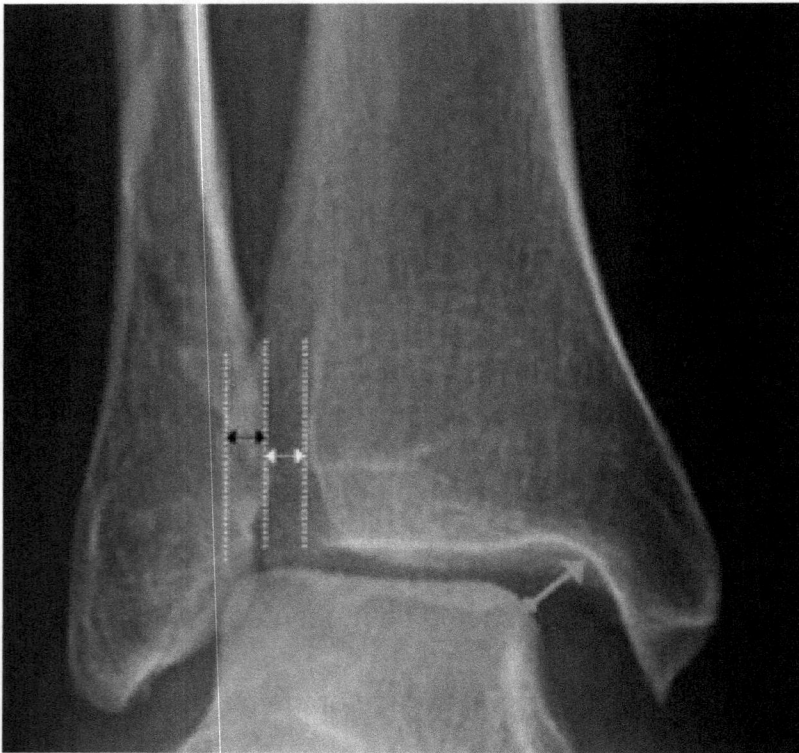

Fig 16: XR of the ankle can be used to assess the syndemosis using the tibio-fibular clear space (white double arrow), tibio fibular overlap (black double arrow) or the medial clear space (arrow). Please refer to the text for normal values.

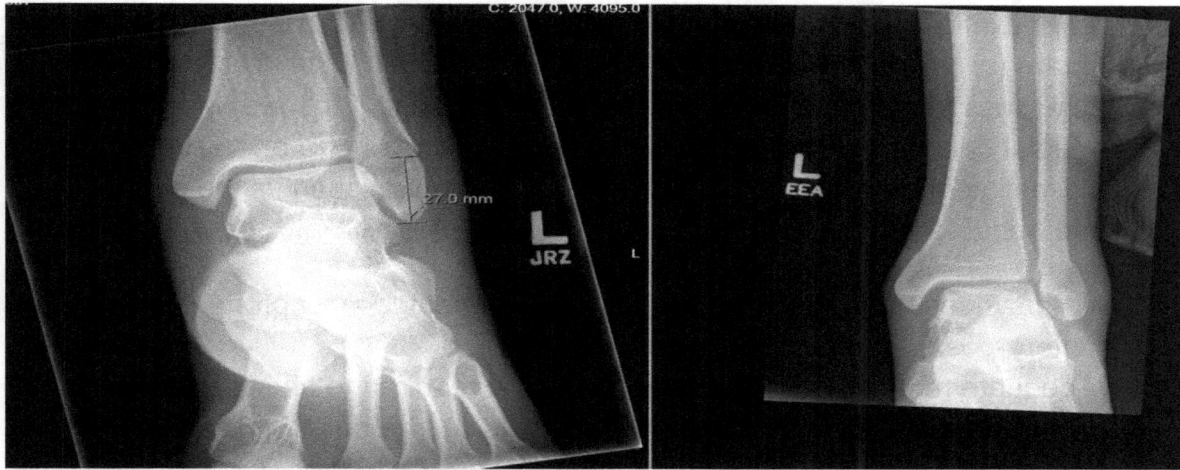

Fig 17: Gravity stress view. XR on the left shows distal fibular fracture (Weber B) with no medial side bony injury. This fracture requires stress view of the ankle to assess deltoid ligament integrity (differentiate between type II and type IV SER). Gravity stress view was done (notice the bolster under the fibula in the XR on the right), the medical clear space had increased with the stress (together with talar shift) indicating SER IV. Without stress (XR on the left) the medial clear space is equal to the superior clear space, while with stess, the medial clear space is wider than the superior clear space.

- Medial ankle tenderness, ecchymosis, and swelling are not reliable findings when trying to determine deltoid competence. *(Question: how to differentiate between SER II and IV?)*
- If stress view shows no medial space widening and no lateral subluxation (SER II): treatment is weight bearing as tolerated in a CAM boot (see before).
- If there indication of syndesmotic injury: widening of the medial clear space (medial clear space measuring > 6 mm or more than 3mm difference between the medial clear space and superior clear space) or lateral talar subluxation indicating deltoid injury (SER IV): fixation of the fibula is needed (to avoid talus translation).
- If primary radiographs shows signs of syndesmotic injury (medical clear space > 6 mm, tibio-fibular clear space more than 5 mm): no need for stress radiographs.
- Most rigid fixation for supination external rotation lateral malleolus fracture is posterior plate (anti-glide mechanism), however this leads to irritation of peroneal tendons. *(Question: what is advantage of lateral plating? (avoid peroneal tendon irritation))*. Lateral plating is the most commonly used method of fixation.

- o After fixation of the fibula fracture, **intra-operative external rotation stress exam** (or lateral pulling of the fibula with towel clip (Cotton Test)) is performed to assess the integrity of the syndesmotic ligament. If there is widening of the medial clear space, syndesmotic fixation is needed. Intra operative assessment of syndesmosis (after fibular fracture fixation) is the most reliable method to detect syndesmotic injury. *(Question: what is the most reliable method of predicting a injury of the tibio-fibular syndesmosis?).*
- o With syndesmotic injury: the fibular displacement is most pronounced in the antero-posterior direction (sagittal plane).
- o Adequate reduction of the fibular fracture is required to obtain syndesmotic reduction. Malreduction of the syndesmosis can be due to fibular mal-reduction.
- o If patient presents with failure (breakage) of the syndesmotic screw without evidence of mal-alignment of the mortise and a pain-free ankle: no need for further surgery (no need for removal of broken screw or insertion of new screw).
- o If patient presents with pain **directly** over the fibular implant: removal of this hardware is indicated.
- o Ankle fracture with syndesmotic widening discovered few weeks/ months post fixation is treated by **revision** surgery with **reduction and fixation of the syndesmosis**. The **medial ankle may have to be explored** (to remove the scarring tissue in the medial side). **Fibular osteotomy** (for distraction and derotation) may be needed to correct fibular shortening or malrotation if the fibula had full healed. *(Scenario: 45 years old, 3 months ago had ORIF of lateral malleolus, with syndesmotic fixation, the syndesmotic screw was removed 9 weeks later, now has pain and limited ROM, XR shows widening of the syndesmosis, treatment?) (Scenario: 40 years old, ankle fracture 4 months ago, having pain, XR syndesmotic widening, treatment?) (40 years old, ankle fracture 16 weeks ago, still in pain, XR shows reduced well fixed medial malleolus fracture with proximal fibular fracture that is not fixed and syndesmotic screw fixation with widening of the syndesmosis, treatment?)*
- o Malunited fibular fracture with subluxation of the talus is treated with corrective osteotomy of the fibula (and possible osteotomy of the medial malleolus). This can improve pain and stability even if there is early arthritis of the joint.
- Diabetic neuropathy patients with acute ankle fracture: treatment is ORIF with increased fixation (for example: addition of cast augmentation) and prolongation of the period of non-weight bearing (usually doubling the period of non-weight bearing).
- For right-side ankle fracture: patient can start driving 9 weeks post operatively (see Rehabilitation chapter).
- Posterior malleolus fracture:
  - o Indication for fixation: >25-30% of the distal articular segment.

- o Fixation can be either by percutaneus screws (postero-anterior or antero-posterior) or by plate applied through posterolateral approach (buttress plate).
  - ▪ Postero lateral approach between FHL (has the most distal muscle belly among muscles crossing the ankle joint (beef to heel muscle)) and peroneii (the peroneal brevis is the muscle close to the fibular).
- Syndesmotic injury without lateral malleolus fracture:
  - o Maissoniave injury (medial malleolus fracture, proximal fibular fracture and syndesmotic injury) is pronation external rotation injury.
  - o If ankle radiographs show medial or posterior malleolus fracture (especially if there associated medial space widening), next step: obtain lower leg (tibia) radiographs to assess possible proximal fibular fracture (Maisonneuve fracture) (see Fig 18).

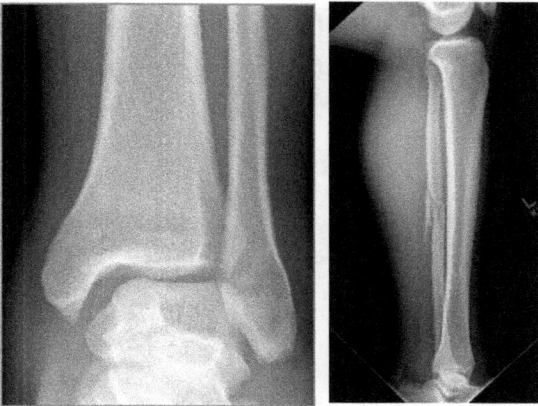

Fig 18: XR of the left ankle of your male who twisted the ankle. XR shows increased medial clear space with no fracture of the lateral malleolus. XR of lower leg showed the fibular fracture in the mid shaft (Maissoniave injury)

Foot Trauma:

Talar Neck Fracture:

- **Classification (Hawkin):**
  - o I: non displaced, II: displaced with subluxation or dislocation of the subtalar joint, III: dislocation of the subtalar and tibio-talar (extruded body of talus), type IV: dislocation of the subtalar, ankle and talo-navicular (the distal part of the talus is also affected).
- Treatment of displaced talar neck is open reduction and internal fixation (even if the displacement is minimal) (NOT closed reduction and percutaneus pinning). *(Scenario: 45 years old with motor cycle, displaced talar neck (grade 3), treatment?)*
  - o Dual incision (antero medial and antero lateral) is needed in cases of high comminution.
  - o The best biomechanical screw construct is posterior to anterior fixation with the entry point at the level of the posterolateral tubercle of the talus.

- o With medial comminution: medial plate helps to prevent varus; other option is to use fully threaded screws (avoid partially threaded screws in these cases as the applied compression can cause varus).
- o Talar body dislocation and extrusion: I&D and re-implantation of the talus (with fracture fixation).
- o If there is nonunion of the talar neck with viable body and no arthritis of the ankle or the subtalar, the treatment is revision ORIF with bone graft. Tibio-talo-calcaneal fusion may be needed if there is AVN of the body.
- Howkin sign: subchondral radiolucency of the talar dome few weeks after talar neck fracture indicating preserved vascularity of the talar body (its presence is a good prognostic factor).
- Most common complication: **subtalar arthritis (not AVN),** most common avoidable complication is malreduciton (varus malunion)
  - o The most important risk factor for development of AVN after fracture neck talus is the amount of initial fracture displacement (not the timing of surgical reduction).

Talar Lateral Process Fracture:
- Common in **snow boarder**, can be easily missed in XR.
- The mechanism of injury is dorsiflexion, axial loading, inversion, and **external rotation**.

Subtalar Dislocation:
- Subtalar dislocation is commonly associated with fracture of the surrounding talar bone
- Treatment is **closed reduction and cast immobilization.**
- Irreducible dislocation:
  - o Lateral: most commonly due to interposition of **posterior tibial tendon** (not anterior tibial) or FHL
  - o Medial: due to interposition of peroneus muscles, EDB or fracture head talus.

Tarsometatarsal Dislocation (Lisfranc Injury):
- Dislocation of the tarsometatarsal joint (the joint between proximal metatarsals and cuneiforms/ cuboid) with injury to **the Lisfranc ligament:**
  - o Lisfranc ligament runs between **medial** cuneiform and **second** metatarsal.
  - o The Lisfranc ligament (oblique interosseous ligament) is the most important stabilizer for tarsometatarsal joint (see anatomy chapter).

- Clinical presentation: Mid foot pain, **plantar ecchymosis**. XR shows possible widening of the 1st-2nd metatarsal bases.
  - CT or XR may show flick sign (Fig 19):
    - The "fleck sign" is a small avulsion fracture at the medial base of the second metatarsal, representing an avulsion of the Lisfranc ligament.
  - If clinical presentation is suggestive of Lisfranc injury with negative XR, the next step is **weight bearing (or simulated standing) XR.**
- Treatment is **open reduction and internal fixation (+/- primary fusion).** *(Scenario: 20-year-soccer player sustains a hyperextension injury, unable to bear weight, tenderness in midfoot with swelling and plantar ecchymosis. XR negative. Next step?) (Scenario: 25 years, foot injury, pain, XR widening between the 1st and the 2nd Metatarsal base, treatment?) (Scenario: Athlete, another player fell on his flexed and planted foot, XR shows 2 mm widening between 1st and 2nd tarsometatarsal joints, treatment?)*
  - Non-reducible dislocation may be due to tibialis anterior entrapment.
  - Primary fusion leads to less reoperation rate than open reduction without fusion.
  - Fusion is preferred treatment for delayed cases or if there is marked comminution of the articular surface.
  - For pure ligamentous injury, fusion may be preferred (controversial).
  - No need for fusion of the lateral column in cases of Lisfranc injury (reduction and K wire fixation for 4-6 weeks is sufficient). Fusion of the lateral 2 rays will result in inferior clinical results.
- Cuboid compression fracture can be associated with homolateral Lisfranc injuries (nutcracker injury). *(Scenario: twisting injury, mid foot pain, XR shows cuboid fracture, what is the associate injury)*
- Posttraumatic arthritis leading to chronic foot pain is the most common complication after open reduction internal fixation of this injury.
  - Chronic foot pain after Lisfranc injury (with radiographic evidence of advanced arthrosis of the first and second tarsometatarsal joints): start with non-operative treatment (NSAIDs, orthotics (rocker button sole); if this fail: mid foot (tarso-metatarsal) fusion. *(Scenario: 50 years old, Lisfranc injury 3 years ago, now complaining of increasing pain in the foot. non operative treatment failed to control symptoms, management?)*

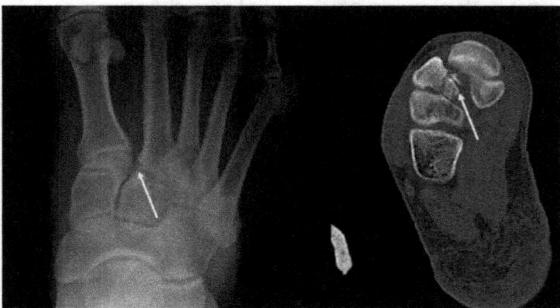

Fig 19: XR and CT of Lisfranc injury showing the "fleck sign" (arrows) representing avulsion of the Lisfranc ligament from the base of the 2nd metatasus.

Navicular Stress Fracture:

- **Pathology**: common in the central third of the bone (central one third is the watershed zone of navicular vascularity).
- Clinical presentation: Common in runner, the patient will have gradual onset of mid foot pain and localized tenderness on the medial side of the dorsum of the foot.
- Lesion may be missed in XR; CT will better show the fracture line.
- MRI will show edema (which could be a stress reaction, stress fracture, or osteonecrosis).
- Treatment depends on CT scan results:
  - Initial treatment is non-weight bearing cast for 6 weeks. If this fails (or patient cannot tolerate NWB), internal fixation +/- bone grafting. *(Scenario: runner, pain for 2 months, tenderness over dorsal medial foot, MRI shows edema, next step? (CT), treatment?)*
  - Surgical treatment is preferred in athletes having the pain for long duration.
  - According to the CT findings:
    - Navicular stress **reaction** (edema in the MRI with no fracture line seen CT), treatment is NWB in cast or boot. Surgery is not needed.
    - If fracture line extends across both cortices, or CT scan shows cystic changes: surgical treatment is preferred.

Calcaneus fracture:

- Relative indications of surgery: mild to moderate comminution (Sanders II and III) displaced intra-articular calcaneal fractures in healthy adults who are nonsmoker and do not have multiple medical co-morbidities (e.g. diabetes), are better treated by open reduction and internal fixation.
  - Young (less than 40 years), nonsmoker, unilateral, females, in non-labor jobs, non-worker's compensable injuries have the best results with surgical treatment of calcaneus fracture.
  - Poor outcome: obese, smoker, male, worker, worker's compensable injuries, diabetic.
  - Surgery treatment is by delayed open reduction and internal fixation.
    - After injury: the limb is elevated, and the surgery is delayed for about 2 weeks until "**wrinkles**" can be seen on the lateral aspect of the calcaneus "indicating decreased swelling".
  - The stable fragment: the medial fragment (sustentaculum tali) which usually does not displace with the fracture. The reduction is "built" to this fragment and fixation should extend to include the stable fragment (screws should capture this piece).

- Long screws that are distal (inferior) to the stable medial fragment will affect FHL (runs underneath the sustentaculum tali).
- o There are two main incisions for the ORIF: sinus tarsi (does not require raising of a flap) and extensile lateral approach (include raising of a flap). Extensile lateral approach can give better anatomical reduction but has the disadvantage of possible extensive skin complication (see approaches in anatomy chapter)
- o Surgical treatment has the advantages of decreased incidence of post traumatic arthritis and better subtalar joint range of motion and earlier returns to work.
  - Most common early post-operative complication is **skin dehiscence** and secondary infection (20-40%) (with better surgical techniques, this percentage had markedly dropped).
  - Most common complication of non-operative treatment of calcaneal fracture is development of subtalar arthirits.
  - Nonsurgical treatment of displaced calcaneal fracture is a risk factor for eventual need for a subtalar arthrodesis.
  - Bone block fusion (Subtalar distraction arthrodesis): if there is anterior ankle impingement (see foot and ankle chapter for more details and scenarios.)
  - Non-surgical management of displaced calcaneus fracture with lateral wall blowout can result in lateral hindfoot pain due to peroneal tendons irritation from lateral subfibular impingement (the displaced expanded lateral wall subluxates the peroneal tendons against the distal tip of the fibula). Treatment: lateral wall exostectomy. (*Scenario: 40 years old, calcaneus fracture one year ago, treated non-operatively, now has lateral hindfoot pain, CT scan show evidence of a lateral wall blowout with no evidence of subtalar arthritis, non-operative treatment failed, treatment?*)
- Open calcaneal fracture: if the open wound is medial (type 1 and 2 open fractures), no increase in incidence of infection after ORIF. The treatment is debridement and wound care followed by ORIF through lateral wound when the swelling had decreased, and medial wound is closed. Lateral open wounds have increased risk for infection and complications.
- Avulsion of the calcaneal tuberosity: needs urgent surgical repair to avoid skin necrosis (Fig 20) (the surgery is better to be done by closed reduction and percutaneous fixation if possible).

Calcaneus Stress Fracture:
- Patient will complain of heel pain with weight bearing, foot is NOT grossly swollen.

- Exam: compression of the calcaneus (by examiner hand) will cause severe pain. Diffusely tender over the lateral, plantar, and medial hindfoot.
- The radiograph (lateral view XR) may show dense condensation of bone. In most cases, XR will be normal.
- MRI will show increased signal affecting on the T2-weighted images (edema).
- Treatment: protect the weight bearing until resolution of symptoms.

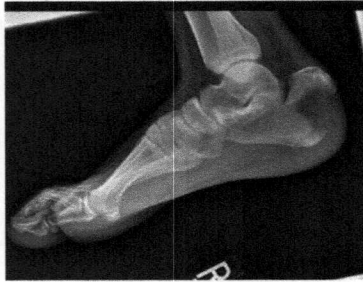

Fig 20: Avulsion of the calcaneal tuberosity. Notice that avulsed piece of the calcaeal tuberosity is compressing against the skin on the posterior aspect of the heel and may cause pressure necrosis.

Fracture of The Proximal Part of 5th Metacarpal:

- Types (See Fig 21-22):
  - Pseudo- Jones (avulsion fracture): The fracture will exit in the TMT joint. Treatment is weight bearing as tolerated with hard sole shoe or CAM boot (casting is not needed).
  - Jones fracture (metaphysio-diaphyseal area, fracture line ends at the 4-5 intermetatarsal articulation). Treatment is a strict non-weight-bearing short leg cast or surgical.
    - High performance athletes: intra medullary fixation is preferred (intra medullary screw with a minimum size 4.5mm non-cannulated screw). *(Scenario: collegiate basketball player, had 5th MT fracture, XR shows the fracture in the metaphysio-diaphyseal area, treatment?) (Bank teller, fall down, Jones fracture, treatment?)*
    - In non-athletes: short leg non weight bearing cast for 6 weeks. If after 6 weeks, no healing with obvious gap: internal fixation by IM screw (no need for open reduction). *(Scenario: 20 years, Jones, treated in cast, 6 weeks XR shows fracture with no healing, next step?).*
    - Refracture and failure of implant after internal fixation is mainly related to **return to activity before radiographic healing and early unprotected weight bearing**.
  - **Stress fracture of the 5th MT (Fig 22):**
    - Stress fracture of the 5th metatarsus may be associated with hind foot varus deformity and possible cavus deformity (subtle cavus deformity with secondary hind foot varus). This may need to be addressed at the

time of surgical repair of the fracture. *(What pathology associated with 5th MT stress fracture?)*

- Needs internal fixation +/- repair of the varus and/or cavus deformity.

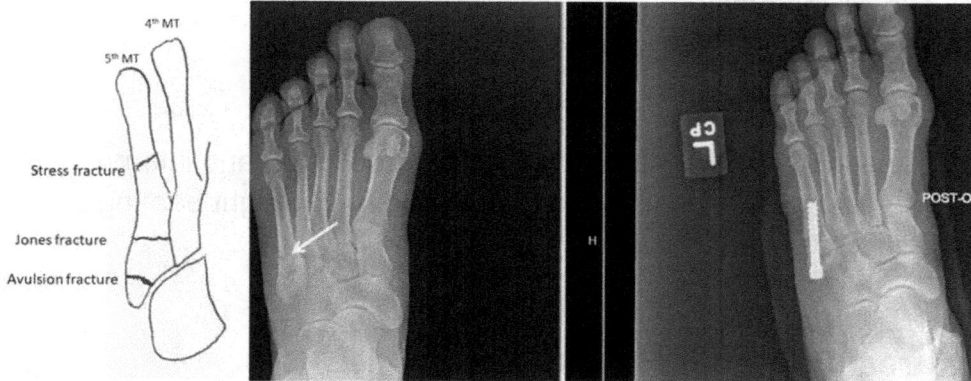

Fig 21: Drawing showing the types of 5th MT fracture. Fractures which exit at the 4-5th MT articulation are considered true Jones. XR shows Jones fracture (arrow) in young adult nurse who could not tolerate cast treatment; IM screw was applied.

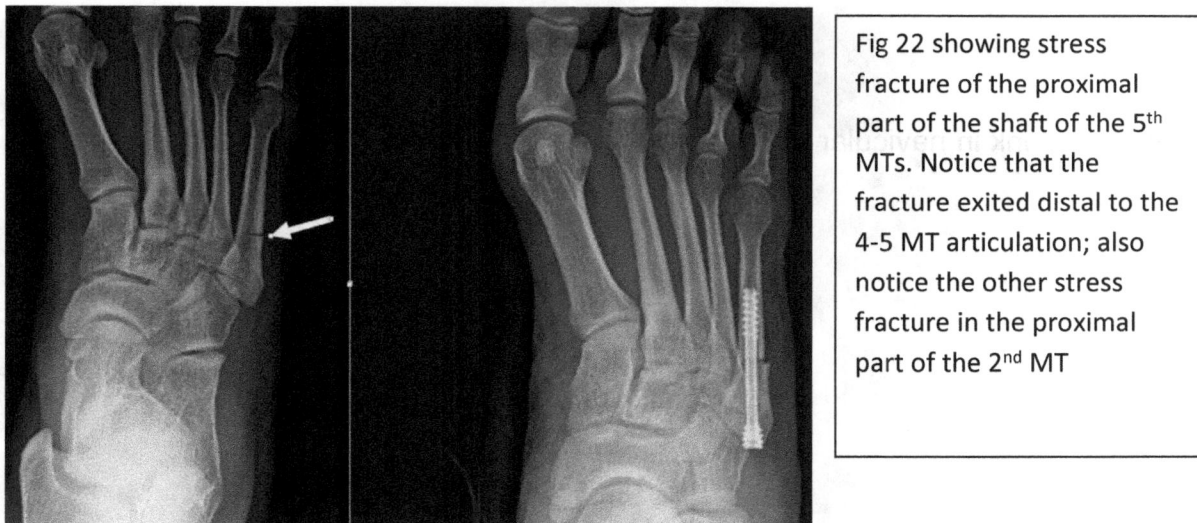

Fig 22 showing stress fracture of the proximal part of the shaft of the 5th MTs. Notice that the fracture exited distal to the 4-5 MT articulation; also notice the other stress fracture in the proximal part of the 2nd MT

Stress Fracture of The Second MT:

- Risk factors:
  - hallux valgus, hallux rigidus (transfer of load to the second metatarsal head)
  - Long second metatarsal (increased duration of contact during push-off in the stance phase).

    o Ballet dancing (most common stress fracture in ballet dancers).
- Treatment: is CAM boot immobilization and weight bearing as tolerated (no need for NWB cast in most cases) with activity modification (same treatment for stress fracture of the 3rd and 4th metatarsus).

1st Metatarsal Shaft Fracture:

- The treatment of displaced 1st MT shaft fracture is open reduction and internal fixation because 1st metatarsus is exposed to high load during weight bearing and malunion can cause transfer metatarsalgia.

Phalangeal Fractures (Same for Hand):

- Fractures of the distal phalanx with bleeding from nail fold are considered open fractures. Antibiotic and irrigation and debridement should be done.
- Seymour's fracture:
  - Fracture of the base of the distal phalanx in which the germinal matrix is entrapped in the fracture
  - Require open reduction and internal fixation (see pediatric chapter).

Tips:

- Runners: think in navicular stress fracture or compression of the Baxter nerve.

References/ Suggested Readings

- Lieberman, J. R. (Ed.). (2009). AAOS comprehensive orthopaedic review. American academy of orthopaedic surgeons.
- Mark D. Miller MD , Stephen R. Thompson MD MedRCSC, Jennifer Hart PA-C ATC (2012). Review of Orthopaedics, 6th edition (Miller Review of Orthopeadics).
- Green, D. P. (2010). Rockwood and Green's fractures in adults. Lippincott Williams & Wilkins.
- Flynn, J. M., Skaggs, D. L., & Waters, P. M. (2014). Rockwood and Wilkins' fractures in children. Lippincott Williams & Wilkins.
- White, T. O., Mackenzie, S. P., & Gray, A. J. (2015). Mcrae's Orthopaedic Trauma and Emergency Fracture Management. Elsevier Health Sciences.
- Wiesel, S. W. (2012). Operative techniques in orthopaedic surgery. Lippincott Williams & Wilkins.
- AAOS Clinical Practice Guidelines, retrieved from https://www.aaos.org/cpg/?ssopc=1.
- AAOS Self-assessment Books, retrieved from https://www.aaos.org/self_assess/.